Clinical and Statistical Considerations in Personalized Medicine

Chapman & Hall/CRC Biostatistics Series

Chapman & Hall/CRC Biostatistics Series

Clinical and Statistical Considerations in Personalized Medicine

Edited by

Claudio Carini
Pfizer
Cambridge, Massachusetts, USA

Sandeep Menon
Pfizer
Cambridge, Massachusetts, USA

Mark Chang
AMAG Pharmaceuticals, Inc.
Waltham, Massachusetts, USA

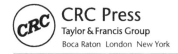

CRC Press
Taylor & Francis Group
Boca Raton London New York

CRC Press is an imprint of the
Taylor & Francis Group, an **informa** business

A CHAPMAN & HALL BOOK

CRC Press
Taylor & Francis Group
6000 Broken Sound Parkway NW, Suite 300
Boca Raton, FL 33487-2742

First issued in paperback 2019

© 2014 by Taylor & Francis Group, LLC
CRC Press is an imprint of Taylor & Francis Group, an Informa business

No claim to original U.S. Government works

ISBN-13: 978-1-4665-9386-2 (hbk)
ISBN-13: 978-0-367-37876-9 (pbk)

Library of Congress Cataloging-in-Publication Data

Clinical and statistical considerations in personalized medicine / Claudio Carini, Sandeep M. Menon, Mark Chang, editors.
       pages cm. -- (Chapman & Hall/CRC biostatistics series)
     Summary: "Personalized medicine has the potential to change the way we think about, identify, and manage health problems. In the pharmaceutical industry, it is already having an exciting impact on both clinical research and patient care. This impact will continue to grow as our understanding and technologies improve. With contributions from well-known industry leaders in clinical development, this book covers the practical aspects of personalized medicine, focusing on issues that have direct application in the industry. Topics include designs for targeted therapy, adaptive designs, evidence-based adaptive statistical decisions, and design strategies for maximizing the efficiency of clinical oncology"-- Provided by publisher.
     Includes bibliographical references and index.
     ISBN 978-1-4665-9386-2 (hardback : acid-free paper) 1. Pharmacogenetics--Statistical methods. 2. Pharmacogenetics--Mathematical models. 3. Pharmacogenomics--Statistical methods. 4. Pharmacogenomics--Mathematical models. I. Carini, Claudio. II. Menon, Sandeep M., editor of compilation. III. Chang, Mark, editor of compilation.

RM301.3.G45C58 2014
615.7072'7--dc23   2014001313

Visit the Taylor & Francis Web site at
http://www.taylorandfrancis.com

and the CRC Press Web site at
http://www.crcpress.com

Contents

Preface

The successful utilization of biomarkers in clinical development and, indeed, realization of personalized medicine require a close collaboration among different stakeholders: clinicians, biostatisticians, regulators, commercial colleagues, and so on. For this reason, we invited experts from different fields of expertise to address the opportunities and challenges and discuss recent advancements related to biomarkers and their translation into clinical development. The first four chapters discuss biomarker development from a clinical perspective ranging from introduction to biomarkers to recent advances in RNAi screens, epigenetics, and rare disease as targets for personalized medicine approaches. Chapters 5 through 10 are devoted to considerations from a statistical perspective, and the last chapter addresses the regulatory issues in biomarker utilization.

A biomarker is a characteristic that can be objectively measured and evaluated as an indicator of a physiological as well as pathological process or response to a therapeutic intervention. Although there is nothing new about biomarkers such as glucose for diabetes and blood pressure for hypertension, the current focus on molecular biomarkers has taken the center stage in the development of molecular medicine. Molecular diagnostic technologies have enabled the discovery of molecular biomarkers and are assisting in the definition of the pathogenic mechanism of diseases. Biomarkers represent the basis of the development of diagnostic assays as well as the target for drug discovery. Biomarkers can help monitoring drugs' effect in clinical trials as well as in clinical practice.

There is a tremendous amount of literature about biomarkers and their utility and potential in clinical development, but there is no comprehensive source of information that integrates and blends the clinical and statistical components together. Of the thousands of biomarkers that are being discovered, very few are being actually validated. This book, which covers a wide spectrum of personalized medicine-related topics, is an overview of the state-of-the-art techniques and advances in the application of biomarkers in drug discovery and development. It represents an important source of information for clinical developers such as biostatisticians, clinicians, scientists, and those involved in drug discovery and development.

The utilization of biomarkers provides great opportunities and tremendous challenges in statistics. One of the major challenges, among many, is the control of false-positive rates due to multiple testing. Multiple testing comes from a larger number of hypotheses tests involving different genes, biomarker subgroup analyses, multiple endpoints, and biomarker adaptive designs. Failing to handle this issue adequately will either increase the likelihood of the false-positive findings in the studies or result in the studies losing their utility and efficiency to the extent that the value of biomarker utilization is completely nullified.

Chapter 1 gives a bird's-eye view of the history, life cycle, and types and applications of biomarkers along with an overview of patient stratification for personalized medicine. Chapter 2 discusses the RNAi screen triumphs and tribulations in the context of drug target development. Chapter 3 presents one of the most exciting and fastest-expanding fields of biology, that is, epigenetics, which is frequently described as a phenomenon of heritable changes in gene expression in the absence of changes in the DNA sequence. Today, human disorders are thought to be driven by combinations of genetic and epigenetic abnormalities. It is the epigenetic component that proves to be most relevant to all aspects of personalized medicine. Chapter 4, which is the final clinical chapter, focuses on rare diseases, which are now becoming targets for personalized medicine approaches, owing to the view that individual susceptibility might now be explained by the subject genetic background and by epigenetic changes. Chapter 5 discusses the new biomarker-informed adaptive design, providing guidance when biomarkers may be used to increase the efficiency of clinical trials. Chapter 6 discusses an adaptive dose-finding design, in which the "dose-arms" are actually different doses potentially efficacious to one subgroup enrolled in the study. Thus, the goal is to select the best dose for this subgroup identified by the genomic marker. Chapter 7 discusses the use of predictive biomarkers in adaptive design. Chapters 8 and 9 present the multiplicity issues in biomarker identification at different stages of clinical trials. Chapter 10 discusses the importance of the patient-report outcomes (PROs) in personalized medicine, where the PRO may be very different for patients with different genomic markers. Chapter 11 addresses the regulatory issues in the utilization of biomarkers for drug development with case studies.

We would like to extend our sincere gratitude to all the authors and reviewers for their sincere tireless effort and time to help us make this project a reality. We would like to thank David Grubbs and Stephanie Morkert from CRC Press for their guidance and coordination. Finally, we would like to dedicate this book to our colleagues in the scientific community and our family and friends.

Editors

Dr. Claudio Carini, **MD, PhD, FRCPath**, has been involved in biomedical research for over 20 years, and his experience includes all stages of biomedical research from bench experimentation to clinical research. Dr. Carini is board certified in internal medicine, pathology, respiratory medicine, and clinical immunology. Dr. Carini obtained his MD in Italy. Later, he earned his PhD in immunology from the University College London (UCL), University of London, and subsequently an FRCPath in immunology from the Royal College of Pathologists, London, and Specialist Diplomas in clinical immunology and in respiratory medicine at the University of Rome.

Currently, Dr. Carini is serving at Pfizer as "Global Clinical Immunology and Biomarkers Lead," being responsible for the immunology/biomarkers strategy for the entire Biosimilars portfolio and other projects. In addition, Dr. Carini holds a honorary faculty position at King's College, School of Medicine, University of London.

Dr. Carini is also serving in several national and international scientific boards:

NIH Biomarkers Consortium Immunology Steering Committee

NIH Biomarkers Consortium "Rheumatoid Arthritis Working Group" Steering Committee

NIH Biomarkers Consortium "SLE Working Group" Steering Committee

NIH Biomarkers Consortium "Ankylosing Spond." "Working Group" Steering Committee

Medical Research Council (MRC, UK) "Inflammation/Immunology Initiative–UK" Rheumatoid Arthritis Consortium, Steering Committee

"Innovation Medicine Initiative, ABIRISK, European Union/EFPIA" Board of Directors

The PML Consortium, Board of Directors

The ISAC "Immuno-Safety Advisory Council," Board of Directors

The Generation Scotland Precision Medicine Initiative University of Scotland (UK), Board of Directors

The Immunogenicity Council, Board of Directors

The Grand Challenge Inflammation & Precision Medicine, University of Glasgow, Board of Directors

Dr. Carini spent several years at:

University College London (UCL), University of London
University of Rome "La Sapienza,"
Johns Hopkins University, Baltimore
Harvard University, Boston

where he served in different faculty roles and was involved in teaching and research focusing on the molecular–cellular immune response.

Dr. Carini has gathered experience in clinical research at:

Wyeth, Novartis, Roche, MDS, Fresenius, and Pfizer

where he held numerous senior positions and was responsible for overseeing the planning, the designing, and the execution of many projects in different therapeutic areas. Dr. Carini has been focusing his research interest in translational medicine covering all the therapeutic areas of interest, and focusing on early and late clinical translational models, biomarkers for decision making, pharmacogenomics, proteomics, clinical assays, and human biobanks.

Dr. Carini has also served on strategic, business development, due diligence, and licensing committees.

Dr. Carini has over 200 publications in national and international peer-reviewed journals. Dr. Carini has spoken in many venues in several national and international meetings, and has been the recipient of meritorious scientific research awards and fellowships.

Dr. Carini is the coeditor of one of the first textbooks on biomarkers, *Biomarkers in Drug Development: A Handbook of Practice, Application and Strategy* published in 2010 by John Wiley & Sons, recently chosen by the British Medical Association (2011) as "Highly Commended" in the pharmacology category.

Dr. Carini is coeditor of a book on personalized medicine, *Clinical and Statistical Considerations in Personalized Medicine*, CRC Press, 2013.

He is also a member of various national and international societies and has served as an ad hoc reviewer for numerous scientific journals.

Sandeep Menon is executive director and head of biostatistics at the Biotherapeutics Research at Pfizer and also an adjunct assistant professor of biostatistics at Boston University, where he teaches intermediate and advanced courses in biostatistics including adaptive designs in clinical trials. Professor Menon has been working in the clinical trials area for almost a decade. He is a regular invited speaker and expert panelist in academic forums and FDA/industry conferences. His research interests are in the area of personalized medicine and adaptive designs. He has received multiple awards for academic excellence. He is also on the thesis committee for multiple doctoral students all of whom focused on the area of adaptive designs. He received his medical degree from the University of Bangalore, India, and later completed his master's and PhD in biostatistics from Boston University.

Mark Chang is vice president of biometrics at AMAG Pharmaceuticals and an adjunct professor at Boston University. Professor Chang is a co-founder of the International Society for Biopharmaceutical Statistics and an elected fellow of the American Statistical Association. He serves on the editorial boards of a statistical journal and has published six books on various topics, including paradoxes in scientific research, adaptive clinical trial designs, modern issues and methods in biostatistics, and Monte Carlo simulations in the pharmaceutical industry.

Contributors

Alexandre Akoulitchev
Oxford BioDynamics
Oxford, United Kingdom

Demissie Alemayehu
Pfizer Inc.
New York, New York

Robert A. Beckman
Center for Evolution and Cancer
Helen Diller Family Cancer Center
University of California at San
    Francisco
San Francisco, California

and

Oncology Clinical Research
Daiichi Sankyo Pharmaceutical
    Development
Edison, New Jersey

Joseph C. Cappelleri
Pfizer Inc.
Groton, Connecticut

Claudio Carini
Pfizer Inc.
Cambridge, Massachusetts

Aloka G. Chakravarty
Division of Biometrics VII
Office of Biostatistics, CDER, FDA
Silver Spring, Maryland

Mark Chang
AMAG Pharma
Waltham, Massachusetts

and

Boston University
Boston, Massachusetts

Cong Chen
Biostatistics and Research
    Decision Sciences
Merck & Co. Inc.
North Wales, Pennsylvania

Alex Dmitrienko
Quintiles
Durham, North Carolina

Candida Fratazzi
Boston Biotech Clinical
    Research, LLC
Cambridge, Massachusetts

Ewan Hunter
Oxford BioDynamics
Oxford, United Kingdom

Fredrick Immermann
Pfizer Inc.
Pearl River, New York

Ilya Lipkovich
Quintiles
Durham, North Carolina

Lingyun Liu
Cytel Inc.
Cambridge, Massachusetts

Sandeep Menon
Pfizer Inc.
Cambridge, Massachusetts

and

Boston University
Boston, Massachusetts

Attila Seyhan
Translational Research Institute for
   Metabolism and Diabetes
Florida Hospital
and
Diabetes and Obesity Research
   Center
Sanford-Burham Medical Research
   Institute
Orlando, Florida

and

Department of Chemical
   Engineering
Massachusetts Institute of
   Technology
Cambridge, Massachusetts

Jing Wang
Department of Biostatistics
Boston University
Boston, Massachusetts

Joseph Wu
Department of Biostatistics
Boston University
Boston, Massachusetts

1

Biomarkers for Drug Development: The Time Is Now!

Claudio Carini and Attila Seyhan

CONTENTS

1.1 Introduction

The practice of medicine today remains largely empirical. Physicians generally rely on pattern matching to establish the diagnosis based on a combination of the patient's medical history, physical examination, and laboratory data. Thus, the treatment is often based on the physician's past experience with similar patients, so typically a blockbuster drug gets prescribed for the typical patient for that specific disease. According to this paradigm, treatment decision is driven by a trial-and-error approach. Thus, the patient becomes the victim of side effects for a drug that works in the majority of people affected by that specific disease. The use of biomarkers (BMs) is going to enable a significant paradigm shift from empirical medicine to precision medicine. It is conceivable that in the immediate future, we will be moving away from the concept of "one size fits all" but rather will be shifting to a precision medicine approach where the right medicine, for the right patient, at the right dose, and at the right time, will be prescribed. As a result of it, we will improve patient care and reduce the health-care cost and potential side effects.

The scientific community is well aware that the use of a specific treatment varies across the targeted population. It has been extensively reported that patients may differ based on different parameters: (1) the early versus late stage of the disease; (2) slow versus fast metabolizers; and (3) good responders versus poor responders. Of course, those are just some of the multiple parameters that one can evaluate.

However, what is driving more and more the acceptance of precision medicine within the scientific community is the need to reduce health-care costs. Payers have increased costs; the pharmaceutical industry has a decreased market share, and patients and physicians are demanding drugs that are more efficacious and safer. This has generated a sense of urgency in the pharmaceutical community that trial and error is not anymore a viable approach. Precision medicine may indeed represent the solution to those problems by improving diagnosis, treatment, and prognosis. A growing body of evidence shows that precision medicine will definitively bring value to the industry by reducing health-care cost and ensuring a more efficacious and safer treatment. Many examples in the literature support this statement proving that targeting therapeutic intervention in a well-characterized population, as is the case for HER2, UGT1A1, can drastically reduce the cost of a patient's treatment.

A few years ago, a report from the Drug and Market Development Publications projected that the revenues for BM-related products and services would expand more than sixfold from an estimate of $452 million in 2003 to 2.9 million in 2008 and even more in 2012. Based on this assessment, the potential savings derived by biomarker (BM) strategy and investments is a must. The same report estimated that 10–20% of pharmaceutical research and development was going to be enhanced by post-genomic BMs (i.e., those relying on genomics, proteomics, or metabonomics), thus cutting the cost for those projects by 15%. By 2008, the same report predicted that half of the projects would be implementing BM in their strategy, resulting in a potential saving of approximately 45%. However, the counterargument is that by the time a marker or a panel of markers are discovered and validated, it can be too late for them to play a role in the decision-making process. However, the real question that remains to be answered before adopting a BM on par to the clinical research is how much the selected BM is intrinsically related to the biology of the disease. Computer models have been applied to published data. However, this can present some risks. It has been recently reported that incorporating results from the published database in order to assess the validity of a chosen BM has raised questions on the accuracy of a nonvalidated and inaccurate database. One of the most relevant issues in designing a translational strategy is to find a BM(s) that has been transferred from animal models to humans. However, it should be taken into consideration that inhibiting an enzyme in an animal model may have a dramatic effect on that animal model, whereas inhibiting the corresponding enzyme in humans may not have a clinical impact, either because the pathway has diverged or because humans have some compensatory mechanism. A treatment may affect a BM but be irrelevant to a specific disease. Thus, it is a must that a BM has to be intrinsically related to the pathogenesis of the disease since we are treating a disease, not a BM. One way of discovering the relevance of a BM is to look for differences between the groups of patients that respond to a specific treatment versus those that do not. Computational biology and mathematical models such as multivariate analysis can reveal differences that would allow members of one group to be separated from another within the sample size utilized for the clinical study. Given some variables, this model should be able to discriminate by chance the treated group from the control with misleading statistical significance. In contrast, when this model will get translated to a wider population with many more variables, the result is definitively a failure. Others may argue that by using SNPs and statistics, we may separate nonresponders from responders. However, the fundamental challenge for the BMs remains to understand how a BM reflects the disease pathogenesis and how it is part of this pathogenesis. Without understanding the pathogenesis of a disease, it is difficult to figure out what is the best BM to be used. Until now, Pharma has pursued for many years the wrong notion that once they discover a difference in response between the control and the treated group, the job is done. The real problem is that they are neglecting to integrate this information with the biology of the disease. When it is not clear what the etiopathogenesis of the disease is, it is hard to figure out what is the right BM to be chosen. However, the real question is that unless a BM is identified as intrinsically related to the pathogenesis of the disease in question, it is very hard to know whether it is linked to the specific disease or simply the indirect expression of poor health. What people would generally do is to take the top few BMs, accordingly to the statistical analysis, and link them to the biological question to be addressed. Unfortunately, as it is often the case, there is little or poor correlation between the BM chosen and the disease studied. For instance, if someone is investigating the potential BM for SLE and Alzheimer versus control, the same set of BMs keep popping up as potential differentiators between those two entities. However, the real question is whether those specific BMs could differentiate SLE from Alzheimer and if the plethora of BM selected is meaningless. Drug companies are obsessed with the idea that a BM needs to be validated before it can be used for decision making. Unfortunately, there are as yet no clear criteria according to which BM is considered validated and reliable. Drug companies have been setting criteria to be satisfied before a BM can be used at the different stages of drug development. However, the rigor on how to use a BM to kill a compound is still exclusively in the hands of pharmaceutical companies. The lack of a standardized process across the pharmaceutical industry, regulatory agencies, and academia and the risk of using the wrong BM or selecting it improperly may lead to the wrong decision of damping a good drug because the selected BM did not work or was wrongly selected.

To overcome this problem, pharmaceutical companies tend to rely for their strategy on several BMs, often too many. This is based on the notion that clusters of variables can be used to differentiate responders from nonresponders. The risk of throwing too many BMs for the same strategy is not only costly but renders the data difficult to be interpreted. Thus, the best strategy for supporting decision making is to select a few BMs with complementary predictive properties.

1.2 History of BMs

The history of biological and pathological processes has been monitored in health and disease. BMs have been one of the pillars of medicine since the times of Hippocrates and even more in recent times. When clinical laboratories became well established in the middle of the twentieth century, many components of body fluids and tissues were analyzed. The uses of blood glucose levels as a marker for diabetes and later of Her2 expression levels as the indicator of treatment response for breast cancer were recognized as some of the markers indicative of a pathological state and disease. Hundreds of BMs are now used in modern medicine for the prediction, diagnosis, and prognosis of disease and therapeutic interventions. The aim of medicine is to now select BMs that are relevant for monitoring therapeutic intervention. Although we think of genes and proteins as BMs, there are many other forms of BMs that have expanded our understanding of, for instance, cardiovascular diseases. In 1733, Stephen Hales first measured blood pressure (Hamilton and Richards, 1982). Subsequent to his initial discovery, many investigators found blood pressure to be elevated in some disorders and reduced in others. Over many years, the meaning of blood pressure, as a surrogate marker for disease, has become ingrained in current clinical practice. Upon first discovery, however, blood pressure had about the same meaning as C-reactive protein (CRP) might have today as a marker for inflammation.

Another early example is the discovery of the electrocardiogram (ECG) by Waller and its refinement by Einthoven in 1887 (Katz and Hellerstein, 1982). These scientists could not have imagined the value ECG has brought to cardiology since that time. ECG is an excellent example of a passive BM that indicates disease but does not participate in the pathologic process. Today's research is focused on chemical or even more molecular markers rather than electrical or physiological markers, but it is important to appreciate the contribution of these early discoveries to the process we use today in searching for newer and more sensitive measures of early disease.

Modern concepts of BMs for vascular disease very likely began with the correlation of blood cholesterol with coronary disease. The best known of modern vascular disease BMs emerged during the cholesterol risk study, the Framingham Heart Study, in which correlations between cholesterol and coronary disease were first reported in 1961. These studies exemplified how a BM was thought to be related to disease and how animal studies can be confirmed after longitudinal studies in large populations.

TABLE 1.1

Candidate BMs for Early Atherosclerosis

C-reactive protein	Leukocyte count
Fibrinogen	Interleukin-6
Tumor necrosis factor alpha	Complement
Cell adhesion molecules	IgG, A, or M
Serum amyloid A	Neopterin
Phospholipase A2	IgE

The relation between cholesterol and coronary disease has stood many challenges, and we are now refining the lipid measures to include more sensitive markers for coronary and other vascular diseases. We now routinely examine high-density lipoprotein (HDL), low-density lipoprotein (LDL), and triglycerides as adjunct BMs for vascular disease. The shift from total cholesterol to LDL cholesterol as a risk factor followed the discovery of the contribution of LDL to the atherosclerotic process.

What are the next BMs? Current interest is focused on markers of inflammation. CRP is a BM that provides information on the presence of inflammation (Ridker et al., 1997, 2003). Although CRP is a standard marker for any inflammation, in the absence of known sources of inflammation, CRP has been considered a marker of inflammation present in several diseases, such as cardiovascular diseases and autoimmune disease. Clearly, any BM needs to stand the test of time in large clinical trials and long-term population studies before it gets widely accepted. In addition, a BM like CRP must be reliably measured. Clinical laboratories must therefore be able to reproduce the measure, and national standards must be established so that measures from different laboratories can be interpreted in the same way (i.e., be standardized) (Pearson et al., 2003).

Other inflammatory BMs are also of interest. The table from Lind (2003) (Table 1.1) provides a list of some other BMs of inflammation that might be useful in predicting coronary disease. Like blood pressure, these BMs would be targets for drugs that block their action and thereby reduce the risk for disease. Other BMs are not directly involved in the disease process, but are indicators of the process. These are similar to ECG in that they would be important indicators of disease, but would not be direct targets for drugs to block their action.

1.3 The Life Cycle of a BM

BMs do not come to preclinical or clinical practice fully formed, fully validated, applicable across all patient populations, and with the guidance as to when to use or not use a specific marker. The tests are introduced poorly characterized with limited directions for understanding their limitations, potential, and applicability, much like an infant enters the life cycle. Over time, the BM can become a powerful tool to be utilized in drug development or patient care. In addition to the biological component of the BM requiring nurturing, there is a need to develop a reliable testing platform to measure the specific BM ready to be utilized for patient care. However, it is often the case in the early stages of a BM implementation that an unreliable and not well-tested platform gets utilized, which is appropriately labeled as "exploratory."

To illustrate the life cycle of a BM, it can be viewed from late maturity, the stage at which most individuals outside of the research laboratory will first encounter the test, working backward to inception. At its most mature stage, an accepted BM is commonly referred to as *"validated,"* meaning the biology is solid and the testing platform is reliable, but for the purpose of making what sort of decision. The term validated also conjures quite varied images in the minds of different people, with the assay's robustness surging to greater steps as one ascends each step of the management ladder. Currently, the concept of *"fit-for-purpose"* is gaining acceptance in the pharmaceutical industry, providing a precise terminology and recognizing the need for a BM. Screening compounds is fundamentally different from deciding dosing escalation in a clinical trial. Indeed, the nature of questions to be asked in different situations varies greatly; however, the real answer of when a given BM is appropriate lies in whether it can reliably provide the necessary information needed to make the right decision. It is mandatory that the risks and benefits of conducting *in vitro* testing of a chemical library, using high-throughput screening, be carefully weighed. It is quite a puzzling process to decide whether a BM *fit-for-purpose* for a specific indication is the real designator of the combinatorial confidence for the proposed action. This approach also takes into account that the magnitude of a decision can be substantially different even when the underlying questions are similar. For example, the acceptable false-positive/false-negative rates for a BM may be higher when one is prioritizing a large number of early stage molecules than when determining whether to terminate a research project on a potential therapeutic target for which only one or two candidate compounds have been identified. The degree of testing can also be affected by the knowledge of similar drugs within the same class or current clinical practice. A BM supporting a new statin with a safety profile comparable to the marketed products is unlikely to require the same degree of characterization as a BM for drugs with a completely new indication (i.e., neovascularization). The potential of a BM to provide actionable information is directly proportional to its maturity, fitness for the intended purpose, and the seriousness of the decision to be made utilizing the information.

The development of a new BM does take at least six to nine months, and can span many years. Testing and building confidence in the biology can strengthen or wane, and the testing platform can improve by becoming smaller, more portable, and more widely available. In many ways, a BM goes through phases similar to the development of a child. The life cycle of a BM can be viewed as progressing from infant to toddler, then to child, pre-teen, adolescent, young adult, independent individual, and finally a mature person.

In 1913, Janeway published a well-documented study where blood pressure was measured via a sphygmomanometer in a large group of patients (Janeway, 1913). This study was made possible because of the blood pressure cuff developed by Scipione Riva-Rocci (1896) and a large relevant patient population (~8000) examined over a nearly 10-year period. Janeway noted that 11% of the patients had systolic blood pressures over 160 mmHg and this group of patients survived for only four to five years after being identified with the condition he named "hypertensive cardiovascular disease" (Janeway, 1913). The underlying physiology of hypertension was poorly understood at this time, and the therapy options were largely limited to rest and reduced salt intake. Extensive research efforts in multiple laboratories led researchers in numerous directions, but it was not until 1939 that the renin–angiotensin–aldosterone system (RAAS) became the coherent focus of primary research (Vertes et al., 1991). Much more bench research and clinical findings, in addition to a consensus opinion of the community, led to the National High Blood Pressure Education Program Task Force I (NHLBI/ NIH); *Report to the Hypertension Information and Education Advisory Committee* in 1973, and the Report of the Joint National Committee (JNC I) (1977) on *Detection, Evaluation, and Treatment of High Blood Pressure* (NIH, 1973). These reports address reference ranges for the BMs of blood pressure, compare recommended therapies and pharmaceutical interventions, and in the most recent release discuss patient stratification. This developing application and acceptance of blood pressure as a BM beyond its original use demonstrates its increasing maturity to the current status as one of the very few accepted surrogate BMs by both clinical practitioners and regulatory agencies. The life cycle of blood pressure is nearly 100 years and continues to grow as knowledge in the field accumulates and scientific and medical confidence in the BM increases.

Further illustrating that BMs are not a new concept and their progression through various stages of development/acceptance can be seen in routine medical practice, the likely tests performed at an annual physical examination include several BMs that have changed over the years, as has the clinical confidence in using them to make decisions. Among the tests administered will be body weight, diastolic/systolic blood pressure, heart rate, and serum lipid profile to provide an initial diagnosis of cardiovascular health. If any of these tests are skewed or abnormal, additional BM measurements would be initiated. Electrocardiogram (EKG or ECG), stress tests, troponins, CRP, and a host of other tests can characterize the presence or absence of heart disease, as well as inform the physician on appropriate therapy. Tests/BMs such as glucose, glycosylated hemoglobin, and alanine aminotransferase (ALT) provide information on other possible clinically important alterations and diseases that may indirectly impact cardiovascular health. Among these BMs, some can be considered "adolescent" (CRP) as "young adult" (prostate-specific antigen), "independent individual" (troponin, stress test, body mass index, glycosylated hemoglobin), and "mature person" (blood pressure, EKG, lipid profile, glucose, ALT).

The two initial reports on hypertension mentioned above can be considered the forerunners of BM initiatives currently underway as consortia between the pharmaceutical industry and the FDA, ILSI/HESI, and NIH. The driver for these present-day programs clearly is the economics of drug development. The process of drug development has grown significantly in cost at the same time as the number of drugs submitted and approved per year has steadily decreased. The decline has resulted from a wide range of causes from the complexity of new disease targets, multifactorial diseases, increased regulatory requirements, and higher expectations of drug safety. As the acute causes of mortality and morbidity have been partially addressed by the medical community, the population now is experiencing the ill effects of more chronic diseases and novel therapeutic targets; thus, new methods have become necessary. Many of these new therapeutic areas are still in need of predictive animal models for early-stage testing, as well as more comprehensive tools for defining the pathological/clinical condition. Owing to the greater uncertainty in these areas, the compound attrition rates have been increasing. Inefficiencies in the drug development process and marketing expenses have also contributed to the increases in drug development costs. The marketplace also has a substantial impact on whether a new drug, even if approved, will actually be distributed to patients. A compound that cannot be sufficiently differentiated from similarly approved molecules in terms of safety, efficacy, or cost is unlikely to be included in the formularies of large insurers or become an approved course of treatment in countries with publicly funded health-care systems. BMs can be used to establish differentiation in class, and this use will likely increase.

In the early-attrition paradigm designed to identify nonviable compounds at the first possible stage of development, many new BMs are being utilized by the pharmaceutical industry to achieve the cost-containment goals. These BMs are only sufficiently characterized to be considered a discovery tool and are generally limited to be used for the prioritization of similar early-stage molecules. Nevertheless, the tests are valuable for proving the viability or proof of nonviability of a therapeutic target or class of compounds. These BMs most often are mechanism-of-action or safety markers. In contrast, disease-related outcome BMs can be difficult to validate in the absence of sizable efforts, like the one for hypertension. Without additional research involving multiple clinical situations, possibly necessitating consortia to share resources, very few BMs currently being developed will go past the point in their lifecycle where they get to be used for internal decision making during pharmaceutical testing.

The time that it takes for a BM to move from discovery to validation and subsequent submission to regulatory authorities may depend on the disease area and the technologies used as well as whether it will be used as a surrogate end point BM or exclusively for dug development. As discussed by Wagner (2002) once candidates of BMs are identified, a decision has to be made whether any of these BMs are useful for downstream decision making and if enough is known about the BM to predict success (Wagner et al., 2007). If the answer is yes to both questions, then the next step is to validate and qualify the specific BM by creating a research plan to be sent to regulatory authorities. Upon completion of the review process, the research plan is executed and the data from the research are sent to the regulators. The regulatory authorities review the data and if the decision is in favor of the qualification as a BM, the qualified BM is used for decision making (Wagner et al., 2007).

1.4 BMs and Decision Making

Traditional clinical trial end points, such as morbidity and mortality, often require extended time frames and may be difficult to evaluate. Imaging-based BMs provide objective end points that may be confidently evaluated in a reasonable time frame. In affected joints, as well as in tissues expressing specific receptors, MRI, CT, and PET imaging deliver new information to clinicians and researchers. This aspect of BMs is rapidly developing, requiring close collaboration between basic researchers and physicians treating patients (Figure 1.1). Imaging techniques tend to be expensive, but can be cost effective when used in well-defined situations where subjective assessment has been the only approach available. In Alzheimer's disease, pain, and osteoarthritis, imaging is reshaping clinical trial design.

Historically, BMs have been referred to as analytes in biological samples, or as a measurement that predicts a disease state or response to a specific drug therapy or pathogenic pathway. BMs are valuable drug development tools that provide more accurate or more complete information regarding drug performance and disease activity/progression. The BM concept has evolved over time from single physiological parameters (blood pressure, serum cholesterol, blood glucose) to highly complex multi-marker genomic/proteomic panels and sophisticated imaging technologies.

Developments in genomics and proteomics have renewed the interest in BMs as useful clinical tools. While the speed of developing these technologies has been impressive, the interpretation of data has not reached maturity as yet. Often, the time required to characterize and validate new BMs

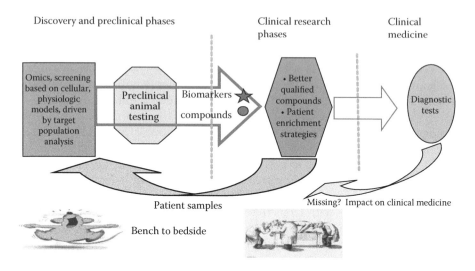

FIGURE 1.1
(See color insert.) BMs connect discovery to clinical research and create a continuous feedback for innovation.

is lagging behind the rapidly evolving technologies. For specific BM panels, the risk is that by the time a BM or a panel of BMs is validated, it may be too late, in the drug development process, to be of value in decision making. Nevertheless, BMs constitute a rational approach that, at its most optimal, reflects both the biology of the disease and the effect of the drug candidate. Proper incorporation of BMs in the drug development strategy enables the concept of "fail fast, fail early," allowing early identification of the extremely high proportion of compounds that fail during drug development. In addition to minimizing human exposure to drugs unlikely to be effective or with safety concerns, substantial cost savings can be achieved by shifting resources to those molecules most likely to become effective new medicines. A properly selected and characterized BM also facilitates the selection of the proper critical path toward approval and can differentiate the new product from approved drugs in a competitive marketplace. The challenge therefore is to identify relevant BMs early enough to implement them for "go, no-go" decisions at critical stages of the development process. However, there is a wide array of considerations that need to be kept in mind when selecting a BM, and which must be balanced against each other, to ensure that the test developed will meet the intended goal. Among the multiple areas that need to be defined, such as the nature and value of the BMs to be used (activity, efficacy, safety, surrogate); the turnaround time requirements to be developed and validated; the reproducibility and sensitivity, and stability and compatibility with the study design.

BMs development forms one of the cornerstones of a new working paradigm in the pharmaceutical industry by increasing the importance of linking diagnostic technologies with the use of drugs. The position of the FDA is rather clear on this. BMs are crucial to generate safe and efficacious drugs and are essential for deciding what patients should receive which treatment. It appears likely that development of pharmaceuticals will also drive the development of BMs as diagnostic probes for clinical decisions and stratification of patients.

1.5 Types of BMs and Their Application

Dictated by the principle of being associated with how they will be used, that is, *fit-for-purpose* (Lee et al., 2006), many different BMs have been developed to assist in the diagnosis and prognosis of specific diseases, disease progress and patient response to treatments, and identification and validation of novel targets, provide insights into the drug mechanism of action, help to characterize disease subpopulations, establish treatments for patients, and predict treatment response (personalized medicine) (Butterfield et al., 2008). Based on the area of application, BMs are classified as:

1. *Predictor BMs:* These are disease-associated BMs that can not only indicate whether there is a threat of disease but can also measure the patient's responsiveness to treatment. For example, serum VEGF and fibronectin can predict clinical response to interleukin-2 (IL-2) therapy of patients with metastatic melanoma and renal cell carcinoma, and high levels of these proteins correlate with lack of clinical response to IL-2 therapy and decreased overall survival of patients (Sabatino et al., 2009). Therefore, serum VEGF and fibronectin are easily measured predictor BMs that could serve to exclude patients unlikely to respond to IL-2 therapy. Additionally, carbonic anhydrase IX-G250MN (CAIX) expression can predict responses to IL-2 in renal cell carcinoma and high CAIX staining of primary renal cell carcinoma tumors correlates with a significantly better survival rate after IL-2 therapy (Atkins et al., 2005).

2. *Diagnostic BMs:* These are the BMs used for diagnosis of an existing disease (Bayele et al., 2010). Examples include cardiac troponin for the diagnosis of myocardial infarction and staging of disease BMs such as brain natriuretic peptide for congestive heart failure and measurements of carcinoembryonic antigen-125 for various cancers (Group, 2001). Auto-antibodies such as anticylic citrullinated peptide (CCP) are detected in patients with RA (Nishimura et al., 2007) while antinuclear antibodies and anti-Ro (SSA) antibodies are also detected in patients with Sjogren's syndrome and other systemic autoimmune diseases (Schulte-Pelkum et al., 2009). Diagnostic BMs

can also be used to stratify patients by disease type and response to treatment. BMs that can reveal the status of the target (e.g., at the level of receptor expression, genetic polymorphism, gene expression, somatic mutation, etc.) in individual patients may provide significant predictive value for treatment response. For example, in cancer, gene-expression profiling was successfully used in tumors to evaluate the likelihood of recurrence (e.g., overexpression of Her-2/neu) and the need for adjuvant therapy, leading to the successful use of trastuzumab and imatinib solely in responder patient populations (Woodcock and Woosley, 2008).

3. *Prognostic markers:* These BMs predict the future outcome of a disease in an individual and can predict overall survival rate and clinical benefit from a therapeutic intervention. For example, the type, density, and location of immune cells within the tumor samples is a better predictor of patient survival than the histopathological methods currently used to stage colorectal cancer (Galon et al., 2006) and the presence of intratumoral T cells correlates with improved progression-free survival and overall survival among patients with advanced ovarian carcinoma (Zhang et al., 2003). Moreover, overexpression of Her-2/neu in breast cancer or EGFR expression in colorectal cancer indicates poor prognoses (Woodcock and Woosley, 2008). These BMs are often used to establish inclusion criteria for a clinical trial or to define a patient population.

4. *Mechanistic BMs.* These may inform and validate the mechanism(s) of action of a particular drug or treatment. For example, sequential gene profiling of basal cell carcinomas treated with imiquimod (a Toll-like receptor-7 agonist capable of inducing complete clearance of basal cell carcinoma (BCC) and other cutaneous malignancies) in a placebo-controlled study has revealed the early transcriptional events induced by imiquimod and provided insights about immunological events preceding acute tissue and/or tumor rejection (Panelli et al., 2007).

5. *Pharmacodynamic (PD) BMs.* These BMs are signatures of a certain pharmacological response to an active compound or BMs for monitoring the clinical response to an active compound or intervention. BMs are the "PD" in PK/PD (pharmacokinetic–pharmacodynamic) and, by linking BMs and mechanistic PK/PD models, are critical to understand the relationship between dose and BM response. BMs can provide information during the drug development and decision-making process; therefore, the BM strategy must be integrated with the PK/PD strategy. Since preclinical PK–PD models have to be validated by predicting the dose–efficacy relationship in clinical trials, knowing the extent and duration of target exposure and modulation is necessary to achieve effects during clinical trials. This is

often accomplished by preclinical PK/PD modeling. Such models are obtained by measuring plasma exposure, target occupancy, and PD end points for target activity (e.g., the level of P-kinase or P-substrate for kinase targets) over time and at various doses (Winkler, 2010). To show target engagement, BMs need to be very closely linked to the target (e.g., examining the proximal P-kinase or P-substrate levels for kinase targets should reveal the target engagement by the drug). In addition, linking BMs and the mechanistic PK/PD models can reveal the underlying mechanism of drug action and the relationship between dose and BM response, impact dose-escalation studies on the time course of response, measure the duration of response and lag between plasma drug concentration and response, measure the effect of repeated doses (toleration, sensitization, reflex mechanisms), range of doses, dose separation, and dosing interval (can be a key uncertainty) and form the basis for clinical trial simulations. These all contribute to increased confidence in BMs, leading to go no-go decisions and helping design future studies. Of course, the main objective is not to measure BM response but to make informed decisions. PD BMs can be used in dose selection for Phase II/III trials based on BM PK–PD and the projected therapeutic index since optimal dose selection is one of the most important deliverables in early clinical development. Moreover, PD BMs can help to differentiate the candidate drug from other compounds based on the demonstration of a key response (safety, efficacy). They can also provide valuable feedback to discovery if the mechanism does not translate to humans. To summarize, these BMs are valuable tools for translational PK–PD and the decision-making process. For example, hemoglobin A1C for antidiabetic treatment is used in decision making in early drug development (Wagner et al., 2007). Other examples of these markers are DCEMRI (dynamic contrast-enhanced magnetic resonance imaging) for the detection of changes in the permeability of tumor vasculature, FDG PET (fluorodeoxy-glucose positron emission tomography) for the detection of changes in glucose metabolism, and FLT PET (fluoro-L-thymidine positron emission tomography) for the detection of changes in DNA synthesis (Holmgren, 2008).

6. *Markers as a surrogate end point.* These may yield information on the clinical benefit/survival at earlier stages as opposed to prolonged disease-free or overall survival analysis (Butterfield et al., 2008). For example, if a treatment affects the BM, the BM will serve as a surrogate end point for evaluating clinical benefit (e.g., hemoglobin A1C) (Wagner et al., 2007). Other examples include the response rate or progression-free survival in oncology or bone mineral density in osteoporosis prevention and treatment. If validated, a surrogate BM

may serve as a primary end point in a registration study (Zwierzina, 2008). Another example is the HIV viral load as a measure of probable clinical benefit with later confirmation of a mortality benefit (Hughes et al., 1998).

7. *Safety BMs.* These BMs can predict at the time of the patient's enrollment her/his likelihood of suffering major toxicity from a specific therapy (Butterfield et al., 2008).

Efforts to expand the safety BM capabilities for drug development have not been as productive as to develop BMs for assessing drug–target engagement, disease progression, and drug efficacy (Sistare et al., 2010). In spite of these shortcomings, there is renewed interest recently in the development and qualification of safety BMs. In addition, recent advances in analytical multi-omics technologies and animal models have raised the utility of these BMs in drug development (Sistare et al., 2010). This interest has been realized and supported by several Predictive Safety Testing Consortium (PSRC) working groups formed to focus on qualifying safety BMs for different organs (e.g., kidney, liver, vascular system, carcinogenesis, and myopathy) and drug-induced injuries (Mattes et al., 2010). From such collaborative efforts, albumin, total protein, B2-microglobulin, cystatin C, Kim-1, and TFF3 have been selected from earlier studies as BMs of drug-induced kidney injuries (Sistare et al., 2010). Given its significance in the ultimate "go" or "no go" decision-making process, no other BM is more important to drug testing than drug safety BMs.

Nonetheless, the development and use of BMs must be dictated by the principle of being associated with how they will be used; that is, *fit-for-purpose* (Lee et al., 2006). Because BMs provide insightful information during the drug development and decision-making process, the BM strategy must be integrated into various phases of drug development from early discovery to late clinical drug development. Linking BMs and mechanistic PK–PD models early in the preclinical phase of drug development can provide the underlying mechanism of drug action, establish a relationship between dose and response to treatment, impact dose-escalation studies on the time course of response, measure the duration of response and lag between plasma drug concentration and response, measure the effect of repeated doses (toleration, sensitization, reflex mechanisms), help to identify the range of doses and dosing interval, and form the foundation for clinical trial simulations. Moreover, BMs can not only guide dose selection for phase II/III studies based on BM PK/PD and the projected therapeutic index but can also help to differentiate candidate drug from competitors based on the demonstration of a key response (safety, efficacy).

To have any utility, assays for BMs must be validated so that anytime, anywhere, and by anyone they are reliable and reproducible. After validation, a

BM can be used to diagnose disease risk, to make a prognosis, or to establish treatments for the patients.

However, the ultimate goal of a BM is to be used for making informed decisions so that all contribute to increase confidence in the BM(s) to make go/no-go decisions and help design future studies.

1.6 Patient Stratification for Personalized Medicine

Patient stratification strengthens traditional medicine by associating an individual patient with a specific therapy. Patient stratification is already practiced in several contexts, though often after first-line empirical treatment proves unsatisfactory because of poor efficacy or intolerable toxicity. Examples can be seen in antibiotics that are matched to specific resistant infections, or the often protracted process of selecting the appropriate medicine for patients with schizophrenia. BMs enable the progression from empirical therapy to stratification therapy linking patient subsets with therapies that have an increased likelihood of success. In breast cancer, patients with different levels of receptor tyrosine kinase HER2 expression characterize not only their cancer type, but also their candidacy for receiving treatment. Similarly, HIV therapies that are tailored to the viral variant present and the oncology treatment regimes prioritize agents based on histological and molecular tests. In the absence of a BM, patient stratification may not be possible. For instance, the lack of accepted BMs in depression that are reflective of disease status or progression often results in patients receiving several different therapies to identify one that leads to a satisfactory response. At present, the treatment for depression remains limited to empirical, trial-and-error therapy.

Patient's stratification has considerable economic impact on the model of the pharmaceutical industry and society. By identifying the populations most likely to benefit from a new therapy, drug development costs can be reduced at the same time as treatment of people unlikely to respond is minimized. Exposure to drugs that do not address a patient's underlying disease is minimized, thereby also reducing the likelihood of adverse events in those for whom the compound does not provide help. Overall, the risk–benefit assessment is substantively refined when the potential for adverse drug–drug interactions is reduced, and the process enhanced when BM data enabling patient stratification are available. Patient compliance also will be improved as treatment becomes more closely linked with disease resolution in a higher proportion of the individuals treated. Ultimately, better targeting of specific disease and responsive patient through BMs can reshape clinical practice by providing clinicians with new opportunities for better patient care (Figure 1.2).

In traditional clinical trial designs, the assumption is that a relative homogenous group of patients with a specific disease will be randomly

Choose the RIGHT DRUG at the RIGHT DOSE for the RIGHT PERSON

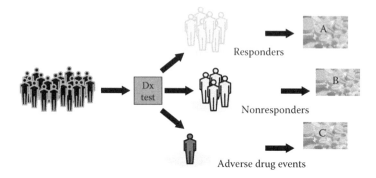

FIGURE 1.2
(**See color insert.**) Personalized medicine concepts foresee greater use of diagnostics in therapeutic decision making. Classical treatments assume a homogenous patient before testing a new drug.

selected to prevent bias. The goal of random sampling is to ensure that the general population is well represented. In reality, the groups are heterogeneous with respect to the stage of disease, drug metabolizing capabilities, environmental conditions (e.g., diet, smoking status, and lifestyle), concurrent or previous medication exposures, and often even an underlying cause of the symptomatology. By using BMs to better characterize the biological makeup of the participants in clinical trials, drug developers are streamlining the testing process. The most obvious and often quoted use of patient stratification is to select only patients who would be expected to respond to a given investigational drug based on the mechanism of action of the specific drug. The drug's statistically significant benefits, in this targeted subset of patients, could be shown in a smaller and shorter clinical trial than those needed for randomly selected patients. Under some circumstances, stratification of responders could also be performed retrospectively on the data collected to demonstrate efficacy of a compound in a subpopulation. Though this approach is not generally acceptable for registration, retrospective findings have proven to be important for identifying potentially new therapeutic applications and redirecting programs (e.g., Neurontin® for neuropathic pain, Rogaine® for hair growth, Viagra® for erectile dysfunction). Stratification can certainly speed approval for drug candidates by narrowing down a specific subset of patients, while leaving the door open for further testing and market expansion in the larger population of patients. On the other hand, stratification can unmask a useful therapeutic agent that would otherwise be lost in the noise generated by the nonresponders, as previously described for trastuzumab and gefitinib (Figure 1.3).

However, before even considering patient stratification, the real challenge of testing a new drug entity, especially in chronic diseases like Alzheimer's

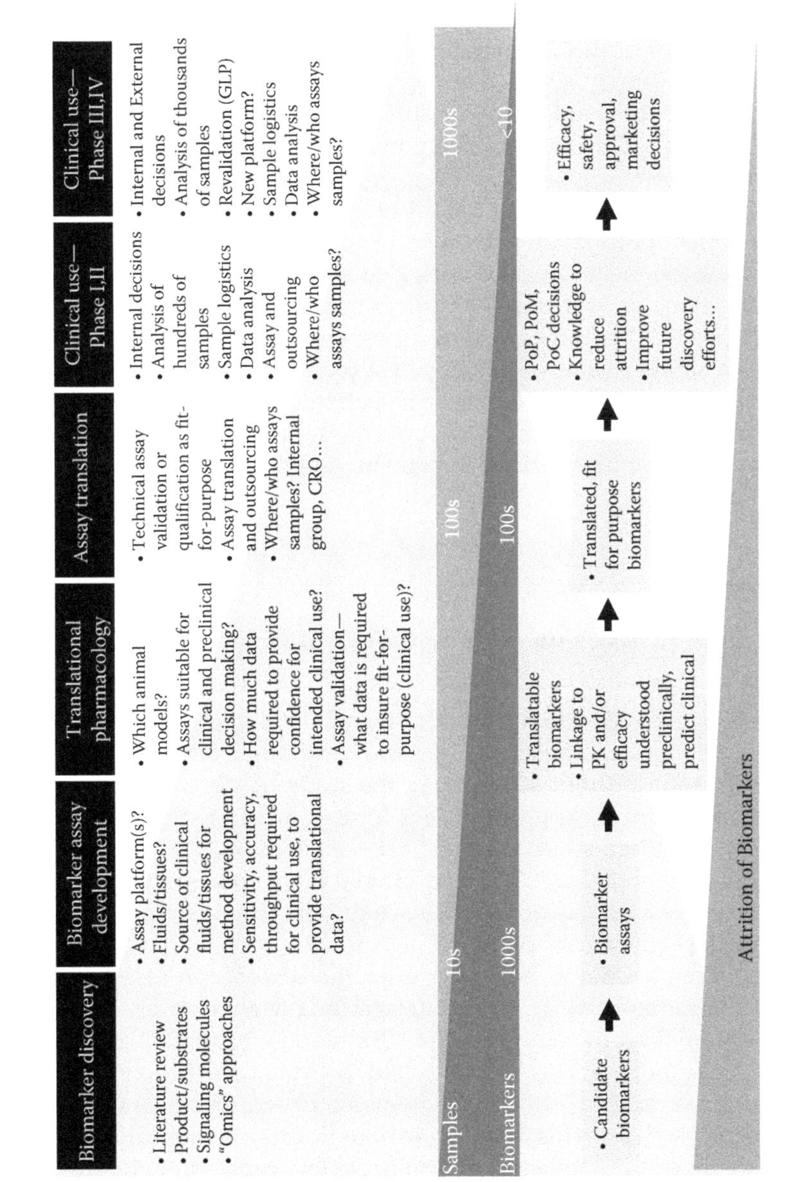

Biomarker discovery	Biomarker assay development	Translational pharmacology	Assay translation	Clinical use—Phase I,II	Clinical use—Phase III,IV
• Literature review • Product/substrates • Signaling molecules • "Omics" approaches	• Assay platform(s)? • Fluids/tissues? • Source of clinical fluids/tissues for method development • Sensitivity, accuracy, throughput required for clinical use, to provide translational data?	• Which animal models? • Assays suitable for clinical and preclinical decision making? • How much data required to provide confidence for intended clinical use? • Assay validation—what data is required to insure fit-for-purpose (clinical use)?	• Technical assay validation or qualification as fit-for-purpose • Assay translation and outsourcing • Where/who assays samples? Internal group, CRO…	• Internal decisions • Analysis of hundreds of samples • Sample logistics • Data analysis • Assay and outsourcing • Where/who assays samples?	• Internal and External decisions • Analysis of thousands of samples • Revalidation (GLP) • New platform? • Sample logistics • Data analysis • Where/who assays samples?

Samples	10s	100s		1000s	
Biomarkers	1000s	100s		<10	

• Candidate biomarkers → • Biomarker assays → • Translatable biomarkers; Linkage to PK and/or efficacy understood preclinically, predict clinical → • Translated, fit for purpose biomarkers → • PoP, PoM, PoC decisions; Knowledge to reduce attrition; Improve future discovery efforts… → • Efficacy, safety, approval, marketing decisions

Attrition of Biomarkers

FIGURE 1.3
(See color insert.) A schematic of a workflow for the discovery and development of a "fit-for-purpose disease-related biomarkers." This process requires a well-planned and executed research plan.

disease (AD), is due to the generally slow progression of the disease and subjective nature of diagnostic tests. Thus, though patient stratification can drastically reduce the length and number of patients selected to assess the efficacy of a new molecular entity, unfortunately, the patient stratification approach and shorter clinical study present some severe limitations: (1) clinical trials need to have a duration of many months to demonstrate statistically significant clinical efficacy; (2) the early-onset form of AD may not predict what will happen in the same population later in their life; and (3) stratification not based on a BM that accurately predicts disease progression will further be problematic.

In conclusion, the goal of patient stratification using BMs is to create subsets within a patient population that yield insightful information about how the patient will respond to a given therapeutic intervention or treatment. Patient stratification can transform a clinical trial from a negative outcome to one with a positive outcome by identifying the subset of the population most likely to respond to a novel therapy. If successful, this can increase the responder population, reduce the size of the patient's samples to be tested as well as the time and cost, but most importantly reduce the attrition rate of drug discovery leading to a positive impact on public health.

1.7 Future Perspectives on BMs and Personalized Medicine

Of the multiple molecular approaches, perhaps none has garnered more attention for BM discovery than genomics using DNA microarrays for surveying global changes in the entire genome. Although DNA microarray studies have led to important advances in the study of global gene expression profiling of autoimmunity, their use is limited owing to the problem of physiologically important splice variants that exist in individual cell populations (Fathman, Soares et al., 2005). An additional problem lies in the fact that a large proportion of mRNAs are not translated into proteins, despite being activated at the level of transcription.

Proteomics offers a unique perspective on the disease process because proteins and their enzymatic functions determine the phenotypic diversity that can arise from a set of common genes (Rifai and Gerszten, 2006). Since posttranslational modifications help regulate the structure, function, localization, maturation, and turnover of proteins and because the entire complement of expressed proteins in their various forms can rapidly change in response to environmental stimuli, the proteome represents the unique collection of proteins that reflects the state of the cell or group of cells at a specific time and space, in a particular context under particular stimuli making the proteome highly dynamic, contrary to the genome (Rifai and Gerszten, 2006).

The proteomics is limited largely by the current technology and the scarcity of high-quality reagents such as monoclonal antibodies and informatics tools as well as the difficulty in identifying low-abundance markers (Rifai, Gillette et al., 2006). Many of the biological molecules relevant to disease are low-abundance proteins. For instance, cardiac markers such as troponin are found in the nanomolar range and insulin in the picomolar range. There are an estimated 10,000 unique proteins found in serum with concentrations spanning a dynamic range of greater than 10 orders of magnitude (Rifai and Gerszten, 2006). Unbiased proteomic approaches have had limited success for studying systemic autoimmune diseases, while array and FACS platforms are limited because it is a bottom-up targeted approach with *a priori* knowledge of target proteins. It is impossible to know which important aspects will be missed owing to the limitations of current arrays or antibodies, etc. (Fathman, Soares et al., 2005).

It is often the target that dictates what assay should be used to assess the target. Drug "targets" are usually part of the cellular pathways or networks that are affected by various downstream and upstream factors of the identified target. Since the state of these targets or pathways may be indicative of drug response in an individual, this reduces the predictive value of a single-target assay (Woodcock and Woosley, 2008).

Another relevant issue is the reproducibility. Many different scientists are conducting their own research with their own samples using their own methods, leading to different outcomes. What is needed is to establish robust, reproducible, and standardized methodologies together with bioinformatics and biostatistics to define the most effective strategies for the discovery of new candidate BMs. Thereby, it is highly recommended to incorporate a team of bioinformatics and biostatisticians into the study from the study design to the data analysis.

The limited or restricted access to disease associated tissues is another limitation. This has led to the wide-scale utilization of peripheral blood as the source tissue for identification of BMs largely in immune diseases. Since the blood is the path where immune cells reach the lymphatic organs, it can be used to identify DNA, RNA, protein, or other small molecule BMs.

In a clinical setting, the peripheral blood is an easily accessible vehicle which has generated great interest in using leukocyte transcript profiling to understand disease processes (Calvano, Xiao et al., 2005; Burczynski and Dorner, 2006). It was shown that differential genomic changes can be observed in distinct blood leukocyte subpopulations in response to the same *in vivo* stimulus (Laudanski, Miller-Graziano et al., 2006). However, the genomic changes seen in the total leukocyte population were skewed in comparison to individual cell subtypes, which led to the practice of leukocyte enrichment to create more homogeneous subpopulations allowing a clearer functional interpretation of gene-expression patterns (Laudanski, Miller-Graziano et al., 2006). Unfortunately, the fractionation of leukocytes into different subpopulations is technically challenging and extremely time consuming. Kotz et al. (2010) developed a microfluidic device that can capture highly enriched (>95%) neutrophils directly from 150 μL of whole blood in 5 min in sufficient quantity and purity for genome-wide microarray and mass spectrometry-based proteomic analysis.

Novel parallel techniques have been used to collect complex BM signatures from unique populations of white blood cells or whole blood, which has led to a better understanding of adaptive immunity. For instance, global gene-expression profiling is now used as a surrogate for biological phenotypes of cell populations within the immune system (Nevins and Potti, 2007).

Although we have learned much from the studies of the discovery of novel BMs in chronic complex diseases, the outcomes and their correlations to disease largely depend on cross-sectional observations (analysis of data gathered from two or more samples at one point in time) that do not clearly define the pathogenesis of the individual disease process. Most of the novel BMs and their correlations with disease have largely been elicited from two or more samples at one point in time. Single measurements rarely capture all the different dimensions of clinical outcomes; thus, a multidimensional and continuous model is needed to replace the single dimension binary model of clinical outcomes for an effective decision-making process. This requires new strategies in the experimental design, including a continuous collection of clinical samples over time.

Since information arising from the population "mean" data may not be applicable to a specific subject, given that the outcomes are related to people rather than the entire population, individual responders rather than population mean analyses should be developed and linked to specific BM status for the implementation of precision medicine. Decreasing the individual differences in drug exposure is therefore critical to reduce the response variability (Woosely and Cossman, 2007; Woodcock and Woosley, 2008).

Development of fit-for-purpose BMs is beginning to allow us to move from empirical medicine to precision medicine, that is, instead of one size fits all, we are beginning to move toward a model that uses the right treatment to the right patient at the right time, as a consequence of availability of improved knowledge on the patient's biology. As stated by Shen and Hwang (2010), precision medicine can lead to (i) improvement of patient care and (ii) facilitate the assessment of clinical utility. For example, patients with a low versus high pretest probability of a condition, early- versus late-stage disease, slow versus fast metabolizers of a drug, or good versus poor medication compliance are among the many other factors that affect the utility of a test or treatment. It is also well known that clinical utility will vary depending on what action to take following a result.

Given that, we believe that targeted therapies will be more widely used. As diseases are subtyped more specifically and therapies better designed, clinical drug trials will be more focused. Precision medicine ensures that patients receive optimal treatment that is personalized and delivered in the most beneficial, cost-effective setting possible.

Attempts to identify specific signatures for complex diseases include inflammatory and autoimmune diseases, which have many overlapping symptoms and associated BMs; it feels like the poem by John Godfrey Saxe (Himmelfarb et al., 2002) where several blinded men are examining the elephant from different angles, except that each of them could assess a little of it, missing the entire picture. Thus, everything being studied and analyzed feels like the different pieces of the puzzle are addressing specific and individual problems. In real terms, we are failing to see how all of the different pieces are interconnected as part of a larger, more cohesive picture (the body of the elephant). This is especially true of multilayer diseases where a new paradigm shift is needed to look at the bigger picture in order to place each signature as a piece of a puzzle into the aforementioned picture (the Elephant) (Figure 1.4).

New approaches in terms of bioinformatics and assay platforms as well as integration of multi-omic platforms need to be developed to study at the same time all the unrelated datasets, including gene, miRNA, and protein expression, and FACS platforms. The use of multi-omic platforms in the analysis of

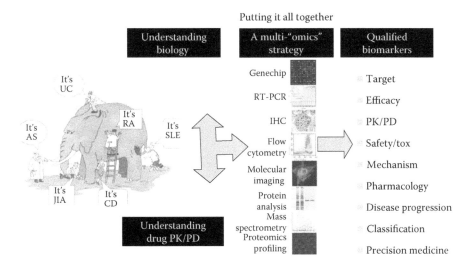

FIGURE 1.4

(**See color insert.**) Putting it all together, a multidimensional and a multi-omics strategy for the discovery of BMs attempting to identify specific signatures for complex diseases including inflammatory and autoimmune disease, which has many overlapping symptoms, begins with understanding the biology of disease as well as understanding the response to drug and finally putting all the pieces together in a unified picture as illustrated. It is also recommended that the correlations largely should derive from cross-sectional observations using a multiomics strategy to develop robust and validated BMs in diseases that do not clearly define the pathogenesis of the individual disease process. (The source of the elephant is: Himmelfarb, J. et al. 2002. *Kidney Int* **62**(5): 1524–1538; doi:10.1046/j.1523-1755.2002.00600.x; Right panel adapted from Rabia Hidi, SGS Biomarkers webinar, 10.07.10) systemic autoimmune diseases will not only identify numerous useful BMs but also will reveal areas for further development and improvement.

Although miRNAs are promising as candidate BMs of diagnosis, prognosis, disease activity, and severity in autoimmune diseases, they need to be validated in larger studies designed specifically for BM validation (Alevizos and Illei, 2010).

In summary, a multidisciplinary approach to study chronic complex diseases is needed for identification of disease BMs that can be translatable to human trials. With the advent of novel approaches and technologies coupled to integrative network biology-based BM discovery efforts, we shall be able to identify robust and reproducible BMs specific for layers of complex multilayered diseases.

Furthermore, coupling BMs to a simple, inexpensive point-of-care diagnostic test can help to stratify patient populations for a specific disease(s) or treatment regimen.

Furthermore, a collaborative effort across different technology experts and disease areas will be required to utilize integrated methodologies for the discovery of robust and validated BMs. Because the development and qualification of new BMs involve many interdisciplinary groups, several consortia have been formed for this purpose (Figure 1.5). For example, The Biomarker Consortium (http://www.biomarkersconsortium.org) was founded by NIH, FDA, and Center for Medicare and Medicaid Services (CMS), along with the private sector organizations PhRMA (the pharmaceutical manufacturers'

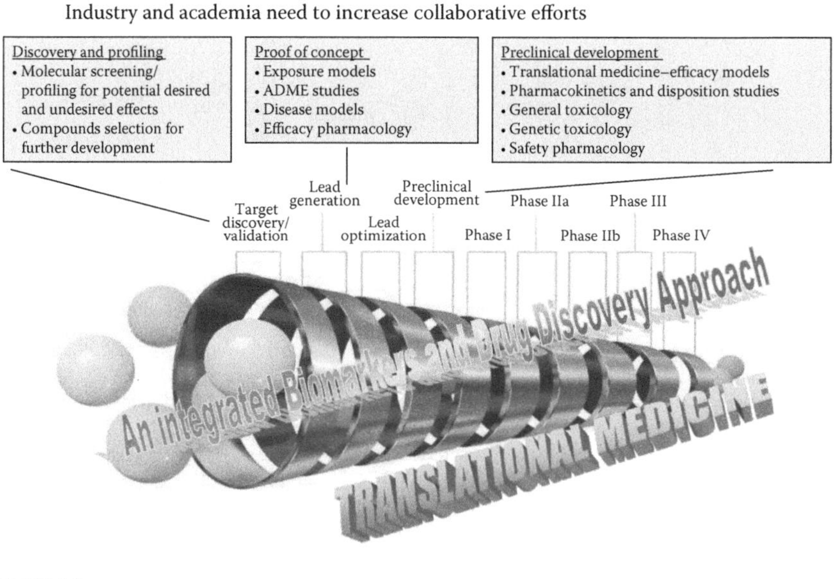
Industry and academia need to increase collaborative efforts
Discovery and profiling
• Molecular screening/ profiling for potential desired and undesired effects
• Compounds selection for further development
Proof of concept
• Exposure models
• ADME studies
• Disease models
• Efficacy pharmacology
Preclinical development
• Translational medicine–efficacy models
• Pharmacokinetics and disposition studies
• General toxicology
• Genetic toxicology
• Safety pharmacology
Target discovery/ validation
Lead generation
Lead optimization
Preclinical development
Phase I
Phase IIa
Phase IIb
Phase III
Phase IV
An integrated Biomarkers and Drug Discovery Approach
TRANSLATIONAL MEDICINE

FIGURE 1.5
(See color insert.) To accelerate the successful drug discovery process and reduce attrition, industry and academia must work collaboratively.

trade organization) and BIO (the Biotechnology Industry Organization), and now includes industrial, academic, and patient group members (Woodcock and Woosley, 2008).

The use of BMs in preclinical and clinical studies can provide information on the efficacy and safety of a new drug in development, which is highly valuable to those responsible for making decisions on the potential therapeutic effect of a new drug under investigation.

These activities will ensure optimal decision making in drug development and will allow the use of BMs and any potential diagnostics (as a consequence of these efforts) in the effective execution of targeted and personalized therapies across complex disease areas.

1.8 Conclusions

BMs serve many purposes in drug development and evaluation of therapeutic intervention and treatment strategies. They can be impactful for the selection of candidate compounds for preclinical and clinical studies. They can play a critical role to characterize subtypes of disease allowing patient stratification for which the most appropriate therapeutic intervention can be aimed at. However, strategies for development have faced many technical challenges, in part, due to the poor experimental design, small sample size, and pharmacogenetic heterogeneity of patients.

Presumably, a more radical strategy is required to warrant future success of BM development and validation. By using the knowledge gained from the earlier studies as well as new strategies for study designs and multiomics technologies to execute them, it is anticipated that we should be able to develop robust BMs. Gathering information and careful design and planning of the study are crucial steps toward the attainment of this goal. As design and planning commence toward the execution phase, other factors and considerations should be evaluated to allow optimization of the process until the objectives are achieved. This process should yield candidate BMs that can be validated and qualified as surrogate markers substituting for clinical end points and help in the decision-making process. Moreover, standardization of sample collection and data analysis and emphasis on computational biology to process large data sets are crucial to facilitate this process.

Finally, robust linkage of a BM with a clinical end point is needed, although it is not needed for the early clinical development where the aim is validation of pharmacologic response or dose and regimen optimization. Realization of the potential benefits of BMs as surrogate end points to facilitate the development of targeted, safe, and precision therapies will require BMs to be linked to clinical end points. To achieve all, it does require a network of collaboration between the academia, pharmaceutical industry, and governmental regulatory agencies and international networks all working toward the same goal.

References

Alevizos, I. and G. G. Illei 2010. MicroRNAs as biomarkers in rheumatic diseases. *Nat Rev Rheumatol* **6**(7): 391–398.

Atkins, M. et al. 2005. Carbonic anhydrase IX expression predicts outcome of interleukin 2 therapy for renal cancer. *Clin Cancer Res* **11**(10): 3714–3721.

Bayele, H. K., A. Chiti et al. 2010. Isotopic biomarker discovery and application in translational medicine. *Drug Discov Today* **15**(3–4): 127–136.

Burczynski, M. E. and A. J. Dorner 2006. Transcriptional profiling of peripheral blood cells in clinical pharmacogenomic studies. *Pharmacogenomics* **7**(2): 187–202.

Butterfield, L. H., M. L. Disis et al. 2008. A systematic approach to biomarker discovery; preamble to "the iSBTc-FDA taskforce on immunotherapy biomarkers". *J Transl Med* **6**: 81.

Calvano, S. E., W. Xiao et al. 2005. A network-based analysis of systemic inflammation in humans. *Nature* **437**7061: 1032–1037.

Fathman, C. G., L. Soares et al. 2005. An array of possibilities for the study of autoimmunity. *Nature* **435**(7042): 605–611.

Galon, J. et al. 2006.Type, density, and location of immune cells within human colorectal tumors predict clinical outcome. *Science,* **313**(5795): 1960–1964.

Hamilton, W. F. and D. W. Richards, 1982. The output of the heart. In: Fishman, A. P. and D. W. Richards (eds). American Physiological Society, Bethesda, MD, 83–85.

Himmelfarb, J., P. Stenvinkel et al. 2002. The elephant in uremia: Oxidant stress as a unifying concept of cardiovascular disease in uremia. *Kidney Int* **62**(5): 1524–1538.

Holmgren, E. 2008. Quantifying the usefulness of PD biomarkers in Phase 2 screening trials of oncology drugs. *Stat Med* **27**(24): 4928–4938.

Hughes, M.D. et al. 1998. CD4 cell count as a surrogate endpoint in HIV clinical trials: A meta-analysis of studies of the AIDS Clinical Trials Group. *AIDS* **12**(14): 1823–1832.

Janeway, H. H. 1913. Intratracheal anaesthesia: A. By nitrous oxide and oxygen. B. By nitrous oxide and oxygen under conditions of differential pressure. *Ann Surg* **58**(6 Suppl): 927–933.

Katz, L. N. and H. K. Hellerstein 1982. Electrocardiography. In: Fishman, A. P., Richards D. W. (eds). American Physiological Society, Bethesda, MD, 83–85.

Kotz, K. T., W. Xiao et al. 2010. Clinical microfluidics for neutrophil genomics and proteomics. *Nat Med* **16**(9): 1042–1047.

Laudanski, K., C. Miller-Graziano et al. 2006. Cell-specific expression and pathway analyses reveal alterations in trauma-related human T cell and monocyte pathways. *Proc Natl Acad Sci USA* **103**(42): 15564–15569.

Lee, J. W., V. Devanarayan et al. 2006. Fit-for-purpose method development and validation for successful biomarker measurement. *Pharm Res* **23**(2): 312–328.

Lind, L. 2003. Circulating markers of inflammation and atherosclerosis. *Atherosclerosis* **169**: 203–214.

Mattes, W. B. et al. 2010. Research at the interface of industry, academia and regulatory science. *Nat Biotechnol* **28**(5): 432–433.

National High Blood Pressure Education Program, Task Force I: Report to the Hypertension Information and Education Advisory Committee. Recommendations for a national high blood pressure data base for effective antihypertensive therapy. 1973. U.S. Department of Health, Education and Welfare Publication No. (NIH) 74-593. Washington, DC: Government Printing Office.

Nevins, J. R. and A. Potti 2007. Mining gene expression profiles: Expression signatures as cancer phenotypes. *Nat Rev Genet* **8**(8): 601–609.

Nishimura, K., D. Sugiyama et al. 2007. Meta-analysis: Diagnostic accuracy of anti-cyclic citrullinated peptide antibody and rheumatoid factor for rheumatoid arthritis. *Ann Intern Med* **146**: 797–808.

Panelli, M.C. et al. 2007. Sequential gene profiling of basal cell carcinomas treated with imiquimod in a placebo-controlled study defines the requirements for tissue rejection. *Genome Biol* **8**(1): R8.

Pearson, T. A., Mensah, G. A. et al. 2003. Markers of inflammation and cardiovascular disease: Application to clinical and public health practice. A statement for healthcare professionals from the Centers for Disease Control and Prevention and the American Heart Association. *Circulation* **107**: 499–511.

Report of the Joint National Committee on Detection, Evaluation, and Treatment of High Blood Pressure (JNC I). 1977. *JAMA* **237**: 255–261.

Ridker, P. M., J. E. Buring, N. R. Cook, N. Rifai 2003. C-reactive protein, the metabolic syndrome, and risk of incident cardiovascular events: An 8-year follow-up of 14 719 initially healthy American women. *Circulation* **107**: 391–397.

Ridker, P. M., M. Cushman, M. J. Stampfer, R. R. Tracy, C. H. Hennekens 1997. Inflammation, aspirin, and the risk of cardiovascular disease in apparently healthy men. *N Engl J Med* **336**: 973–979.

Rifai, N. and R. E. Gerszten 2006. Biomarker discovery and validation. *Clin Chem* **52**(9): 1635–1637.

Rifai, N., M. A. Gillette et al. 2006. Protein biomarker discovery and validation: The long and uncertain path to clinical utility. *Nat Biotechnol* **24**(8): 971–983.

Riva-Rocci, S. 1896. Un nuovo sfigmomanometro. *Gazzetta medica di torino* **47**: 981–996;1001 1017. English translation: Faulconer, A. Jr, Keys, T. E. (eds.) 1965. *Foundations of Anesthesiology*, Vol. 2. Springfield, IL: Charles C. Thomas, 1043–1075.

Sabatino, M. et al. 2009. Serum vascular endothelial growth factor and fibronectin predict clinical response to high-dose interleukin-2 therapy. *J Clin Oncol* **27**(16): 2645–2652.

Schulte-Pelkum, J., M. Fritzler, and M. Mahler 2009. Latest update on the Ro/SS-A autoantibody system. *Autoimmun Rev* **8**(7): 632–637.

Shen, B. and Hwang, J. 2010. The clinical utility of precision medicine: Properly assessing the value of emerging diagnostic tests. *Clinical Pharmacology & Therapeutics* **88**(6): 754–756.

Sistare, F.D. et al. 2010. Towards consensus practices to qualify safety biomarkers for use in early drug development. *Nat Biotechnol* **28**(5): 446–454.

Vertes, V., L. Tobias, and S. Galvin 1991. Historical reflections on hypertension. *Prim Care* **18**(3): 471–482.

Wagner, J. A. 2002. Overview of biomarkers and surrogate endpoints in drug development. *Dis Markers* **18**(2): 41–46.

Wagner, J. A., S. A. Williams et al. 2007. Biomarkers and surrogate end points for fit-for-purpose development and regulatory evaluation of new drugs. *Clin Pharmacol Ther* **81**(1): 104–107.

Winkler, H., 2010. Biomarkers in the development of novel medicines for the treatment of cancer. *Europena Pharmaceutical Review*, **2010**(3).

Woodcock, J. and R. Woosley 2008. The FDA critical path initiative and its influence on new drug development. *Annu Rev Med* **59**: 1–12.

Woosley, R. L. and J. Cossman 2007. Drug development and the FDA's Critical Path Initiative. *Clin Pharmacol Ther* **81**(1): 129–133.

Zhang, L. et al. 2003. Expression of endocrine gland-derived vascular endothelial growth factor in ovarian carcinoma. *Clin Cancer Res* **9**(1): 264–272.

Zwierzina, H. 2008. Biomarkers in drug development. *Ann Oncol* **19 (Suppl 5)**: v33–37.

2

RNAi Screens: Triumphs and Tribulations

Attila Seyhan and Claudio Carini

CONTENTS

2.1 Introduction

Selection of drug targets forms the foundation of a long and risky drug development process with high attrition that can vary among different therapeutic areas and different phases of drug development (David et al., 2009; Fryburg, 2010; Paul et al., 2010). Beginning from the selection of a drug target candidate to regulatory approval, the overall probability of success is less than 1% (Fryburg et al., 2011) and mostly the majority of failures occur in phase II and III because either the efficacy or safety is not achieved (Arrowsmith, 2011; Ledford, 2011). Efficacy failures occur because either: (i) the drug fails to achieve the required pharmacology; or (ii) target and mechanism targeted by the drug did not significantly contribute to the disease or; (iii) target and mechanism represented only in a subset of patient population (i.e., high heterogeneity of patient population) (Laifenfeld et al., 2012).

Since inappropriate target selection is one of the major factors responsible for failure in drug development research (Ledford, 2011) and approximately only one-fifth of the novel targets or mechanisms achieve efficacy in phase II trials (Arrowsmith, 2011), the importance of drug target selection is paramount. This has been demonstrated by recent publications demonstrating that most (75%) pharmaceutical targets published in the literature could not be reproduced in other laboratories (Begleyand Ellis, 2012; Prinz et al., 2011) indicating that the validity of literature data is in question and potential drug targets must be confirmed in house before embarking on assay development, high-throughput (HTP) compound screening campaigns, lead optimization, and animal testing (Prinz et al., 2011). Furthermore, target validation improves the underlying biology about the target and mechanism and the alterations at the molecular level that may be responsible of disease. Therefore, it is imperative to have a better understanding why some compounds are successful in phases II and III and most others are not involving new targets and mechanisms.

Although the annotation of human genome has helped to develop new and better drugs, most of the new drugs developed each year for most of the chronic human diseases are directed against previously identified targets, with only a few drugs licensed against novel targets (Collins and Workman, 2006). This is partly due to the fact that most complex chronic diseases such as many cancer types and autoimmune diseases are polygenic in nature and there is no single gene or mechanism responsible of disease. For example, HER2/EGFR kinase inhibitor drugs have had limited success rate because some tumor cells can develop resistance to drug, suggesting that some compensatory pathways (e.g., TGFbR, integrins, ER signaling, insulin signaling) enable these cells to overcome the direct effect of the drug on its target (Germano and O'Driscoll, 2009; Seyhan et al., 2011). Similarly, multiple mechanisms may be responsible for the development of various autoimmune disease pathophysiology (e.g., rheumatoid arthritis can be driven by TNF, IL6,

IL-21 as well as through activation of B- or T-cell REF needed). Because there may be more than one mechanism and target associated with each disease, developing drugs for a single target or mechanism may not be the best strategy for a successful drug development (Hopkins, 2008).

Since multiple mechanism may be the drivers of various complex diseases and each mechanism may be present only in a subset of patient population, an all-comers approach where a highly heterogeneous patient population is treated with a single compound specific to a single target or mechanism will more likely fail to show desired efficacy and safety in phases II and III trials. Additionally, when heterogeneous patient population is used, the results more likely will not be statistically significant if the patient population is not significantly large. Therefore, a successful drug development research must begin from the selection of a target that is relevant to a human disease and expressed in the diseased tissue of a homogeneous patient population. For example, if breast cancer patients had not been stratified for high HER2 expressers for the phase III clinical trial, the size of the trial had to contain ~11,000 patients to achieve statistically significant results (Woodcock, 2007). It is therefore imperative to select for those patients who are homogeneous for the presence of target or mechanism and the study cohort is sufficiently large enough to achieve statistically significant results.

Pharmaceutical compounds generally exert their therapeutic effects by binding to and subsequently modulating the activity of a particular protein (e.g., enzyme, receptor, membrane proteins, nucleic acid, or other molecular targets, Ohlstein et al., 2000; Zambrowicz and Sands, 2003). Over the years, hundreds of successful targets have been identified (targeted by at least one approved drug) and greater than 1000 research targets (targeted by experimental drugs only) have been identified (Golden, 2003; Imming et al., 2006; Overington et al., 2006; Zheng et al., 2006). A recent study by Zhu et al. (2010) has generated a therapeutic target database (TTD) which has reported 348 successful, 292 clinical trial and 1254 research targets, and 1514 approved, 1212 clinical trial, and 2302 experimental drugs linked to their primary targets (3382 small molecule and 649 antisense drugs with available structure and sequence).

Recent advances in systems-based approaches including genomic, proteomic, structural, functional, and systems studies of the known and novel targets and other disease-associated factors have led to the discovery of drugs, multitarget agents, combination therapies and new targets, analysis of on-target toxicity, and pharmacogenetic responses (Zhu et al., 2010). Additionally, the therapeutic actions of drugs are typically through modulating the activities of their targetes (e.g. proteins, enzymes, receptors) (Yildirim et al., 2007) and up to 14,000 drug-targeted-proteins have been reported in the literature (Wishart et al., 2006). The reported number of primary targets directly related to the therapeutic actions of approved drugs is limited to 324 (Overington et al., 2006). This emphasizes why it is paramount for structural and functional characterization of primary targets and those yet to be discovered to for developing new more specific and efficacious drugs.

2.2 Classical Approaches to Drug Target Development

Target identification and validation is the first step in drug discovery and development hence forms the foundation of new drug development research, and inappropriate target selection is one of the main causes responsible for failure in drug development research (Butcher, 2003; Lindsay, 2003; Sams-Dodd, 2005). A drug target can be any number of biological molecular classes (e.g., proteins, genes, RNAs, sugars) (Sleno and Emili, 2008). Drug target and drug discovery rely on a variety of techniques and sources including target in house identification and validation campaigns, in-licensing and public sourcing based on data published in the literature and data generated from the human genome project. Thus, the validity of candidate targets is critical for pharmaceutical companies when deciding to launch new projects.

A variety of clinical, genetic, biochemical, and molecular approaches have been used for novel drug target identification (Terstappen et al., 2007). Classical genetic approaches (e.g., gene knockouts) traditionally used in target discovery and development are slow and risky, whereas specific inhibitors of a particular protein are limited in scope and their specificity is questionable.

A systems approach based on the use of *clinical and literature data* and *experimental datasets* from *molecular approaches* is the current norm for target development (Lindsay, 2003). Clinical and literature data enables target selection through the study of diseases in whole organisms using information derived from clinical trials and a variety of preclinical studies whereas the *molecular approach*, the mainstream of current target discovery strategy (Butcher, 2003; Sakharkar and Sakharkar, 2007), aims to identify "druggable" targets where activities can be modulated through interactions with candidate pharmaceuticals or biopharmaceuticals.

2.2.1 Data Mining

Steady increase in publicly available biomedical data is providing opportunities for identification of potential drug targets and biomarkers in support of the drug development research (Butcher, 2003). As an example, MEDLINE/PubMed currently contains more than 18 million literature abstracts, and more than 60,000 new abstracts are added monthly and the number of chemical, genomic, proteomic, and metabolic data is rapidly growing and has been estimated to double every 2 years. As discussed by Zhu et al. (2010), several publicly accessible therapeutic targets databases have been developed including drugbank (Wishart et al., 2008), potential drug target database (PDTD) (Gao et al., 2008), and TTD (Chen et al., 2002). These complementary databases provide a global view of target and drug profiles as well as comprehensive drug data with information about drug actions and multiple targets (e.g., drugbank) (Wishart et al., 2008), whereas PDTD contains active-sites and functional information for potential targets with available

3D structures (Gao et al., 2008) (23) and TTD provides information about the primary targets of approved and experimental drugs (Chen et al., 2002).

2.2.2 Data Analysis

Parallel to the growth of collection of a variety of databases, bioinformatics for data and text mining of literature, microarray, proteomic, genomic, and chemogenomic databases and to filter valuable targets by combining biological ideas with computer tools or statistical methods have been grown rapidly to support the discovery and development of novel targets (Sakharkar and Sakharkar, 2007). With the recent development of HTP proteomics and chemical genomics, another two data mining approaches, proteomic and chemogenomic data mining, have emerged. To benefit from the constantly growing scientific data, more efficient data mining and analysis methods must be developed to support target discovery in the postgenomics era (Butcher, 2003).

2.2.3 Data Interpretation, Integration, and Application

To develop targets that are successful and relevant to disease, it is critical to elucidate the underlying biology of target, mechanism, and genetic and molecular alterations in diseased cell or tissue that contributes to disease pathogenesis.

Innovative interrogation, integration, and application of such multidimensional dataset obtained from various sources including clinical and literature data and a variety of molecular approaches can: (i) help identify and prioritize therapeutic targets most likely to succeed; and (ii) help identify patient populations most likely to benefit from treatment.

In recent years, a systems-based molecular approaches have emerged to address this which takes an holistic approach to biological research by integrating information gained from various "omics"-based molecular technologies and building networks and pathways to model biological processes for target identification and disease association. A variety of molecular approaches have been used for target identification and development including human genetics, genomics (transcriptional profiling of a variety of RNA species), proteomics, metabolomics, *in vitro* functional assays, model organisms, and animal models (transgenic, e.g., APP-Tg mouse for Alzheimer's disease; TNF-alpha Tg mouse for rheumatoid arthritis and IBD, knock-out, and knock-in) of disease or condition.

To have pharmaceutical utility, a target must be "druggable," that is, a target must be accessible to candidate drug molecules (e.g., small molecules or biologics) and bind them such a way that a desirable biological effect is inflicted. *Druggable genome* comprises only a fraction of the entire genome hence many key proteins remain "undrugged" either because they are unknown or knowable or they cannot be targeted by current therapeutics.

This in fact provides an opportunity to develop novel therapies that can target the genes and their products that are currently outside of reach with current therapies and reveal novel disease-specific targets or molecular pathways as well as biomarkers to monitor drug efficacy and patient response to treatments. Because of this, novel strategies are needed to facilitate discovery of novel drug targets previously unknown or knowable for a specific disease.

Even the modest number of these genes encode a multitude of proteins. Similarly, a large array of noncoding nucleic acid sequences including microRNAs (miRNAs) and natural antisense sequences and more than 14,000 pseudogenes (Balasubramanian et al., 2011; Gerstein and Zheng, 2006)—some with regulatory functions have functions in a variety of structural, enzymatic processes. Proteins involved in signaling pathways are also interconnected to various molecular networks resulting in a higher order of network resulting in a high order of mechanistic and functional complexity associated with a specific molecular target to disease (Ho and Lieu, 2008). Hence, biological processes are highly complex and dynamic and operate in a multilayered fashion in spatially and temporally and all these processes are impacted by the environmental stimuli and disease state including the effects of drugs (Fishman and Porter, 2005; Janga and Tzakos, 2009; Stelling et al., 2004). Moreover, the target and changes in its expression or modulation must be critical for disease or pathway associated with the disease and safe, that is, its activity can be modulated by a therapeutic agent to inhibit or reverse disease onset or progress.

Furthermore, modulation of a therapeutic target by a candidate drug should alter the levels of biological pathways, crucial "nodes" on a regulatory network and should be monitored and measured by selected disease and treatment response biomarkers. Access to such "surrogate or disease biomarkers" can contribute significantly to a successful drug development research; therefore, development of targets and biomarkers specific to homogeneous patient subpopulation for diseases and treatments is as critical to the successful drug development as the selection of drug targets. Biomarkers are important for drug development and clinical research. If translated into clinical practice, they can be used for diagnosis, treatment risk stratification, early detection, treatment selection, prognostication, and the monitoring for recurrence (Cho and Tapscott, 2007).

2.3 Current State of the Art of Drug Target and Biomarker Discovery

Traditionally, global genomics, transcriptomics, and proteomic strategies have been used for hypothesis generation, rather than hypothesis testing, by identifying sets of genes, RNAs, proteins or gene or protein networks or biological pathways perturbed in a specific disease. Advances in a variety of technologies can now be used to identify molecular targets associated with specific disease onset providing researcher's information on the mechanism-of-action of new drugs. Because of this, mechanism-based (traditional) and genome-based (new strategies) approaches alongside a variety of omics technologies and animal models including the use of gene knockout (deletion), suppression, knock in (replace endogenous gene with new gene with mutation), or ectopic overexpression of a gene of interest while comparing the influence of lead molecules with and without genetic disruption have been used. Information on potential targets is elucidated from increased sensitivity with decreased gene dosage for a certain drug concentration (Seyhan et al., 2011) or by enhanced resistance when a target is overproduced (Brown and Wright, 2005) or its expression inhibited (Seyhan et al., 2012). Consequently, by examining the overlap of gene/RNA/protein interaction networks with the data obtained from chemical genetic sensitivity screens, candidate pathways that are perturbed by drugs can be identified (Giaever et al., 2004; Hughes et al., 2000; Lamb et al., 2006; Parsons et al., 2006; St Onge et al., 2007).

To be a validated target, first the candidate target must be confirmed in preclinical studies *in vitro* and in animal models to confirm the effect of target on mechanism and its link to human disease. In preclinical validation, the target expression or modulation must be shown disease tissue and cell type. The expression level must correlate with disease severity in the human tissue samples. Modulation of the level of activity of target in a cell culture and in animal models must be relevant to disease pathophysiology. Finally, modulation of the level of activity of the target must be associated with disease pathophysiology in humans. This is clinically validated target which is now a molecular target of a known therapeutic agent.

To develop targeted therapies to identify factors responsible of the molecular vulnerabilities of diseased cells or tissue has benefited the initiatives such as the cancer genome atlas, which has enabled systematic characterization of the structural basis of many cancer types by identifying the genomic alterations and vulnerabilities associated with each disease. This has enabled the development of target/mechanism-specific therapies including imatinib (Gleevec™) in chronic myeloid leukemia and gastrointestinal stromal tumors, trastuzumab (Herceptin™) in HER2-positive breast cancer, BCR–ABL translocation for treatment of chronic myelogenous leukemia (CML) with imatinib (Gleevec), estrogen receptor (ER), or progesterone receptor (PR) positivity, which is a prerequisite for treatment of breast cancer with tamoxifen or aromatase inhibitors, somatic mutations in the tyrosine–kinase domain of the epidermal growth factor receptor (EGFR), which have recently been shown to predict a greater efficacy of gefitinib (Iressa), xalkori to treat lung cancer found in patients with a rare genetic abnormality, and CCR5 inhibitors which block HIV entry (Kuritzkes, 2009), and CD20 positivity for treatment of lymphomas with rituximab (Rituxan).

This was accomplished by identifying the genes essential for cancer cell growth, angiogenesis, metastasis, and other changes involved in cancer pathogenesis and tumorigenesis.

Although the development of genotype-specific cancer drugs that are only effective in a cancer-specific genetic context has been the hallmark of the targeted cancer therapies (Hartwell et al., 1997), the number of new and truly validated drug targets to date is few (Quon and Kassner, 2009). This is partly due to the use of classical genetic approaches for the identification of targets which involve the evaluation of the changes in pathway activation status in tumor tissue compared to healthy controls and modeling of compound sensitivity and resistance in the preclinical setting. The number of genes that are consistently altered in cancer or other chronic diseases is limited and patients are highly heterogeneous in their genetic make up and only a faction of those in complex disease category including cancer may display a particular genetic signature and vulnerability to disease (Cobleigh et al., 1999; Vogel et al., 2002) suggesting that not all patients benefit from a specific therapy, and a subset of patients relapse after an initial response. Because of this, cancer and other complex disease research will benefit from a more insightful understanding of disease biology for the development of targeted therapies and development of patient selection biomarkers by identifying potential treatment responders and associate drug targets or molecular pathways.

To develop more efficacious drugs for various chronic diseases, there is a need to identify factors responsible of the molecular vulnerabilities of diseased cells or tissue and biomarkers for patient stratification require novel strategies and technologies. Existing platforms are costly and time consuming and because of this many key cellular targets remain undiscovered or cannot be translated into clinical utility. Therefore, approaches such as genome-wide functional genomic screens may facilitate this process by identifying completely new disease-specific drug targets, molecular pathways, and new classes of drug targets and vulnerabilities of the diseased cell that result from its genetic differences from healthy cells.

2.4 RNAi Functional Genome Screens

Although the completion of the mapping of the human genome was a great achievement in recent history, its societal impact can be put in practice only if genomic information that is associated with various traits of medical importance, such as susceptibility to a disease or response to a drug, can be identified. Consequently, many key targets remain "undrugged." This requires new strategies to accelerate drug target discovery and validation, identify disease-specific targets, and determine the relevance of sequence or isoform variants to the disease of interest. Although progress in genome sequencing and annotation have enabled biological assays to be performed and analyzed in an HTP fashion, this process was further accelerated by the introduction of RNAi technology which led to the development of genome-scale or focused RNAi screens in which the effects of gene silencing on biological phenotypes can be systematically interrogated.

RNAi was first discovered in *Caenorhabditis elegans* and revolutionized the functional genomics field by knocking down the expression of gene(s) of interest. RNAi is an evolutionarily conserved sequence-specific gene silencing phenomenon induced by double-stranded RNA (dsRNA) which can function at both transcriptional and posttranscriptional levels (Chapman and Carrington, 2007; Dykxhoorn et al., 2003; Meister and Tuschl, 2004; Zamore and Haley, 2005) across a wide range of organisms. RNAi may have evolved as a natural defense against viruses or transposons and induced by endogenous miRNAs encoded in the genome, but RNAi can also be triggered by exogenous dsRNAs that have been introduced to the cell in the form of synthetically made or vector-encoded (plasmid or virus) short hairpin RNAs (shRNAs) or small interfering RNAs (siRNAs) (Quon and Kassner, 2009; Seyhan et al., 2005, 2007; Whitehead et al., 2009). In cells, upon the introduction of dsRNAs or shRNAs, these precursor dsRNAs are processed into 21–23 base pair siRNAs by a type III ribonuclease (Dicer). Subsequently, one of the siRNA strands is incorporated into RNA-induced silencing complex (RISC). The strand in the RISC referred as "guide strand" binds to complementary target RNA sequence initiating an RISC-mediated target RNA cleavage or block translation if the guide strand does not have perfect homology with the messenger RNA (mRNA) as in miRNA-mediated gene silencing. The ability of RNAi reagents to inhibit gene expression has provided opportunities for their use as novel therapeutics. There have been more than 30 clinical trials involving 21 different RNA9-based therapeutics for more than a dozen diseases, including various cancers, viruses, and genetic disorders (Burnett et al., 2011; Seyhan, 2011).

Researchers can now use RNAi for such functional screening in a variety of mammalian or insect cells or using *C. elegans* to systematically interrogate the function of each gene in the genome of these model systems in a relatively short period of time (Figure 2.1) (Simpson et al., 2012). Consequently, RNAi has facilitated the discovery and development of novel drug targets in a genome-scale fashion by querying the effects of gene silencing on biological phenotypes systematically (Seyhan and Ryan, 2010; Seyhan et al., 2011, 2012). RNAi technology allows systemic analysis of each gene function either at global scale or in a targeted fashion suing focused collections of RNAi reagents effectively by streamlining the process from the initial target identification to the validation of those candidate targets and development of candidate drugs for those targets (Iorns et al., 2007; Seyhan and Ryan, 2010) or combination drug treatment strategies (Seyhan, 2011) or genetic biomarkers (Seyhan et al., 2012).

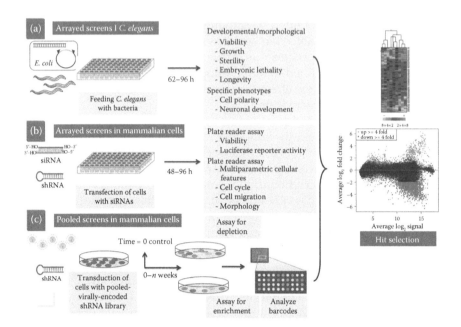

FIGURE 2.1

(**See color insert.**) Arrayed or pooled-RNAi screening g workflows. (a) Screening in *C. elegans*. Feeding *C. elegans* with dsRNA-producing bacteria is accomplished by seeding bacteria into 96 well plates. Developmentally synchronized worms are then added into each well of the 96-well plate and depending on the assay, worms are scored for phenotypic aberrations within 2–4 days. (b) Arrayed RNAi screens. Each RNAi reagent targeting a unique gene is dispensed (or spotted) in each well of a multiwell dish (96-, 284-, or 1536-well plate or spotted on glass slides) and assayed 72–96 h posttransfection. RNAi reagent libraries can comprise synthetic siRNAs, plasmid- or virus-encoded shRNAs. Various assay readouts are used to determine the effect of RNAi on the phenotype of interest such as the measurement of cell viability, luminescent or fluorescent reporter assays as well as high-content image analysis using throughput microscopes may be used to measure cellular phenotypes in screens. (c) Vector-derived RNAi screens in pooled format: Pooled vector libraries can be used to transduce target cell population in a single tissue culture dish using pooled-viral vectors encoding libraries of shRNAs targeting multiple genes or entire genome. Transduced cells are selected and expanded and then assayed for a defined period of time. After selecting for the desired phenotype, genomic DNA is isolated from reference (time = 0) and assayed populations, and analyzed for the identification of genes whose inhibition by RNAi knockdown causes the specific phenotype such as changes in general cell morphology, cell proliferation, or cellular death. The relative abundance of each shRNA or a random 60-mer barcode specific to each shRNA can be identified and quantified by labeling the PCR product with fluorescent dyes (e.g., Cy5 or Cy3). The PCR products are then hybridized to custom designed cDNA microarrays containing barcode or shRNA complementary oligonucleotides. Alternatively, next-generation sequencing can be used to indentify barcode or shRNA sequences responsible for the desired phenotype. The relative abundance of barcodes obtained from the cells that were exposed to selective pressure is compared to that detected in control cells that have been exposed to the same shRNA library, but not to the selective pressure (e.g., drug treatment or genetic mutations). (Adapted from Simpson KJ, Davis GM, Boag PR, 2012. *Nat Biotechnol* **29**(4): 459–470.)

Because genome-scale RNAi screens are a nonhypothesis-driven approach (i.e., there is no requirement for *a priori* knowledge of what types of targets will be discovered), nontraditional targets including those that are not associated with specific pathways or disease or condition can be identified (Quon and Kassner, 2009). RNAi screening is a forward genetic screen that has accelerated the discovery of a large number of novel targets and pathways including the identification novel oncogenes for the development of new therapeutics (Mohr et al., 2010) as well as previously unknown genes involved in cancer drug resistance and viral or bacterial pathogenesis (Seyhan and Ryan, 2010). In principle, RNAi acts like a biopharmaceutical compound; albeit, more specifically and can target entire transcriptome including the druggable and nondruggable genome providing opportunities for the identification of novel targets. RNAi screens also uncover the sequence identity of hit genes identified in the screen immediately after the screen is complete enabling more sophisticated data analyses on previously identified and previously unknown genes (Boutros and Ahringer, 2008; Ledford, 2011). Because of this, RNAi technology enables functional genomics screens to be performed rapidly using loss-of-function (LOF) of a family of genes or pathways or entire genome relatively easily. RNAi-mediated target identification studies have already resulted in the discovery of novel drug targets or genetic biomarkers with clinical implications including the identification novel oncogenes for the development of new therapeutics (Mohr et al., 2010), novel targets for combination drug therapy strategies (Seyhan et al., 2011) as well as previously unknown genes involved in cancer drug resistance (Seyhan et al., 2012), and viral or bacterial pathogenesis (Seyhan and Ryan, 2010). RNAi screens have also been used in other species for which functional genomics would otherwise not be feasible (Mohr et al., 2010).

Although some of the concerns related to false discovery, off-targeting effects, and delivery still exist, recent improvements in reagent design algorithms and statistical tools for data analysis and various improvements in delivery technologies have mitigated some of these problems (Birmingham et al., 2006; Jackson et al., 2006b; Judge et al., 2005; Lin et al., 2005a; Sledz and Williams, 2004a). Additionally, earlier RNAi screening studies provided valuable information that has enabled better screening campaigns with appropriate controls and downstream validation processes (Mohr et al., 2010; Seyhan, 2010; Seyhan and Ryan, 2010). But issues related to false discovery and best methods to validate the "hit" genes remain to be addressed.

In spite of these issues, RNAi screening has proven to be a powerful tool for functional genome-scale studies in a variety of systems. Improved RNAi reagent designs and learnings from the earlier studies with better strategies for validation of the "hit" genes identified in the screens and mapping those hits to specific pathways and molecular networks associated with a disease will facilitate these preclinical findings into clinical research benefiting drug development and translational medicine (Kaelin, 2012).

2.5 RNAi Reagent Formats

As illustrated in Figure 2.1, mainly two types of RNAi reagent libraries are used in the screens: (i) synthetic siRNAs that are transfected directly into cells in an arrayed format using multiwell plates; and (ii) vector-encoded shRNAs (or siRNAs that are expressed from opposing RNA polymerase III promoters in the form of siRNAs) (Seyhan et al., 2005) that can be used to transduce target cells either in an arrayed format in multiwell plates or in a pooled format where a collection of individual shRNA expression vectors are used to transduce target cells as pools (Seyhan and Ryan, 2010). It is common that the cell type and duration of the screen are the main determinants on the type of RNAi reagents that can be used in a screen. Because the gene silencing mediated by siRNAs is transient, they are used in screens that are limited to only 2–5 days. When longer-term gene silencing is desired, viral or plasmid vectors are the method of delivery of RNAi reagents. Cell types also determine what type of delivery options can be used. If cells are not amenable to traditional transfection, reagents such as primary or stem cells, electroporation, or viral vectors are the most commonly used strategies in mammalian cells (Mohr et al., 2010; Seyhan and Ryan, 2010).

2.6 RNAi Library Genome Coverage

The type of biological question and the scale of the study dictate the type of screening strategy and coverage to be used. RNAi reagent libraries can have coverage from anywhere from entire genomes of various organisms to a subset of target class gene families, druggable genome (Falschlehner et al., 2010) and the collections can be customized to fit the purpose of a study by focusing on any number of genes, pathways, or particular gene families, that are perceived to be linked to a biological process or disease. This provides a hypothesis-based strategy to systematically examine the role of a particular gene within a cell or system as well as characterization of functional gene clusters and the dissection of cellular signaling networks.

2.6.1 Annotated Genome-Wide Screens

A genome-wide RNAi reagent collections target entire annotated genome which comprises as many as ~24,000 protein-coding genes. Therefore, a genome-scale RNAi screen will uncover functions of all possible regulators of a biological process leading to the discovery of novel modulators, targets, pathways and networks, and drug sensitizer targets as novel targets for combination therapy strategies (Seyhan et al., 2011) or drug resistance genes as potential biomarkers for patient stratification (Seyhan et al., 2012).

2.6.2 Druggable Genome Screens

The concept of the druggable genome first coined by Hopkins and Groom in 2002 (2002) has been used to define a list if genes that can be targeted by existing small molecule and protein-based drugs. The term has been in vogue since the number of genes in the panel is variable as illustrated in Sophic White paper Integrated Druggable Genome Database (sophicalliance. com) and Figures 2.2 and 2.3.

The integrated druggable genome illustrates that this number is dynamic and can range from 3610 (BioLT list) to 4126 (Sophic list), or 6669 (Qiagen list). The list of gene families has been regularly revised and updated (Imming et al., 2006; Overington et al., 2006; Russ and Lampel, 2005; Zheng et al., 2006; Zhu et al., 2010). Information on the druggable genome is dynamic and scattered throughout various databases making it difficult to have a unified perspective about its coverage and annotation. Since the genes are identified

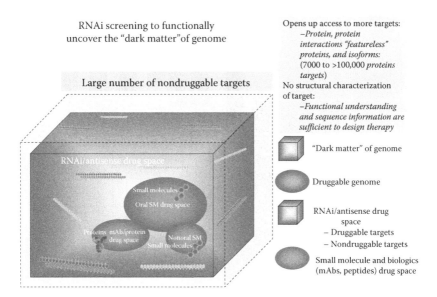

FIGURE 2.2
(See color insert.) RNAi screens can uncover previously unknown and unknowable large number of nondruggable targets and automatically reveal information on their functional activity. RNAi screening provides access to entire genome icluding the noncoding genome which constitutes the majority of genome. It provides opportunities to more previously unknown or knowable targets, molecular pathways and mechanisms, cellular functions, protein–protein interactions, "featureless" proteins, isoforms, and factors contributing to disease the biological and physical manifestations of disease.

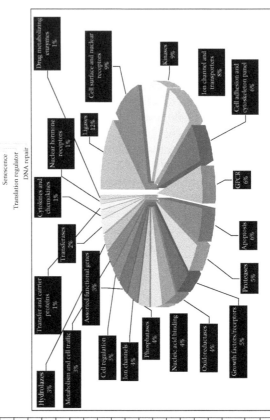

Gene families	No. of genes	% of druggable genome
Ligases	949	13.9
Cell surface and nuclear receptors	722	10.6
Kinases	719	10.6
Ion channel and transporters	639	9.4
Cell adhesion and Cytoskeleton	496	7.3
GPCR	479	7.0
Apoptosis	437	6.4
Proteases	379	5.6
Growth factors/receptors	375	5.5
Oxidoreductases	338	5.0
Nucleic acid binding	310	4.6
Phosphatases	293	4.3
Ion channels	285	4.2
Assorted functional genes	228	3.3
Cell regulation	227	3.3
Metabolism and cell traffic	217	3.2
Hydrolazes	204	3.0
Transferases	184	2.7
Cytokines and chemokines	106	1.6
Transfer and carrier proteins	71	1.0
Nuclear hormone receptors	46	0.7
Drug-metabolizing enzymes (CyP450, etc.)	54	0.8
Drug transporters		
Total	6809	100

FIGURE 2.3

mostly through text mining, they have not been fully curated or validated making this a needed research area using RNAi as a means to delineate the functions of each gene in the druggable genome panel.

As illustrated in Figure 2.2, the majority of "druggable" genome comprises kinases, ligases, cell surface and nuclear receptors, ion channels, and transporters and G-protein-coupled receptors (GPCRs). Because the biological mechanisms of diseases are rather complex, the task is not only to identify, prioritize, and select "druggable" targets but also to understand the cellular interactions underlying disease phenotypes, to provide predictive models and to construct biological networks for human diseases (Lindsay, 2003).

Currently a variety of RNAi reagent libraries targeting specific cellular functions and pathways within the druggable genome is available (Figure 2.2) commercially enabling researchers to study the function of individual genes in a specific mechanism or cellular function or entire entire pathways and cellular functions or druggable genome. Since the functions of genes are well-annotated and there are currently drugs available to these targets, this allows for the development of novel drugs for previously unknown targets as well as development of combination therapies using existing drugs which accelerates drug development process (Seyhan et al., 2011).

2.6.3 Focused or Targeted Genome Screens

The "focused" or "targeted" screening offers an opportunity to study the function of a panel of genes in a specific pathway or cellular function that is hypothesized to exist, but whose molecular identity is not well understood. This strategy has been used most effectively in smaller-scale RNAi screens than the genome-wide screens. As illustrated in Figure 2.2, the focused gene families may include druggable genome or genes involved in specific cellular processes (e.g., kinases, phosphatases, apoptosis, GPCRs, ion channels,

---

FIGURE 2.3
(**See color insert.**) Human druggable genome that can be studied using RNAi. The table illustrates number of genes that can be targeted by RNAi reagent collections that permit the study of the function of entire pathway, specific gene families, pathways, mechanisms, and specific cellular functions. For example, drug-metabolizing enzymes (DMEs) and drug transporters (DTs) are molecular determinants of pharmacokinetic property of a drug and their expression is controlled by nuclear receptors (NRs). Due to the complex nature of studying the function of individual DMEs, DTs, and NRs, RNAi can be used in addition to chemical inhibitors and inhibitory antibodies to characterize their specific roles in drug metabolism and transport, gene regulation, and drug–drug interactions. Additionally, RNAi may be employed to modulate DT expression to overcome multidrug resistance. Top right panel illustrates human druggable genome and gene classification. Bottom right panel illustrates percentage of gene families within druggable genome that can be probed by RNAi reagent collections. (Adapted from Hopkins AL, Groom CR, 2002. *Nat Rev Drug Discov* **1**(9): 727–730; Wishart DS et al. 2008. DrugBank: A knowledgebase for drugs, drug actions and drug targets. *Nucleic Acids Res* **36** (Database issue): D901–906.), Selectbiosciences.com, SigmaAldrich. com, and Dharmacon.com.

transcripton factors, nuclear receptors, cell cycle regulators, apoptosis, signaling molecules, proteases, ion channels, transporters, membrane traffic proteins, and ligases).

Several reports in the literature have shown the utility of this approach. For example, a small panel of retroviral-derided shRNAs targeting 55 deubiquitinating (DUB) enzymes identified the DUB enzyme responsible for removing ubiquitin from the Fanconi anemia D2 protein (Bernards et al., 2006). Similarly, a focused siRNA library targeting 510 kinase family genes (known and predicted) identified novel factors that modify cellular sensitivity to TRAIL-induced apoptosis including DOBI, a gene required for progression of the apoptotic signal through the intrinsic mitochondrial cell death pathway, and MIRSA, a gene that acts to limit TRAIL-induced apoptosis and confirmed the known factors involved in apoptosis (Aza-Blanc et al., 2003). Another siRNA screen targeted against known and predicted human tyrosine kinome identified the G2/M checkpoint protein WEE1 as a potential therapeutic target (Murrow et al., 2010).

2.6.4 Noncoding Genome

It has been estimated that only less than 1% of the human genome code for proteins while at least a half of the human genome is transcribed (Birney et al., 2007; Carninci et al., 2005), and the 80% of disease-associated variants that are located outside of protein-coding genes (Manolio et al., 2009). However, there are still many unknowns about the so-called "dark matter" of genome (Derrien et al., 2011) making it potential drug targets. Significant progress has been made to annotate the noncoding regions of the genome including the ones termed as "pseudogenes" either by interpreting the functional genomics data or comparative sequence analysis (Alexander et al., 2010; Balasubramanian et al., 2011). Recent data suggest that noncoding regions of genome (Gerstein and Zheng, 2006; Gerstein et al., 2007) represent a historical record of the genome but also contain the control elements for coding regions and some noncoding regions are functional and are ubiquitously transcribed and most disease-associated mutations (e.g., GWAS hits) are found in noncoding regions (Gerstein and Zheng, 2006; Gerstein et al., 2007). Currently there are no drugs against noncoding genome possibly with the exception of oligonucleotides.

While genes are described as protein-coding loci, pseudogenes are described as protein-coding loci that may have lost their functionality (dying genes) due to incorporation of nonsense single-nucleotide polymorphisms (SNPs) or SNPs that affect splicing sites. The definitions of the terms "gene" and "pseudogene" are discussed in detail elsewhere (Gerstein and Zheng, 2006; Gerstein et al., 2007). Pseudogenes are among those noncoding intergenic elements and there are estimated 14,000 pseudogenes which only ~900 of them are transcribed as noncoding RNAs (ncRNAs). Transcribed pseudogenes may play regulatory functions (miRNA) via acting as miRNA decoys

(PTEN), (Swami, 2010) preventing degradation of parents mRNA (makorin), or acting as endogenous siRNAs (Gerstein and Zheng, 2006; Gerstein et al., 2007) or inhibiting degradation of parent's mRNA (Poliseno et al., 2010). SNP-mediated LOF can impact only one individual, leading to the inactivation of an essential gene which may lead to a disease whereas some LOF mutations become more common in the population and are retained (MacArthur and Tyler-Smith 2010) and may retain some or all of their function; still others may be either on the way to pseudogenization or as nonfunctional relics of evolution and have regulatory functions as described.

A variety of ncRNAs including long noncoding RNAs (lncRNAs), PIWI-associated ncRNAs, and siRNAs have been identified (Heuston et al., 2011). LncRNAs are modestly conserved and lack functional open reading frames (ORFs) and appear to negatively and positively regulate protein coding gene expression, in *cis* and *trans* and involve in diverse mechanisms of action including regulation of transcription (Derrien et al., 2011) (see for reviews Ponting et al., 2009; Nagano and Fraser, 2011). Additionally, ncRNAs function as regulators of cell cycle progression, proliferation, and fate and their deregulation has been shown to be linked to various human diseases including cancer (Derrien et al., 2011) representing a new frontier in human disease genomics. Although many lncRNAs have been identified in mammals, few have been functionally characterized which suggest that these RNAs are key regulators of epigenetic regulation in mammalian cells. Therefore, new methods to predict functions based on the functional screens will help to generate annotated catalog of transcribed ~900 pseudogenes and ~15,000 lncRNAs with functional predictions to integrate these data into existing functional genome database and infer possible roles in human diseases.

There is no *a priori* method for the prediction of pseudogenes and other no-coding RNAs function based on sequence alone, contrary to proteins where protein function can be assumed by analysis of the amino acid sequence. It has been estimated that there are ~15,000 new lncRNA transcripts (Derrien et al., 2011). To address this question, large-scale functional screens targeting pseudogenes and other ncRNAs should be done to uncover functions for these genes that have not been identified, unknown, or unknowable via conventional annotation methods. A recent siRNA screen conducted in mouse embryonic stem (ES) cells to identify the function of such intergenic noncoding RNAs (lincRNAs) showed that knockdown of several of lincRNAs causes either exit from the pluripotent state or upregulation of lineage commitment programs (Guttman et al., 2011). The results showed that knockdown of dozens of lincRNAs screen study causes either exit from the pluripotent state or upregulation of lineage commitment programs. LincRNA genes are regulated by key transcription factors and that lincRNA transcripts bind to multiple chromatin regulatory proteins to affect shared gene expression programs (Guttman et al., 2011) suggesting that lincRNAs have key roles in the circuitry controlling ES cell state.

Because of their association with epigenetic regulations, the analysis of protein-binding partners of these RNAs and advances in bioinformatics annotation of RNA structures (Torarinsson et al., 2006; Parker et al., 2011) will add another layer of information on the function of these RNAs and infer possible roles in human diseases. Many ncRNAs have been implicated in a variety of human diseases including cancer and neurodegeneration, emphasizing the importance of this emergent field. It has been suggested that many pseudogene LOF will result in phenotypes associated with loss of olfactory factors (smell), or color blindness (personal communication with Mark Gerstein).

2.7 RNAi Screening Formats

As illustrated in Figure 2.1, RNAi libraries are primarily used in two screening formats: (i) arrayed screening either in mammalian or insect cells or in *C. elegans* in multiwell format which highlights the breadth of applications of this technology; or (ii) in a pool-based screening, collections of shRNA expression vectors are used to transduce target cells in bulk and the library of cells are selected for the phenotype of interest.

Both siRNAs and vector-derived shRNAs can be used for arrayed screens, whereas only the vector-derived shRNAs can be used in pool-based screens followed by the measurement of phenotypic changes induced by RNAi several days after the beginning of screen.

Although much simpler in data deconvolution, the logistics involved in arrayed screening is much more complicated and requires more resources.

Conversely, pooled screens, once optimized are much easier to use and hence have the potential to greatly increase the number of large-scale analyses that can be performed without the requirement of laboratory automation. Additionally, viral RNAi constructs enable the generation of cell lines that express RNAi reagents from constitutive or inducible promoters, allowing constitutive or regulatable, and long-term silencing of gene expression. This enables the analysis of many relevant biological questions for a longer time period in cell lines as well as primary and stem cells that are not amenable to conventional transfection methods. Following the transduction of cells with the vector library, the cell population is subjected to a selective pressure for a period of time to permit the RNAi-mediated LOF of gene expression to reveal specific cell phenotypes or change of growth patterns or viability, followed by the identification of RNAi reagents that are either enriched or depleted from the population.

RNAi screens with genome and species coverage have been successfully conducted with in both arrayed or pooled formats (Berns et al., 2004, 2007; Brummelkamp et al., 2006; Kolfschoten et al., 2005; Luo et al., 2008; Ngo et al.,

2006; Schlabach et al., 2008; Silva et al., 2008; Westbrook et al., 2005a). RNAi libraries with whole genome, a particular pathway, or a subset of gene families or cellular functions using retroviral (Berns et al., 2007; Schlabach et al., 2008; Silva et al., 2008) or lentiviral (Luo et al., 2008; Root et al., 2006) vectors have been used resulting in the identification of novel targets and biomarkers (Seyhan et al., 2011, 2012).

In addition to their capacity to identify genes involved in cell survival in cancer, this type of screen can be used to identify genes involved in susceptibility to drug treatment (Brummelkamp et al., 2006; Seyhan et al., 2011), comparison of genotypic variation (Berns et al., 2004), or comparison of distinct cancer subgroups (Ngo et al., 2006). Several reports showed that focused or genome-wide RNAi screens can identify genetic interdependencies in human cancer (Bernards et al., 2006; Downward, 2004; Ngo et al., 2006; Scholl et al., 2009; Westbrook et al., 2005b) or synthetic lethal interactions in cancer cells harboring mutant KRAS (Scholl et al., 2009). In another study, whole-genome RNAi screen identified genes involved in cell survival in two distinct diffuse large B-cell lymphoma subtypes (Ngo et al., 2006).

The pooled RNAi screens have been most successfully employed in positive selection screens where RNAi-mediated gene silencing results in a phenotype that is easily identifiable, such as cell survival under lethal concentrations of a cancer drug (Seyhan et al., 2012), colony formation or growth in soft agar (Berns et al., 2004; Hattori et al., 2007; Kolfschoten et al., 2005; Westbrook et al., 2005a), cell rescue from cytotoxic or cytostatic influence, cellular proliferation, membrane bound or intracellular protein modification, or activation or suppression of a pathway (i.e., promoter activation measured by expression of a reporter gene) (Berns et al., 2007; Kolfschoten et al., 2005; Westbrook et al., 2005a). Another study showed the utility of RNAi screen to identify the mechanisms that control the cell surface expression of the pro-apoptotic Fas receptor in Fas receptor-negative, K-Ras positive NIH 3T3 cells (Westbrook et al., 2005a).

On the contrary, negative selection or depletion screens rely on a system in which the RNAi reagents that are lost from the populations of transduced cells must be identified. To do this, a molecular barcoding strategy has been used. Toward this, a unique 60-mer barcode sequence expressed in cis to each shRNA (Seyhan et al., 2012). Alternatively part of the shRNA sequence itself can be used to identify cell-lethal or drug-sensitive RNAi reagents that are depleted (Schlabach et al., 2008; Silva et al., 2008) or enriched (Berns et al., 2007; Brummelkamp et al., 2006) in screens. The identities of genes are then identified by competitive hybridization of oligonucleotide barcodes before and after selection or before and after treatment in a microarray (Luo and Elledge, 2008; Schlabach et al., 2008; Silva et al., 2008; Whitehurst et al., 2007). For instance, positive selection barcode screens have identified novel drug targets, probed the drug–host interaction, and identified genes and pathways that resulted in resistance or sensitivity to a specific agent (Brummelkamp et al., 2006; Luo et al., 2008; Seyhan and Ryan, 2010; Seyhan et al., 2012; Westbrook et al., 2005a). Similar RNAi screens have also been employed to identify host factors involved in a variety of viral and bacterial pathogenesis including HIV (Brass et al., 2008; Zhou et al., 2008), HCV (Li et al., 2009; Randall et al., 2007; Tai et al., 2009), influenza (Hao et al., 2008), WNV (Krishnan et al., 2008), and brucella (Qin et al., 2008).

The next-generation sequencing (NGS) which has become widely available eliminates the concerns of probe-cross-hybridization as is the case for microarray technology and it does not suffer from dynamic range compression at extreme levels of barcodes or shRNAs. The cDNA library generated from the shRNA or barcode library can be directly sequenced. It is recommended that the coverage should be 500–2000 fold to represent entire library and to deconvolve the library accurately (Hu and Luo, 2012).

2.8 Endpoint Assay Readout Systems

Outcome of functional screens depend on methods for detecting the altered and desired phenotype, easily, robustly, and in an HTP fashion. The readout system must be robust to avoid background noise, but sensitive enough to detect subtle changes induced by RNAi reagents. Readout systems must involve a selectable alteration in cell phenotype such as *cell viability* or *cell proliferation, apoptosis,* or *altered expression of a protein* that can be detected by *flow cytometry* (i.e., a surface marker expressed through activation of a promoter or a signaling pathway, a florescent reporter activated by promoter activation, or splicing of a reporter gene), *enzymatic assays* (e.g., ELISAs), or *high-content image analysis*. Additionally, protein–protein associations can be measured by fluorescence resonance energy transfer, and changes in phosphorylation status can be monitored with phosphorylation-specific antibodies (Echeverri and Perrimon, 2006; Moffat and Sabatini, 2006; Perrimon and Mathey-Prevot, 2007). In addition, any combination of these assays can be performed to address different biological questions (e.g., RNAi and drug synthetic lethal screens). Many readout systems have been adopted from HTP compound screens and have been successfully used in RNAi screens (Falschlehner et al., 2010).

2.8.1 Cellular Proliferation, Viability, and Apoptosis

Several readily available assays based on the detection of fluorescence, or luminescence can be used in large-scale RNAi screens in an HTP fashion using a variety of plate readers rapidly and conveniently. Cellular viability is often measured by quantifying ATP levels (e.g., CellTiter-Glo), esterase activity and membrane integrity (e.g., Calcein-AM), or cellular redox potential (e.g., WST-1/MTT).

2.8.2 Cell Morphology

Cell morphology measured by immunofluorescent staining of cellular features such as cytoskeleton, DNA, and different organelles enables parallel and automated analysis of various cellular features with image analysis software. The clustering of high-content phenotypic data allows generation of phenotypic signatures or "phenoprints" that characterize the individual knockdowns. High-content image analysis and flow cytometry are examples of this method.

2.8.3 Reporter and Enzymatic Assays

A variety of cell-based reporter or enzymatic assays have been used for screening including measuring ATP levels, transcriptional activity, and protein stability using luciferase or fluorescence or chemiluminescence readouts to study the activity of signaling pathways or biological networks (Seyhan, 2010; Seyhan and Ryan, 2010). A reporter gene driven by a pathway specific promoter or a chimeric reporter gene with a transcription factor-binding site for a pathway-specific transcription factor driven by a minimal promoter can be used as reporters in cells transfected or transduced with RNAi reagents. Examples are promoter activation, enzymatic assays (ELISAs), and flow cytometry. Additionally, a wide variety of functional assays (e.g., caspase activity, Ca^{2+} signaling) can be used to assess different cellular events and can be based on different readouts.

2.8.4 High-Content Image Analysis

The emergence of high-content imaging technology has enabled the capture of multiple readouts of various different fluorescent or other visual markers simultaneously providing opportunities to probe cellular and subcellular changes after the screen. The images obtained in high-content image-base screening rely on automated solutions to capture and identify phenotypes induced by RNAi reagents. Many tens of different features can be identified from screen image datasets and then used to define or identify phenotypes that are relevant to the study. The availability of real-time imaging involving time-lapse imaging with live cells opens new opportunities and challenges specifically regarding the acquisition time of large datasets and analysis of data.

2.8.5 Phenotypic Assays

In a *pooled RNAi screen*, the "readout" must confer a selectable change in cell phenotype, cell viability, or proliferation, or altered expression of a protein that can be detected by flow cytometry as described above. Cells that show the desired phenotype are analyzed to determine if any genes silenced by RNAi are responsible for producing the phenotype. A variety of phenotypic assays induced by a drug, infectious pathogen, or environmental stress to discover modifiers of the phenotype normally induced upon exposure to that treatment or chemosensitizer or chemoresistor screens in combination with RNAi reagents (Mohr and Perrimon, 2011; Seyhan and Ryan, 2010; Seyhan et al., 2011, 2012). To study the phenotypic changes at the individual cell level, fluorescence-assisted cell sorting (FACS) has been used in arrayed screens to measure the relative levels of DNA and other few markers (Mohr and Perrimon, 2011). Because the method is slow and limited in number of markers that can be studied by using various fluorescent-labeled dyes, probes, or antibodies, platforms such as laser-scanning cytometers can facilitate this process.

2.9 Experimental Design Considerations

As illustrated in Figure 2.1 and outlined in Figure 2.4, RNAi screen begins with the type of biological question and disease and the cell type of interest. This often dictates the selection of suitable experimental system, choosing the screening format (arrayed RNAi reagents or pooled vector-derived RNAi screens) and genome coverage (genome-wide or a more focused screen), readout assays, the use of proper controls (e.g., positive, negative, and nonsilencing), addressing cell culture assay-related artifacts (e.g., well, plate, and edge effects), the choice of statistical methods for data analyses, and criteria for candidate "hit" ranking and validation of hit genes in appropriate cell types, such as cells obtained from patient samples or animal models (Figure 2.4). A robust large-scale screening assay must have a robust signal-to-noise ratio and low inter- and intraplate and -assay variation. A careful planning of the screen and assay optimization is the foundation of a successful screen.

Many of the siRNAs will have some effect in a genome-scale RNAi screen. Since cells are controlled by dynamic actions of many genes interacting with one another in a complex gene networks, the LOF of any gene by RNAi may affect other genes, pathways or the entire network or signaling cascade (Zhao et al., 2005). Because of these reasons and some other RNAi specific and nonspecific off-targeting effects which can lead to the false discovery results, a pilot study must be conducted where every variable in the screen is measured and optimized.

During the optimization, efficacy, specificity, and potency of a small panel of RNAi reagents and transfection reagents and end point readout assays are assessed. Other factors such as duration of screen, tissue culture conditions (cell densities, plate formats, 96-well, or 384-well), number of assay replicates, and any other assay variables are evaluated to optimize assay conditions (Sharma and Rao, 2009). Predefined housekeeping genes (e.g., GAPDH) and negative control RNAi reagents (multiple nontargeting RNAi reagents)

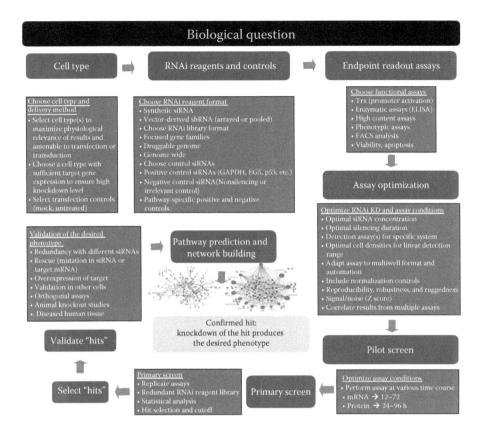

FIGURE 2.4

(See color insert.) Guideline for a successful pilot study for RNAi screen. RNAi screening workflow begins with choice of diseases to target, choice of cell type, choice of delivery and screening method as well as RNAi reagent format and genome-coverage, followed by experimental design (scope, redundancy, throughput, controls), selection or development of a cell-based assays to monitor RNAi effect, such as phenotypic assays (growth advantage, cell viability, mobility, etc.), reporter-based assays (GFP, labeled antibodies, fluorescent dyes), transcriptional and enzymatic assays (luciferase), antibody and microscopy-based assays (e.g., protein modification (phospho-specific abs). This is followed by primary screen with appropriate controls and data analysis and statistical tools for hit selection. After the primary screen, candidate genes are mapped into pathways and gene networks to provide better understanding of the functions of these genes in biological system. Finally, the candidate-hit genes are validated using a variety of approaches. Assay optimization and a pilot screen is necessary to optimize the conditions and identify issues before embarking on the primary screen. Additionally, analytical and statistical tools must be identified or developed for proper analysis of large data sets, hit selection, gene annotation, pathway prediction, and gene network building.

should be tested to determine baseline, signal, and standard deviation (s.d.) values for the system as well as mock treated and untreated cells must be tested during the optimization process.

After the optimization phase, pilot screen in which several tens of targets (low hundreds) alongside appropriate controls are tested. In the pilot screen, assay conditions are assessed to evaluate the overall performance, reproducibility, and robustness of the screen. Once the confidence is in place, the primary screen is conducted preferably in triplicates.

The raw data are analyzed to calculate quality control parameters, such as outliers between replicate measurements, plate effects and other variables, and to identify the measurements for downstream analysis (Boutros and Ahringer, 2008) and normalized to a control or set of controls and "hits" are identified based on predefined criteria such as the significance of the phenotypes compared with positive or negative controls (Boutros and Ahringer, 2008). Various data analysis packages (e.g., cellHTS, Spotfire/Tibco) can be used to normalize data, correct for plate position effects and batch-to-batch variations and to identify "hit" genes (Falschlehner et al., 2010). Because many RNAi collections now contain four or more siRNA/shRNA per target gene, this is also used as an additional feature to rank "hits" based on number of RNAi reagents showing the same phenotype (e.g., two or more).

The general quality of the screen and noise in large datasets can be monitored. This is achieved by Z' factors, as a measure of the statistical power of the assay to discriminate between positive and negative hits (Zhang et al., 1999) before hits are ranked on the basis of predefined thresholds. The calculation of the Z' factor requires several replicates of the assay with positive and negative controls. A Z' factor of > 0.5 (ideally > 0.7) indicates a suitable difference between signal and background values; therefore, a Z'-factor 0.5–1 is considered excellent (Boutros and Ahringer, 2008); although, a Z' factor 0.5 is considered acceptable for RNAi screens since many more variables influence the screen.

2.10 Off-Target Effects and Strategies to Mitigate Them

RNAi screens are impacted by false-positive and false-negative hits (Mohr and Perrimon, 2011) contributed by a variety of factors including the variable siRNA/shRNA effect as illustrated in Figure 2.5. Meta analyses of many screens have shown a poor correlation between or among related screens (Bushman et al., 2009; Muller et al., 2008; Snijder et al., 2012). The lack of concordance between screens is due to the use of different screening designs, reagents, cell lines, isogenic cells, cellular phenotype which is different than the tissue environment or whole organism due to dynamic adaptations to the microenvironment of individual cells (Snijder et al., 2012), screening duration, end-point readouts, and both false-positive and false-negative results. False discovery can be due to sequence-dependent (targeting sequences other than intended) and independent effects including activation of toll-like receptors (TLR), induction of an interferon response and general toxicity induced by the delivery method or reagent (Echeverri et al., 2006; Echeverri and Perrimon, 2006), and competition with the endogenous miRNA pathway (Pan et al., 2011).

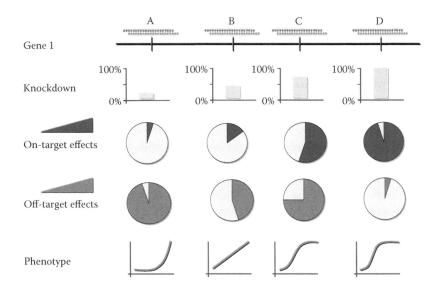

FIGURE 2.5
(See color insert.) Examples of variables that impact RNAi screens. For a phenotypic RNAi screen involving X number of genes, the ranking of any one gene will be influenced by the knockdown efficiencies of the RNAi reagents (e.g., knockdown efficiency siRNAs D > C > B > A for that gene), their off-target effects (A > C > D > B), and on-target effects (D > C > B > A), and the dose-response curves linking the activity of that gene and the phenotype being measured (e.g., loss of viability). (Adapted from Kaelin WG, Jr, 2012. *Science* **337**(6093): 421–422.)

Off-targeting effects can occur because: (i) sequence of RNAi reagent is identical or nearly identical to a sequence of an irrelevant mRNA, leading to a phenotype or production of a false-positive result (Jackson et al., 2003); (ii) RNAi sequences that are identical to "seed" sequences of the natural miRNAs and may pair with a complementary sequence in the 3′-untranslated region (3′-UTR) of an unrelated mRNA (Birmingham et al., 2006; Jackson et al., 2006b; Lin et al., 2005a); (iii) RNAi reagent activates the antiviral type I interferon response in a sequence-independent fashion (e.g., PKR signaling) (Sledz et al., 2003) especially when saturating concentrations of siRNAs are used (Sledz and Williams, 2004a), and (iv) RNAi reagent activates TLR (Agrawal and Kandimalla, 2004) or other cellular signaling pathways which has been caused by the presence of GU-rich motifs in the siRNA or shRNA (Judge et al., 2005) (e.g., 5′-UGUGU-3′ or 5′-GUCCUUCAA-3′) and has only been observed with primary peripheral blood leukocytes and plasmacytoid dendritic cells. Careful choice of the siRNAs and designing siRNA sequences devoid of any of the abovementioned sequences minimize or eliminate this type of off-targeting effects.

Off-targeting effects mediated by *sequence-independent* effects can be mitigated by optimizing the reagent delivery methods for the specific cell type or organism (Falschlehner et al., 2010). A recent *Drosophila* cell-based RNAi screen study has shown the utility of using proper number of reagents and replicates to reduce false-negative discovery (Booker et al., 2011). *Sequence-dependent* false-positive results have been more challenging because RNAi reagents either target of transcripts other than the intended target or they compete with endogenous miRNA pathways. Coexpressing miRNA pathway associated factors (e.g., Dicer 2) has been suggested as a strategy to improve the efficiency of long dsRNAs in *Drosophila* (Dietzl et al., 2007). Similar approaches have been used to express Exportin 5, which has been involved in trafficking of endogenous miRNAs to the cytoplasm (Grimm et al., 2006) and expression of shRNAs causes toxic effects due to competition with endogenous miRNA trafficking and other endogenous cellular RNAi factors including the four members of the human Argonaute (Ago) proteins as downstream factors involved in saturation of endogenous cellular RNAi, all of which interact with delivered or expressed shRNAs in cells and mice (Grimm et al., 2010). A better strategy may be to use weaker RNA polymerase III or RNA polymerase II promoters or inducible promoters to minimize and control the level of shRNA expression like the one used in our recent studies (Seyhan et al., 2012).

Additional factors such as poor knockdown efficacy of RNAi reagents can be improved by using improved siRNA designs and more redundant RNAi reagents per target (e.g., 10 or more has been suggested). To avoid potential off-targeting effects by siRNAs, new siRNA or shRNA design strategies have been used such that RNAi reagents are devoid of any sequences that may have identical or nearly identical sequences to other mRNA and "seed" regions (nucleotides 2–8 from 5′-end of the guide strand) of the endogenous miRNAs (Birmingham et al., 2006; Jackson et al., 2003, 2006a, b; Lin et al., 2005b).

Careful choice of the siRNA duplex sequence and designing siRNA sequences devoid of any of the abovementioned sequences minimize or eliminate this type of off-targeting effects.

To further minimize or eliminate the detrimental RNAi reagent and methodology-induced off-targeting effects, multiple nontargeting or scrambled RNAi reagent sequences should be used extensively in the RNAi screens. In addition, interferon responses and cell activation and/or differentiation that might be induced by the delivery methods or reagents used for the RNAi reagent delivery to target cells must also be examined to identify the source of any off-targeting effect during the optimization and pilot screen phase of screens.

In addition to the inherent characteristics of siRNA design that leads to false discovery in RNAi screens, suboptimal experimental design or application can contribute to false discovery in large-scale RNAi screens. Other factors that may contribute to the false discovery are: use of poorly designed RNAi reagents, lack of appropriate controls and insufficient number of replicates, inappropriate tissue culture practices including issues related to well, and edge and other tissue culture-related factors, or lack of statistical analyses for the specific screen performed (Mohr et al., 2010). Several strategies have been developed to mitigate these problems including experimental validation of the primary screen hits.

To further reduce the activation of the antiviral type I interferon response in a sequence-independent fashion, which is usually exacerbated when saturating concentrations of siRNAs are introduced to cells (Sledz and Williams, 2004b) and may compete with endogenous miRNA function, we will "titrate down" the amount of siRNA while achieving the highest level of inhibition.

Suboptimal experimental design can also result in false positives and false negatives in large-scale RNAi screens. There are several options to mitigate this problem by conducting an appropriate number of replicates and applying appropriate statistical analyses. Many approaches have been proposed or used to address the false discovery. To characterize a functional gene is a true hit, assays that are complementary (orthogonal) to those used in the primary screen should be used including small-molecule inhibitors, dominant negative mutational analysis, or inhibiting antibodies (Iorns et al., 2007; Sharma and Rao, 2009).

Another method for limiting false discovery rate is the careful analysis of multiple parameters extracted from high-content image data which can lead to a subset of parameters that are most representative of the gene knockdown phenotype (Collinet et al., 2010; Kummel et al., 2010).

To address the off-targeting effects, a recent study employed a triple parallel genome-scale RNAi screens to study endocytosis (Collinet et al., 2010). The researchers used two siRNA libraries and a third endoribonuclease-prepared siRNA (esiRNA, in total, 161,492 si/esiRNAs representing 7–8 si/esiRNAs per gene) and developed a multivariate image analysis method to capture phenotype induced by siRNA and esiRNA to limit off-targeting effects. They used comprehensive image analysis algorithms to capture diverse number of phenotypes that result following gene inhibition (e.g., number or distribution in cellular space and changes in endosome size) and to delineate multiple parameters of endosomal morphology and organization and to derive a "phenoscore." The authors then calculated the most probable on-target RNAi-specific signatures (the mode of the posteriori joint probability distribution) by compounding RNAi "pheno-scores" by considering all individual siRNA/esiRNA profiles for each gene. By this method, the authors were able to select for those phenotypes to limit the contribution of off-targeting effect to a gene profile.

This study illustrates how multiparametric data analysis capturing multiple phenotypic signatures can improve the data analysis, reduce false discovery, and provide improved information about the architecture of signaling networks and how different aspects or morphological regulation are controlled temporally and spatially (Bakal et al., 2007; Gunsalus et al., 2005; Sonnichsen et al., 2005). The study also demonstrates that the protein products of two genes with highly correlated phenotypic signatures are more likely to be present in the same signaling pathway (Collinet et al., 2010; Gunsalus et al., 2005).

To further improve the selection criteria and eliminate false positives, the hits from the screening can be compared to transcriptome data (Boettcher and Hoheisel, 2010).

Furthermore, comparison of the screen data with pathways or networks captured from the literature or large-scale proteomics datasets is yet another approach for limiting false discovery (Collins, 2009) such that false positives can be eliminated by identifying screen hits that do not corroborate with the orthogonal datasets. Conversely, false negatives can be retested by including genes that did not emerge as positives from the screen but are components of specific pathways or cellular function to the secondary analyses (Brass et al., 2008).

The use of multiple nonoverlapping RNAi reagents per gene is considered the most practical strategy for initial confirmation of primary screen results. In addition, by testing for comparable effects *in vivo* in the same species or testing for comparable effects in cells or *in vivo* in another species can be used to verify that effects are gene specific (Mohr and Perrimon, 2011). It is argued that the ultimate validation whether the phenotype is RNAi specific is rescue experiments using a genomic fragment, cDNA, or ORF construct designed to evade RNAi silencing through mismatch mutations (Kittler et al., 2005; Kondo et al., 2009; Langer et al., 2010; Lassus et al., 2002; Poser et al., 2008; Sarov and Stewart, 2005; Schulz et al., 2009; Stielow et al., 2008; Yokokura et al., 2004, 142–150). Confidence in results is further improved when results are verified using other molecular genetic methods (Mohr and Perrimon, 2011).

Furthermore, extensive use of statistical tests that are sensitive to the unique dynamics of RNAi screens and standards for performing and reporting screening data will improve robustness of the screens and will further reduce false discovery rates.

These examples illustrate how a genome-wide RNAi screen performed in a rigorous fashion can inform us on fundamental cellular process.

2.11 Data Analysis and "Hit" Identification

In an RNAi screen, the ranking of the hit genes will be influenced by a variety of factors including the knockdown efficiencies of the RNAi reagents, their off-target effects, and the dose–response curves linking the activity of that gene and the phenotype being measured (e.g., cell proliferation, changes in cell viability, reporter gene activity) (Kaelin, 2012). Because of these variables, RNAi screens designed to achieve the same end points such as cell death induced by a particular pathogen or cancer-relevant mutation but using different RNAi libraries, cell types, siRNA concentrations, duration of screening, and different ranking algorithms can produce different results

(Kaelin, 2012). One approach to mitigate this issue is to conduct pilot screens involving fewer genes (a few hundred) with appropriate controls (positive and negative knockdown as well as other related controls), to identify weak spots, and issues early on before embarking on larger screens. Pilot screens should be conducted such that siRNA dose, duration of optimal silencing, and measurement of endpoint readouts can be optimized.

After the primary screen, the data are analyzed to identify candidate gene "hits" that show the desired phenotype in an arrayed screen or identifying phenotypes that conferred resistance or those that are under- and/or overrepresented in the experimental set(s) as compared with the reference in pool-based screens (Mohr et al., 2010). A variety of analytical and statistical methodologies are used for data analysis (Birmingham et al., 2009). Many of these have been adopted from HTP compound screening protocols which may include: (i) performing at least one replicate preferable triplicate screen; (ii) including an appropriate type and number of "no treatment"; (iii) appropriate positive, negative, or nontargeting siRNA controls; (iv) controls to test assay conditions, plate, and well effect; (v) data normalization; (vi) determining appropriate thresholds for hit identification; and (vii) setting appropriate cutoff values for significant results (Mohr et al., 2010).

After the primary screen is completed, the goal is to identify high-scoring genes, annotate the hits, and determine which biological processes are represented by these genes. A variety of data analysis programs are available to search for gene ontology (GO) categories that are enriched for high-scoring genes such as the *bioconductor category* package (Boutros et al., 2006). The program compares the distribution of scores of genes in a category with the overall distribution and identifies those categories that separate from the mean plot; which have both a large difference in means as well as a small P value.

Traditionally, a "hit" is identified when assay replicates are beyond 2–3 standard deviation (s.d.) (hits with an s.d. of > 5 from the mean should be excluded from the analysis as to not to skew the calculated mean values) values from the mean or beyond a predetermined phenotypic threshold (for screens that assess morphology or other parameters that cannot be readily quantified). This is termed the Z-score and defined as a measure of the distance in standard deviations of a sample from the mean (Boutros and Ahringer, 2008). Although mean and s.d. values are often computed with positive and negative and nontargeting RNAi reagent controls, the entire RNAi library as *de facto* nonfunctional control or negative controls can be used as a sample-based approach. Since sample-based normalization uses more experimental data points which do not contribute to the desired phenotype, it can provide more accurate data analysis. Especially if robust controls are not available, the sample-based approach should be used as a negative control (Birmingham et al., 2009). It is critical to conduct screens at least in triplicate, to minimize false discovery (Luo et al., 2008; Ngo et al., 2006).

Many problems associated with false discovery and validation of hit genes remain as challenges. It is possible that statistical and better designed and controlled screens can minimize the problem. Sources contributing to false discovery are extensively discussed here and elsewhere (Mohr and Perrimon, 2011; Seyhan, 2010).

2.12 Hit Validation

The validation of hits in a screen constitutes one of the most important steps of any screen. Usually the validation is performed by another set of RNAi reagents, preferably with different sequence features targeting the same gene.

To validate that the RNAi effect is directly responsible for the phenotype, "recue" and "redundancy" experiments should be conducted (Echeverri et al., 2006) by using independent set of RNAi reagents (i.e., from different vendors) targeting different sites on the same gene or reversing the phenotype induced by the RNAi by expressing a cDNA that has a mismatch mutation with the RNAi reagent-binding site of the mRNA which abolishes RNAi-mediated target cleavage by RISC complex. However, confirmation of a large panel of hits in this fashion is impractical and cDNA overexpression can lead to aberrant effects (Lord et al., 2009). Alternatively, siRNAs targeting the the 3'-UTRs of target mRNAs can be used to rescue the phenotype such that the rescue construct can then be designed without the 3'-UTR, becoming resistant to the siRNAs (Falschlehner et al., 2010). Redundancy usually sufficient to confirm knockdown specificity since multiple RNAi reagents targets different sites of the same gene provided that these RNAi reagents are functionally efficient to generate the same phenotype (at least two or more siRNA/shRNA per taget).

Redundancy is more widely accepted approach to confirm if the phenotype is due to RNAi effect. To accomplish this, it is recommended to use multiple RNAi reagents targeting different sites of the same hit gene mRNA other than the one used in the screen. In fact, many RNAi reagent libraries have a redundancy built into the collection (Seyhan et al., 2011).

If a library of pooled siRNAs (e.g., four siRNAs per well targeting the same gene) is used in the screen, the candidate pools must be validated as individual siRNAs after the screen to identify the most potent siRNA(s) that is responsible for the phenotype. From the screen, at least two siRNA molecules in the pool should confer the phenotype, and there should be a clear correlation between mRNA, protein depletion, and phenotypic severity.

RNAi knockdown by a single siRNA should be confirmed at the RNA (qRT-PCR), protein (Western), and correlating the results with the observed phenotype where the candidate gene phenotypes should be reproducible with at least two or more independent RNAi reagents (Falschlehner et al., 2010).

Additionally, different assays as endpoint readout and different cells that contain or lack of the target expression should be used to confirm that hits are true. Concomitant RNAi silencing and cDNA overexpression can be used to assess if two genes selected in the screen are in the same pathway. To establish a physical interaction among candidate proteins, coimmunoprecipitation or tandem affinity purification as well as gene network analysis can be used to establish network relationships among a set of candidate genes (Lord et al., 2009).

The novel targets, metabolic and regulatory networks, and disease-relevant pathways must be validated to translate these findings into druggable targets. Bioinformatically, RNAi-induced phenotype should represent the disease phenotype that is being studied by mapping disease-associated regions, mutations, and amplifications through gene and pathway validation (Mohr et al., 2010) and by examining protein–protein interactions. For example, coimmunoprecipitation, mass spectrometry, and yeast two-hybrid screens can often reveal physical interactions among newly identified proteins (Mohr et al., 2010).

To establish network relationships among a set of genes identified from the screen, database mining and bioinformatics are commonly used (e.g., Ingenuity™) (Lord et al., 2009). Hits may be grouped by end points themselves or grouped by hierarchical clustering or principal-components analyses. For screens that test multiples for each gene, these methods allow detection of off-targeting effects through clustering. An siRNA that results in an off-targeting effect will induce a different set of phenotypes and therefore fall into a separate cluster from the other siRNAs targeting the same gene (Haney, 2007). The candidate genes in a pathway should be investigated further to elucidate their exact mechanism of action in the respective signaling pathway(s). To confirm if two genes selected in the screen are in the same pathway, concomitant knockdown experiments should be conducted in combination of RNAi reagents and these results should be captured by analyzing the information generated from diseased tissue samples and healthy controls or samples from treated samples. Correlation of the expression levels of the selected genes to either treatment response or disease outcome can facilitate the validation of the RNAi "hits." Another area of improvement may include the correlation of different types of large-scale genomic datasets with the RNAi screening data to select those targets that are truly important for the biological phenotype under investigation (Haney, 2007).

Since validation of hit genes is often complex and requires more resources and time than the primary screen itself, bioinformatics and statistical tools (e.g., Ingenuity) should be used which subject the candidate genes to pathway prediction analysis to determine whether a number of hits from the screen cluster into the same biological pathway or have a well-established physical or functional interaction.

Ultimately, genetic analysis is required to test the effects of mutations of gene hits in whole animals for validating the phenotype in an *in vivo* system.

In addition, the results should be compared with list of validated candidate genes that are available in open access databases or published literature (Campeau and Gobeil, 2011; Seyhan et al., 2012) for an independent confirmation of the screening hits or to elucidate their mechanism(s) of action. To support this, a vast amount of HTP data is now available online, including data from microarrays, proteomic and interactome studies, genetic networks, and small molecule and RNAi screens, as well as through various online computational resources such as gene ontology (GO, 2001).

2.13 Challenges and Future Directions

RNAi screens have demonstrated their value for the identification of novel targets and pathways providing better understanding about individual genes, pathways, and molecular networks toward the development of novel therapies. However, false discovery and validation of hits are the main challenges and translating *in vitro* functional data into *in vivo* systems often results in poor correlation of *in vitro* phenotype to *in vivo* systems and disease. This is partly due to the lack of correlation of screening data to diseased tissue or patient data as well as limited understanding of the underlying biology of the disease onset and due to several technical issues related to RNAi reagents, assay design and screening methods, and analytical and statistical methods used for hit identification.

The RNAi "hits" or "phenotype" results from a screen must be validated to establish the biological effect independent of the cellular context and under the influence of the complex *in vivo* environment. It is critical that the cell type used in the screen is directly relevant to the disease under investigation and recombinant or transformed cell lines such as HeLa, or HEK293 traditionally employed screens are not suitable to study the biology of different diseases including cancer, pathogen–host interactions, or receptor signaling.

The performance of genome-scale screens will further improve by incorporating integrative and multiplexed strategies such as parallel screening using different RNAi libraries, screening of multiple cell types or lines, pathogens, active compound treatments as in synthetic lethal screens and assays, and capture multiple assay readouts per screen. Furthermore, RNAi reagent library enhancements including increasing the number of siRNA/shRNAs per gene (10 or more shRNA per target) which increases RNAi reagent redundancy into the library potentially eliminating the need for extensive validation of hit genes and eliminating siRNA/shRNA empirically found to produce false positives across multiple screens, and the use of algorithms that take into consideration of siRNA/shRNA knockdown efficiencies, and incorporation of orthogonal datasets such as data from genomic studies or chemical screens will further improve the performance of RNAi screens and reduce false discovery. In the meantime, greater attention must be paid when analyzing RNAi screen data and better bioinformatics tools to reduce the validation of the candidate hits provided that primary screen data is robust.

As for the arrayed screens, high-density RNAi screens can be performed in 1536 well plates or on microarray chips. This can greatly increase the throughput permitting replicate screens to be conducted rapidly and cost effectively (Pfeifer and Scheel, 2009). This strategy also allows the use of greater genome coverage in a few plates or chips enabling ultra-throughput screens with a variety of compounds of interest (Borawski and Gaither, 2010).

Besides these improvements, the main challenge that still remains is to better integrate data generated by different systems biology studies (Neumuller and Perrimon, 2011). The integration of phenotypic data with protein localization, protein–protein interaction, and posttranslational modification data should significantly improve the interpretation of the complex genotype–phenotype relationships. Much needed proteomics data has been fueled by the recent advances in genome-scale protein localization and affinity purification studies conducted in yeast (Gavin et al., 2006; Huh et al., 2003).

2.13.1 Screening in Multicell Cultures or in Cells Grown in Three Dimension

A major challenge in cell biology is to understand how cells and molecular processes function and operate together as systems and to translate *in vitro* functional data into *in vivo* systems. This is usually very challenging and often results in poor correlation of *in vitro* phentotype to *in vivo* systems. The poor *in vitro* and *in vivo* correlation of gene hits identified in some screens may be due in part to the inability of monolayer or two-dimensional (2-D) cell culture systems to reproduce *in vivo* conditions.

Large-scale RNAi screens are often conducted in monolayer or 2-D cell culture system that does not perfectly capture the true *in vivo* environment with interactions between cells mediated via tissue architecture and the vascular system being absent.

In addition, the scientific question in mind relates to a tissue or whole organism instead of a specific cell type. Therefore, RNAi screens undertaken in a system that resembles the three-dimensional (3-D) environment of an actual tissue would be an ideal system. Performing RNAi screens using cells obtained from tumor samples of patients should produce results that correlate with *in vivo* systems better than the results obtained from the screens of 2-D monocultures (Stein, 2010).

Since large-scale screens may be challenging using these systems, another strategy is to validate the candidate-hit genes in cocultured cells or in 3-D cell culture systems to recreate complex, functional tissue *ex vivo* environment (Stein, 2010).

3-D cell culture systems can uncover genes that are required for unique phenotypes such as anchorage-independent growth of cancer cells that 2-D cell culture may not capture since anchorage-independent growth of tumor cells grown in soft agar in a 3-D environment closely matches those of xenograft assays (Freedman and Shin, 1974). Since HTP soft-agar assays have already been demonstrated (Anderson et al., 2007; Thierbach and Steinberg, 2009), focused RNAi screens in 3-D soft agar systems can be applied to identify new targets and pathway validations whose inhibition results in a suppressed tumor growth representing a more physiologically relevant phenotype than cells grown in 2-D systems as monocultures (Borawski and Gaither, 2010). Hit validation process should also include cells from patient samples or animal models.

For orthogonal validation of hits, if kinases or other enzymes are identified in the screen, inhibitors of those enzymes should be used to confirm phenotype or if transcription factors are identified, they should be examined to see if they alter transcription of relevant genes important in the pathway studied in the screen (Lord et al., 2009).

Since validating individual genes can take much more time and resources, than the actual screen itself, bioinformatics can play an important role to improve the target identification and validation process lending confidence that the effects are real.

In one example, the candidate genes can be used in pathway prediction analysis to determine if a number of genes from the screen can be categorized within the same biological pathway or have a well-established physical or functional interaction suing tools such as Ingenuity.

However, this approach is only appropriate for whole-genome RNAi screens since focused screens already are biased toward particular pathways and this approach is only as good as the quality of the data.

2.13.2 RNAi Screening *In Vivo*

Although results obtained from RNAi screens performed in cell lines or panels of cocultured cells are close match to the microenvironment of a tissue or tumor, they do not represent the true *in vivo* results clinical response and many complex phenotypes cannot be captured in cell-based assays. It is therefore critical to confirm the gene function *in vivo*. RNAi screen has been used in various model organisms and in an increasing number of other species (Mohr and Perrimon, 2011) and is benefitting from the development of sophisticated new tools, reagents, and data analysis and statistical, and software tools for collecting and analyzing large set of data.

Recently, several *in vivo* RNAi screens in whole organisms have been performed, mostly in *C. elegans* (Fraser et al., 2000; Gonczy et al., 2000) and *Drosophila melanogaster* (Bartscherer et al., 2006; Boutros et al., 2004; Neumuller and Perrimon, 2011) and related *Melanogaster* libraries (Dietzl et al., 2007; Kambris et al., 2006). Populations of virus-transduced cells have been proposed as a way to reintroduce libraries of cells into mice and select for loss- or gain-of-function or phenotype (e.g., cell intrinsic factors) or control the activity (e.g., differentiation, function, and homing) of cells in an organism (Sharma and Rao, 2009).

As examples, pools of shRNA-transfected cells have been introduced into mice, an approach referred to as *ex vivo* screening particularly in cancer-based studies, in which transduced cells can be assayed for their ability to contribute to tumor formation following introduction into the host animal (Bric et al., 2009; Meacham et al., 2009).

The utility of this approach has also been demonstrated in mice using a small panel of lentiviral-shRNA library targeting a small subset of genes (Bric et al., 2009; Dickins et al., 2007; Zender et al., 2008). However, his approach has been mostly employed for validation of candidate-hit genes including tumor suppressors (Bric et al., 2009; Xue et al., 2008; Zender et al., 2008). In another study, lentiviral-shRNAs were introduced into mice to knockdown the gene encoding the immunomodulatory receptor CTLA-4 to compare hypomorphic phenotypes resulting from partial knockdown with the severer phenotypes produced by complete gene deletion (Chen et al., 2006).

Additionally, inducible expression vectors that can be introduced into ES cells, facilitating regulatable RNAi in ES cells or production of transgenic mice for *in vivo* RNAi, have been explored (McJunkin et al., 2011; Premsrirut et al., 2011); or lentivirus-mediated transduction of skin facilitates *in vivo* RNAi (Beronja et al., 2010; Williams et al., 2011). Designer lentiviral vectors for *in vivo* studies should help *in vivo* studies in mice in the future (Meerbrey et al., 2011).

In vivo RNAi screening also termed as *ex vivo* functional screening provides a path for screening a phenotype of interest in a tissue and stage-specific manner in an organism which has been exemplified in organisms including *Lepidoptera* (Terenius et al., 2010) and other insects (Belles, 2010); ticks (de la Fuente et al., 2007); hydra (Lohmann et al., 1999); planarians (Reddien et al., 2005); a variety of plants (Gilchrist and Haughn, 2010; McInnis, 2010); and pathogens such as *trypanosomes* (Baker et al., 2011; Schumann Burkard et al., 2011) and mice (Mohr and Perrimon, 2011).

This approach also has been used successfully to examine the vulnerabilities of primary leukemia cells from 30 patients using a focused siRNA library that individually assesses targeting of each member of the tyrosine kinase gene family (Tyner et al., 2009). Therefore, the direct functional *ex vivo* screening of cells obtained from patients could, in principle, identify novel targets, pathways, and vulnerabilities that can be translated directly into humans.

2.14 Conclusions

RNAi-mediated functional genomics screens have been widely recognized as a powerful technology by researchers for the discovery of novel genes that encode molecules with previously unknown functions in a biological system. As demonstrated in literature (Falschlehner et al., 2010; Seyhan and Ryan, 2010; Sharma and Rao, 2009), the application of RNAi screening technology has been successful in examining important biological questions and to identify novel, important insights into individual genes and the associated molecular networks that can be explored for therapeutic intervention. Consequently, many of the RNAi screens have resulted in the identification of novel modulators, alternative signaling and disease pathways, and drug targets and biomarkers in areas including cancer, general cell biology, RNA biology, and viral pathogenesis (Seyhan and Ryan, 2010).

Combining RNAi screening results with the data obtained from other genomic, transcriptomic, and proteomic data can further improve our understanding of the biological relevance of the newly discovered targets, pathways and networks to biological processes, and disease pathogenesis.

Because of the challenges related to false discovery, RNAi reagent designs, assay design and screening methods, and the biological model systems used to interrogate the scientific question, the hits identified in the screens still require a comprehensive validation to establish a relationship to the *in vivo* biological effect independent of the cellular context.

Despite of these issues, the advances in RNAi reagent designs and use of powerful statistical tools to minimize false discovery should improve the quality of results obtained from such screens leading to the identification of novel drug targets, pathways and gene networks associated with biological processes or disease as well as disease or treatment-response biomarkers that can impact basic science as well as translational medicine.

2.14.1 Review Criteria

PubMed and Internet were used to identify research and review articles published on the subject discussed in this review. Following search terms used to identify relevant articles: "drug" and "pharmaceutical target identification," "biomarker identification," "RNA interference" and "RNAi screens and screening" were used. The search was restricted to the recent studies involving RNAi and all searches were limited to articles published in English.

Biography

After receiving his PhD in microbial biochemistry and biotechnology from Michigan Technological University (MTU), Houghton, MI on a NATO (North Atlantic Treaty Organization) Science Fellowship, Dr. Attila Seyhan moved to Paris, France, for his postdoctoral studies in Professor Bernard Grandchamp's lab at Xavier Bichat Hospital, University of Paris VII. There he studied regulation of ferritin gene during erythroid differentiation and cell proliferation with Dr. Carole Beaumont on a postdoctoral fellowship from the National Institute of Health and Medical Research of France (INSERM). He did his second postdoctoral fellowship with Professor John Burke at University of Vermont studying hairpin ribozyme biochemistry and their use as antigene and antiviral agents. He later joined SomaGenics, Inc. to develop self-ligating hairpin ribozymes (RNA LassoTM) for *in vitro* and *in vivo* target modulation and as diagnostics and then on RNAi and methods for generating RNAi libraries and their application as antigene and antiviral (HIV, hepatitis C virus, and Semliki Forest virus) therapeutics. He then moved to Dharmacon, Inc. and OpenBiosystems (both part of Thermo Scientific) to develop lentiviral miRNA-based siRNA libraries, lentiviral-shRNAmir libraries, and lentiviral human and mouse miRNA mimic libraries. Thereafter, he joined Wyeth Pharmaceutical as the Head of Functional Genomics group to lead the RNAi and compound library screening efforts for novel drug target discovery and development across different disease areas. Later, as Senior Leader in translational Medicine of Inflammation and Immunology at Pfizer Global Biotherapeutics, he led the genomics biomarker discovery and development efforts to advance various pharmaceutical programs from late preclinical to clinical research and managed several external alliances to support clinical research. He is an MIT research affiliate at the Chemical Engineering Department, Massachusetts Institute of Technology.

In addition, Dr. Seyhan is currently an Associate Investigator/Faculty at the Translational Research Institute for Metabolism and Diabetes and an advisor to the Biomarker Discovery and Development Unit (BDDU) at Florida Hospital, Orlando, FL and Adjunct Professor at Sanford Burnham Medical Research Institute, Diabetes and Obesity Research Center, Metabolic Disease Program, Orlando, FL. His research focuses on the Translational Research to develop personalized medicine and patient stratification strategies to segment disease and patient populations associated with metabolic diseases including obesity and diabetes with a particular focus on beta cell destruction and dysfunction in pathogenesis and pathophysiology of T1 and T2 diabetes.

References

Agrawal S, Kandimalla ER, 2004. Role of toll-like receptors in antisense and siRNA [corrected]. *Nat Biotechnol* **22**(12): 1533–1537.

Alexander RP, Fang G, Rozowsky J, Snyder M, Gerstein MB, 2010. Annotating noncoding regions of the genome. *Nat Rev Genet* **11**(8): 559–571.

Anderson SN, Towne DL, Burns DJ, Warrior U, 2007. A high-throughput soft agar assay for identification of anticancer compound. *J Biomol Screen* **12**(7): 938–945.

Arrowsmith J, 2011. Trial watch: Phase II failures: 2008–2010. *Nat Rev Drug Discov* **10**(5): 328–329.

Aza-Blanc P, Cooper CL, Wagner K, Batalov S, Deveraux QL, Cooke MP, 2003. Identification of modulators of TRAIL-induced apoptosis via RNAi-based phenotypic screening. *Mol Cell* **12**(3): 627–637.

Bakal C, Aach J, Church G, Perrimon N, 2007. Quantitative morphological signatures define local signaling networks regulating cell morphology. *Science* **316**(5832): 1753–1756.

Baker N, Alsford S, Horn D, 2011. Genome-wide RNAi screens in African trypanosomes identify the nifurtimox activator NTR and the eflornithine transporter AAT6. *Mol Biochem Parasitol* **176**(1): 55–57.

Balasubramanian S, Habegger L, Frankish A, MacArthur DG, Harte R, Tyler-Smith C, Harrow J, Gerstein M, 2011. Gene inactivation and its implications for annotation in the era of personal genomics. *Genes Dev* **25**(1): 1–10.

Bartscherer K, Pelte N, Ingelfinger D, Boutros M, 2006. Secretion of Wnt ligands requires Evi, a conserved transmembrane protein. *Cell* **125**(3): 523–533.

Begley CG, Ellis LM, 2012. Drug development: Raise standards for preclinical cancer research. *Nature* **483**(7391): 531–533.

Belles X, 2010. Beyond Drosophila: RNAi *in vivo* and functional genomics in insects. *Annu Rev Entomol* **55**: 111–128.

Bernards R, Brummelkamp TR, Beijersbergen RL, 2006. shRNA libraries and their use in cancer genetics. *Nat Methods* **3**(9): 701–706.

Berns K, Hijmans EM, Mullenders J, Brummelkamp TR, Velds A, Heimerikx M, Kerkhoven RM et al. 2004. A large-scale RNAi screen in human cells identifies new components of the p53 pathway. *Nature* **428**(6981): 431–437.

Berns K, Horlings HM, Hennessy BT, Madiredjo M, Hijmans EM, Beelen K, Linn SC et al. 2007. A functional genetic approach identifies the PI3K pathway as a major determinant of trastuzumab resistance in breast cancer. *Cancer Cell* **12**(4): 395–402.

Beronja S, Livshits G, Williams S, Fuchs E, 2010. Rapid functional dissection of genetic networks via tissue-specific transduction and RNAi in mouse embryos. *Nat Med* **16**(7): 821–827.

Birmingham A, Anderson EM, Reynolds A, Ilsley-Tyree D, Leake D, Fedorov Y, Baskerville S et al. 2006. 3′ UTR seed matches, but not overall identity, are associated with RNAi off-targets. *Nat Methods* **3**(3): 199–204.

Birmingham A, Selfors LM, Forster T, Wrobel D, Kennedy CJ, Shanks E, Santoyo-Lopez J et al. 2009. Statistical methods for analysis of high-throughput RNA interference screens. *Nat Methods* **6**(8): 569–575.

Birney E, Stamatoyannopoulos JA, Dutta A, Guigo R, Gingeras TR, Margulies EH, Weng Z et al. 2007. Identification and analysis of functional elements in 1% of the human genome by the ENCODE pilot project. *Nature* **447**(7146): 799–816.

Boettcher M, Hoheisel JD, 2010. Pooled RNAi screens—Technical and biological aspects. *Curr Genomics* **11**(3): 162–167.

Booker M, Samsonova AA, Kwon Y, Flockhart I, Mohr SE, Perrimon N, 2011. False negative rates in Drosophila cell-based RNAi screens: A case study. *BMC Genomics* **12**: 50.

Borawski J, Gaither A, 2010. The evolution of RNAi technologies in the drug discovery business. *Eur Pharm Rev* **5**(5): 35–39.

Boutros M, Ahringer J, 2008. The art and design of genetic screens: RNA interference. *Nat Rev Genet* **9**(7): 554–566.

Boutros M, Bras LP, Huber W, 2006. Analysis of cell-based RNAi screens. *Genome Biol* **7**(7): R66.

Boutros M, Kiger AA, Armknecht S, Kerr K, Hild M, Koch B, Haas SA, Paro R, Perrimon N, 2004. Genome-wide RNAi analysis of growth and viability in Drosophila cells. *Science* **303**(5659): 832–835.

Brass AL, Dykxhoorn DM, Benita Y, Yan N, Engelman A, Xavier RJ, Lieberman J, Elledge SJ, 2008. Identification of host proteins required for HIV infection through a functional genomic screen. *Science* **319**(5865): 921–926.

Bric A, Miething C, Bialucha CU, Scuoppo C, Zender L, Krasnitz A, Xuan Z et al. 2009. Functional identification of tumor-suppressor genes through an *in vivo* RNA interference screen in a mouse lymphoma model. *Cancer Cell* **16**(4): 324–335.

Brown ED, Wright GD, 2005. New targets and screening approaches in antimicrobial drug discovery. *Chem Rev* **105**(2): 759–774.

Brummelkamp TR, Fabius AW, Mullenders J, Madiredjo M, Velds A, Kerkhoven RM, Bernards R, Beijersbergen RL, 2006. An shRNA barcode screen provides insight into cancer cell vulnerability to MDM2 inhibitors. *Nat Chem Biol* **2**(4): 202–206.

Burnett JC, Rossi JJ, Tiemann K, 2011. Current progress of siRNA/shRNA therapeutics in clinical trials. *Biotechnol J* **6**(9): 1130–1146.

Bushman FD, Malani N, Fernandes J, D'Orso I, Cagney G, Diamond TL, Zhou H et al. 2009. Host cell factors in HIV replication: Meta-analysis of genome-wide studies. *PLoS Pathog* **5**(5): e1000437.

Butcher SP, 2003. Target discovery and validation in the post-genomic era. *Neurochem Res* **28**(2): 367–371.

Campeau E, Gobeil S, 2011. RNA interference in mammals: Behind the screen. *Brief Funct Genomics* **10**(4): 215–226.

Carninci P, Kasukawa T, Katayama S, Gough J, Frith MC, Maeda N, Oyama R et al. 2005. The transcriptional landscape of the mammalian genome. *Science* **309**(5740): 1559–1563.

Chapman EJ, Carrington JC, 2007. Specialization and evolution of endogenous small RNA pathways. *Nat Rev Genet* **8**(11): 884–896.

Chen X, Ji ZL, Chen YZ, 2002. TTD: Therapeutic target database. *Nucleic Acids Res* **30**(1): 412–415.

Chen Z, Stockton J, Mathis D, Benoist C, 2006. Modeling CTLA4-linked autoimmunity with RNA interference in mice. *Proc Natl Acad Sci USA* **103**(44): 16400–16405.

Cho DH, Tapscott SJ, 2007. Myotonic dystrophy: Emerging mechanisms for DM1 and DM2. *Biochim Biophys Acta* **1772**(2): 195–204.

Cobleigh MA, Vogel CL, Tripathy D, Robert NJ, Scholl S, Fehrenbacher L, Wolter JM et al. 1999. Multinational study of the efficacy and safety of humanized anti-HER2 monoclonal antibody in women who have HER2-overexpressing metastatic breast cancer that has progressed after chemotherapy for metastatic disease. *J Clin Oncol* **17**(9): 2639–2648.

Collinet C, Stoter M, Bradshaw CR, Samusik N, Rink JC, Kenski D, Habermann B et al. 2010. Systems survey of endocytosis by multiparametric image analysis. *Nature* **464**(7286): 243–249.

Collins I, Workman P, 2006. New approaches to molecular cancer therapeutics. *Nat Chem Biol* **2**(12): 689–700.

Collins MA, 2009. Generating "omic knowledge": The role of informatics in high content screening. *Comb Chem High Throughput Screen* **12**(9): 917–925.

David E, Tramontin T, Zemmel R, 2009. Pharmaceutical R&D: The road to positive returns. *Nat Rev Drug Discov* **8**(8): 609–610.

de la Fuente J, Kocan KM, Almazan C, Blouin EF, 2007. RNA interference for the study and genetic manipulation of ticks. *Trends Parasitol* **23**(9): 427–433.

Derrien T, Guigo R, Johnson R, 2011. The long non-coding RNAs: A new (P)layer in the "Dark Matter". *Front Genet* **2**: 107.

Dickins RA, McJunkin K, Hernando E, Premsrirut PK, Krizhanovsky V, Burgess DJ, Kim SY et al. 2007. Tissue-specific and reversible RNA interference in transgenic mice. *Nat Genet* **39**(7): 914–921.

Dietzl G, Chen D, Schnorrer F, Su KC, Barinova Y, Fellner M, Gasser B et al. 2007. A genome-wide transgenic RNAi library for conditional gene inactivation in Drosophila. *Nature* **448**(7150): 151–156.

Downward J, 2004. Use of RNA interference libraries to investigate oncogenic signalling in mammalian cells. *Oncogene* **23**(51): 8376–8383.

Dykxhoorn DM, Novina CD, Sharp PA, 2003. Killing the messenger: Short RNAs that silence gene expression. *Nat Rev Mol Cell Biol* **4**(6): 457–467.

Echeverri CJ, Beachy PA, Baum B, Boutros M, Buchholz F, Chanda SK, Downward J et al. 2006. Minimizing the risk of reporting false positives in large-scale RNAi screens. *Nat Methods* **3**(10): 777–779.

Echeverri CJ, Perrimon N, 2006. High-throughput RNAi screening in cultured cells: A user's guide. *Nat Rev Genet* **7**(5): 373–384.

Falschlehner C, Steinbrink S, Erdmann G, Boutros M, 2010. High-throughput RNAi screening to dissect cellular pathways: A how-to guide. *Biotechnol J* **5**(4): 368–376.

Fishman MC, Porter JA, 2005. Pharmaceuticals: A new grammar for drug discovery. *Nature* **437**(7058): 491–493.

Fraser AG, Kamath RS, Zipperlen P, Martinez-Campos M, Sohrmann M, Ahringer J, 2000. Functional genomic analysis of *C. elegans* chromosome I by systematic RNA interference. *Nature* **408**(6810): 325–330.

Freedman VH, Shin SI, 1974. Cellular tumorigenicity in nude mice: Correlation with cell growth in semi-solid medium. *Cell* **3**(4): 355–359.

Fryburg DA, 2010. Do technical and commercial biases contribute to the pharmaceutical industry's productivity problems? An analysis of how reordering priorities can improve productivity. *Drug Discov Today* **15**(17–18): 766–772.

Fryburg DA, Song DH, de Graaf D, 2011. Early patient stratification is critical to enable effective and personalised drug discovery and development. *Drug Discovery World Summer Issue* 47–56.

Gao Z, Li H, Zhang H, Liu X, Kang L, Luo X, Zhu W, Chen K, Wang X, Jiang H, 2008. PDTD: A web-accessible protein database for drug target identification. *BMC Bioinform* **9**: 104.

Gavin AC, Aloy P, Grandi P, Krause R, Boesche M, Marzioch M, Rau C et al. 2006. Proteome survey reveals modularity of the yeast cell machinery. *Nature* **440**(7084): 631–636.

Germano S, O'Driscoll L, 2009. Breast cancer: Understanding sensitivity and resistance to chemotherapy and targeted therapies to aid in personalised medicine. *Curr Cancer Drug Targets* **9**(3): 398–418.

Gerstein M, Zheng D, 2006. The real life of pseudogenes. *Sci Am* **295**(2): 48–55.

Gerstein MB, Bruce C, Rozowsky JS, Zheng D, Du J, Korbel JO, Emanuelsson O, Zhang ZD, Weissman S, Snyder M, 2007. What is a gene, post-ENCODE? History and updated definition. *Genome Res* **17**(6): 669–681.

Giaever G, Flaherty P, Kumm J, Proctor M, Nislow C, Jaramillo DF, Chu AM, Jordan MI, Arkin AP, Davis RW, 2004. Chemogenomic profiling: Identifying the functional interactions of small molecules in yeast. *Proc Natl Acad Sci USA* **101**(3): 793–798.

Gilchrist E, Haughn G, 2010. Reverse genetics techniques: Engineering loss and gain of gene function in plants. *Brief Funct Genomics* **9**(2): 103–110.

Gene Ontology Consortium, 2001. Creating the gene ontology resource: Design and implementation. *Genome Res* **11**: 1425–1433.

Golden JB, 2003. Prioritizing the human genome: Knowledge management for drug discovery. *Curr Opin Drug Discov Devel* **6**(3): 310–316.

Gonczy P, Echeverri C, Oegema K, Coulson A, Jones SJ, Copley RR, Duperon J et al. 2000. Functional genomic analysis of cell division in *C. elegans* using RNAi of genes on chromosome III. *Nature* **408**(6810): 331–336.

Grimm D, Streetz KL, Jopling CL, Storm TA, Pandey K, Davis CR, Marion P, Salazar F, Kay MA, 2006. Fatality in mice due to oversaturation of cellular microRNA/ short hairpin RNA pathways. *Nature* **441**(7092): 537–541.

Grimm D, Wang L, Lee JS, Schurmann N, Gu S, Borner K, Storm TA, Kay MA, 2010. Argonaute proteins are key determinants of RNAi efficacy, toxicity, and persistence in the adult mouse liver. *J Clin Invest* **120**(9): 3106–3119.

Gunsalus KC, Ge H, Schetter AJ, Goldberg DS, Han JD, Hao T, Berriz GF et al. 2005. Predictive models of molecular machines involved in *Caenorhabditis elegans* early embryogenesis. *Nature* **436**(7052): 861–865.

Guttman M, Donaghey J, Carey BW, Garber M, Grenier JK, Munson G, Young G et al. 2011. lincRNAs act in the circuitry controlling pluripotency and differentiation. *Nature* **477**(7364): 295–300.

Haney SA, 2007. Increasing the robustness and validity of RNAi screens. *Pharmacogenomics* **8**(8): 1037–1049.

Hao L, Sakurai A, Watanabe T, Sorensen E, Nidom CA, Newton MA, Ahlquist P, Kawaoka Y, 2008. Drosophila RNAi screen identifies host genes important for influenza virus replication. *Nature* **454**(7206): 890–893.

Hartwell LH, Szankasi P, Roberts CJ, Murray AW, Friend SH, 1997. Integrating genetic approaches into the discovery of anticancer drugs. *Science* **278**(5340): 1064–1068.

Hattori H, Zhang X, Jia Y, Subramanian KK, Jo H, Loison F, Newburger PE, Luo HR, 2007. RNAi screen identifies UBE2D3 as a mediator of all-trans retinoic acid-induced cell growth arrest in human acute promyelocytic NB4 cells. *Blood* **110**(2): 640–650.

Heuston EF, Lemon KT, Arceci RJ, 2011. The beginning of the road for non-coding RNAs in normal hematopoiesis and hematologic malignancies. *Front Genet* **2**: 94.

Ho RL, Lieu CA, 2008. Systems biology: An evolving approach in drug discovery and development. *Drugs R D* **9**(4): 203–216.

Hopkins AL, 2008. Network pharmacology: The next paradigm in drug discovery. *Nat Chem Biol* **4**(11): 682–690.

Hopkins AL, Groom CR, 2002. The druggable genome. *Nat Rev Drug Discov* **1**(9): 727–730.

Hu G, Luo J, 2012. A primer on using pooled shRNA libraries for functional genomic screens. *Acta Biochim Biophys Sin* **44**: 103–112.

Hughes TR, Marton MJ, Jones AR, Roberts CJ, Stoughton R, Armour CD, Bennett HA et al. 2000. Functional discovery via a compendium of expression profiles. *Cell* **102**(1): 109–126.

Huh WK, Falvo JV, Gerke LC, Carroll AS, Howson RW, Weissman JS, O'Shea EK, 2003. Global analysis of protein localization in budding yeast. *Nature* **425**(6959): 686–691.

Imming P, Sinning C, Meyer A, 2006. Drugs, their targets and the nature and number of drug targets. *Nat Rev Drug Discov* **5**(10): 821–834.

Iorns E, Lord CJ, Turner N, Ashworth A, 2007. Utilizing RNA interference to enhance cancer drug discovery. *Nat Rev Drug Discov* **6**(7): 556–568.

Jackson AL, Bartz SR, Schelter J, Kobayashi SV, Burchard J, Mao M, Li B, Cavet G, Linsley PS, 2003. Expression profiling reveals off-target gene regulation by RNAi. *Nat Biotechnol* **21**(6): 635–637.

Jackson AL, Burchard J, Leake D, Reynolds A, Schelter J, Guo J, Johnson JM et al. 2006a. Position-specific chemical modification of siRNAs reduces "off-target" transcript silencing. *RNA* **12**(7): 1197–1205.

Jackson AL, Burchard J, Schelter J, Chau BN, Cleary M, Lim L, Linsley PS 2006b. Widespread siRNA "off-target" transcript silencing mediated by seed region sequence complementarity. *RNA* **12**(7): 1179–1187.

Janga SC, Tzakos A, 2009. Structure and organization of drug-target networks: Insights from genomic approaches for drug discovery. *Mol BioSyst* **5**(12): 1536–1548.

Judge AD, Sood V, Shaw JR, Fang D, McClintock K, MacLachlan I, 2005. Sequence-dependent stimulation of the mammalian innate immune response by synthetic siRNA. *Nat Biotechnol* **23**(4): 457–462.

Kaelin WG, Jr, 2012. Molecular biology. Use and abuse of RNAi to study mammalian gene function. *Science* **337**(6093): 421–422.

Kambris Z, Brun S, Jang IH, Nam HJ, Romeo Y, Takahashi K, Lee WJ, Ueda R, Lemaitre B, 2006. Drosophila immunity: A large-scale *in vivo* RNAi screen identifies five serine proteases required for Toll activation. *Curr Biol* **16**(8): 808–813.

Kittler R, Pelletier L, Ma C, Poser I, Fischer S, Hyman AA, Buchholz F, 2005. RNA interference rescue by bacterial artificial chromosome transgenesis in mammalian tissue culture cells. *Proc Natl Acad Sci USA* **102**(7): 2396–2401.

Kolfschoten IG, van Leeuwen B, Berns K, Mullenders J, Beijersbergen RL, Bernards R, Voorhoeve PM, Agami R, 2005. A genetic screen identifies PITX1 as a suppressor of RAS activity and tumorigenicity. *Cell* **121**(6): 849–858.

Kondo S, Booker M, Perrimon N, 2009. Cross-species RNAi rescue platform in Drosophila melanogaster. *Genetics* **183**(3): 1165–1173.

Krishnan MN, Ng A, Sukumaran B, Gilfoy FD, Uchil PD, Sultana H, Brass AL et al. 2008. RNA interference screen for human genes associated with West Nile virus infection. *Nature* **455**(7210): 242–245.

Kummel A, Gubler H, Gehin P, Beibel M, Gabriel D, Parker CN, 2010. Integration of multiple readouts into the z′ factor for assay quality assessment. *J Biomol Screen* **15**(1): 95–101.

Kuritzkes DR, 2009. HIV-1 entry inhibitors: An overview. *Curr Opin HIV AIDS* **4**(2): 82–87.

Laifenfeld D, Drubin DA, Catlett NL, Park JS, Van Hooser AA, Frushour BP, de Graaf D, Fryburg DA, Deehan R, 2012. Early patient stratification and predictive biomarkers in drug discovery and development: A case study of ulcerative colitis anti-TNF therapy. *Adv Exp Med Biol* **736**: 645–653.

Lamb J, Crawford ED, Peck D, Modell JW, Blat IC, Wrobel MJ, Lerner J et al. 2006. The Connectivity Map: Using gene-expression signatures to connect small molecules, genes, and disease. *Science* **313**(5795): 1929–1935.

Langer CC, Ejsmont RK, Schonbauer C, Schnorrer F, Tomancak P, 2010. *in vivo* RNAi rescue in Drosophila melanogaster with genomic transgenes from *Drosophila pseudoobscura*. *PLoS One* **5**(1): e8928.

Lassus P, Rodriguez J, Lazebnik Y, 2002. Confirming specificity of RNAi in mammalian cells. *Sci STKE* **2002**(147): pl13.

Ledford H, 2011. Translational research: 4 ways to fix the clinical trial. *Nature* **477**(7366): 526–528.

Li Q, Brass AL, Ng A, Hu Z, Xavier RJ, Liang TJ, Elledge SJ, 2009. A genome-wide genetic screen for host factors required for hepatitis C virus propagation. *Proc Natl Acad Sci USA* **106**(38): 16410–16415.

Lin X, Ruan X, Anderson MG, McDowell JA, Kroeger PE, Fesik SW, Shen Y 2005a. siRNA-mediated off-target gene silencing triggered by a 7 nt complementation. *Nucleic Acids Res* **33**(14): 4527–4535.

Lin XY, Ruan X, Anderson MG, McDowell JA, Kroeger PE, Fesik SW, Shen Y 2005b. siRNA-mediated off-target gene silencing triggered by a 7 nt complementation. *Nucleic Acids Res* **33**(14): 4527–4535.

Lindsay MA, 2003. Target discovery. *Nat Rev Drug Discov* **2**(10): 831–838.

Lohmann JU, Endl I, Bosch TC, 1999. Silencing of developmental genes in Hydra. *Dev Biol* **214**(1): 211–214.

Lord CJ, Martin SA, Ashworth A, 2009. RNA interference screening demystified. *J Clin Pathol* **62**(3): 195–200.

Luo B, Cheung HW, Subramanian A, Sharifnia T, Okamoto M, Yang X, Hinkle G et al. 2008. Highly parallel identification of essential genes in cancer cells. *Proc Natl Acad Sci USA* **105**(51): 20380–20385.

Luo J, Elledge SJ, 2008. Cancer: Deconstructing oncogenesis. *Nature* **453**(7198): 995–996.

MacArthur, DG, Tyler-Smith C, 2010. Loss-of-function variants in the genomes of healthy humans. *Hum Mol Genet* **19**(R2): R125–R130.

Manolio TA, Collins FS, Cox NJ, Goldstein DB, Hindorff LA, Hunter DJ, McCarthy MI et al. 2009. Finding the missing heritability of complex diseases. *Nature* **461**(7265): 747–753.

McInnis K, 2010. RNAi for functional genomics in plants. *Brief Funct Genom* **9**: 111–117.

McJunkin K, Mazurek A, Premsrirut PK, Zuber J, Dow LE, Simon J, Stillman B, Lowe SW, 2011. Reversible suppression of an essential gene in adult mice using transgenic RNA interference. *Proc Natl Acad Sci USA* **108**(17): 7113–7118.

Meacham CE, Ho EE, Dubrovsky E, Gertler FB, Hemann MT, 2009. *In vivo* RNAi screening identifies regulators of actin dynamics as key determinants of lymphoma progression. *Nat Genet* **41**(10): 1133–1137.

Meerbrey KL, Hu G, Kessler JD, Roarty K, Li MZ, Fang JE, Herschkowitz JI et al. 2011. The pINDUCER lentiviral toolkit for inducible RNA interference *in vitro* and *in vivo*. *Proc Natl Acad Sci USA* **108**(9): 3665–3670.

Meister G, Tuschl T, 2004. Mechanisms of gene silencing by double-stranded RNA. *Nature* **431**(7006): 343–349.

Moffat J, Sabatini DM, 2006. Building mammalian signalling pathways with RNAi screens. *Nat Rev Mol Cell Biol* **7**(3): 177–187.

Mohr S, Bakal C, Perrimon N, 2010. Genomic screening with RNAi: Results and challenges. *Annu Rev Biochem* **79**: 37–64.

Mohr SE, Perrimon N, 2011. RNAi screening: New approaches, understandings, and organisms. *Wiley Interdiscip Rev RNA* **3**(2): 145–158.

Muller P, Boutros M, Zeidler MP, 2008. Identification of JAK/STAT pathway regulators—Insights from RNAi screens. *Semin Cell Dev Biol* **19**(4): 360–369.

Murrow LM, Garimella SV, Jones TL, Caplen NJ, Lipkowitz S, 2010. Identification of WEE1 as a potential molecular target in cancer cells by RNAi screening of the human tyrosine kinome. *Breast Cancer Res Treat* **122**(2): 347–357.

Nagano T, Fraser P, 2011. No-nonsense functions for long noncoding RNAs. *Cell* **145**(2):178-181.

Neumuller RA, Perrimon N, 2011. Where gene discovery turns into systems biology: Genome-scale RNAi screens in Drosophila. *Wiley Interdiscip Rev Syst Biol Med* **3**(4): 471–478.

Ngo VN, Davis RE, Lamy L, Yu X, Zhao H, Lenz G, Lam LT et al. 2006. A loss-of-function RNA interference screen for molecular targets in cancer. *Nature* **441**(7089): 106–110.

Ohlstein EH, Ruffolo RR, Jr., Elliott JD, 2000. Drug discovery in the next millennium. *Annu Rev Pharmacol Toxicol* **40**: 177–191.

Overington JP, Al-Lazikani B, Hopkins AL, 2006. How many drug targets are there? *Nat Rev Drug Discov* **5**(12): 993–996.

Pan Q, de Ruiter PE, von Eije KJ, Smits R, Kwekkeboom J, Tilanus HW, Berkhout B, Janssen HL, van der Laan LJ, 2011. Disturbance of the microRNA pathway by commonly used lentiviral shRNA libraries limits the application for screening host factors involved in hepatitis C virus infection. *FEBS Lett* **585**(7): 1025–1030.

Parker BJ, Moltke I, Roth A, Washietl S, Wen J, Kellis M, Breaker R, and Pedersen JS. New families of human regulatory RNA structures identified by comparative analysis of vertebrate genomes. *Genome Res* **21**(11): 1929–1943.

Parsons AB, Lopez A, Givoni IE, Williams DE, Gray CA, Porter J, Chua G et al. 2006. Exploring the mode-of-action of bioactive compounds by chemical-genetic profiling in yeast. *Cell* **126**(3): 611–625.

Paul SM, Mytelka DS, Dunwiddie CT, Persinger CC, Munos BH, Lindborg SR, Schacht AL, 2010. How to improve R&D productivity: The pharmaceutical industry's grand challenge. *Nat Rev Drug Discov* **9**(3): 203–214.

Perrimon N, Mathey-Prevot B, 2007. Applications of high-throughput RNA interference screens to problems in cell and developmental biology. *Genetics* **175**(1): 7–16.

Pfeifer MJ, Scheel G, 2009. Long-term storage of compound solutions for high-throughput screening by using a novel 1536-well microplate. *J Biomol Screen* **14**(5): 492–498.

Poliseno L, Haimovic A, Christos PJ, Vega YSdMEC, Shapiro R, Pavlick A, Berman RS, Darvishian F, Osman I, 2010. Deletion of PTENP1 pseudogene in human melanoma. *J Invest Dermatol* **131**(12): 2497–2500.

Ponting CP, Oliver PL, Reik W. 2009. Evolution and functions of long noncoding RNAs. *Cell* **136**(4): 629–641.

Poser I, Sarov M, Hutchins JR, Heriche JK, Toyoda Y, Pozniakovsky A, Weigl D et al. 2008. BAC TransgeneOmics: A high-throughput method for exploration of protein function in mammals. *Nat Methods* **5**(5): 409–415.

Premsrirut PK, Dow LE, Kim SY, Camiolo M, Malone CD, Miething C, Scuoppo C et al. 2011. A rapid and scalable system for studying gene function in mice using conditional RNA interference. *Cell* **145**(1): 145–158.

Prinz F, Schlange T, Asadullah K, 2011. Believe it or not: How much can we rely on published data on potential drug targets? *Nat Rev Drug Discov* **10**(9): 712.

Qin QM, Pei J, Ancona V, Shaw BD, Ficht TA, de Figueiredo P, 2008. RNAi screen of endoplasmic reticulum-associated host factors reveals a role for IRE1alpha in supporting Brucella replication. *PLoS Pathog* **4**(7): e1000110.

Quon K, Kassner PD, 2009. RNA interference screening for the discovery of oncology targets. *Expert Opin Ther Targets* **13**(9): 1027–1035.

Randall G, Panis M, Cooper JD, Tellinghuisen TL, Sukhodolets KE, Pfeffer S, Landthaler M et al. 2007. Cellular cofactors affecting hepatitis C virus infection and replication. *Proc Natl Acad Sci USA* **104**(31): 12884–12889.

Reddien PW, Bermange AL, Murfitt KJ, Jennings JR, Sanchez Alvarado A, 2005. Identification of genes needed for regeneration, stem cell function, and tissue homeostasis by systematic gene perturbation in planaria. *Dev Cell* **8**(5): 635–649.

Root DE, Hacohen N, Hahn WC, Lander ES, Sabatini DM, 2006. Genome-scale loss-of-function screening with a lentiviral RNAi library. *Nat Meth* **3**(9): 715–719.

Russ AP, Lampel S, 2005. The druggable genome: An update. *Drug Discov Today* **10**(23–24): 1607–1610.

Sakharkar MK, Sakharkar KR, 2007. Targetability of human disease genes. *Curr Drug Discov Technol* **4**(1): 48–58.

Sams-Dodd F, 2005. Target-based drug discovery: Is something wrong? *Drug Discov Today* **10**(2): 139–147.

Sarov M, Stewart AF, 2005. The best control for the specificity of RNAi. *Trends Biotechnol* **23**(9): 446–448.

Schlabach MR, Luo J, Solimini NL, Hu G, Xu Q, Li MZ, Zhao Z et al. 2008. Cancer proliferation gene discovery through functional genomics. *Science* **319**(5863): 620–624.

Scholl C, Frohling S, Dunn IF, Schinzel AC, Barbie DA, Kim SY, Silver SJ et al. 2009. Synthetic lethal interaction between oncogenic KRAS dependency and STK33 suppression in human cancer cells. *Cell* **137**(5): 821–834.

Schulz JG, David G, Hassan BA, 2009. A novel method for tissue-specific RNAi rescue in Drosophila. *Nucleic Acids Res* **37**(13): e93.

Schumann Burkard G, Jutzi P, Roditi I, 2011. Genome-wide RNAi screens in bloodstream form trypanosomes identify drug transporters. *Mol Biochem Parasitol* **175**(1): 91–94.

Seyhan AA, 2010. RNAi screens for the identification and validation of novel targets: Current status and challenges. *Eur Pharmaceutical Rev* (6): 13–24.

Seyhan AA, 2011. RNAi: A potential new class of therapeutic for human genetic disease. *Hum Genet* **130**(5): 583–605.

Seyhan AA, Alizadeh BN, Lundstrom K, Johnston BH, 2007. RNA interference-mediated inhibition of Semliki Forest virus replication in mammalian cells. *Oligonucleotides* **17**(4): 473–484.

Seyhan AA, Ryan TE, 2010. RNAi screening for the discovery of novel modulators of human disease. *Curr Pharm Biotechnol* **11**(7): 735–756.

Seyhan AA, Varadarajan U, Choe S, Liu Wa, Ryan TE, 2012. A genome-wide RNAi screen identifies novel targets of neratinib resistance leading to identification of potential drug resistant genetic markers. *Mol BioSyst* **8**: 1553–1570.

Seyhan AA, Varadarajan U, Choe S, Liu Y, McGraw J, Woods M, Murray S, Eckert A, Liu W, Ryan TE, 2011. A genome-wide RNAi screen identifies novel targets of neratinib sensitivity leading to neratinib and paclitaxel combination drug treatments. *Mol BioSyst* **7**(6): 1974–1989.

Seyhan AA, Vlassov AV, Ilves H, Egry L, Kaspar RL, Kazakov SA, Johnston BH, 2005. Complete, gene-specific siRNA libraries: Production and expression in mammalian cells. *RNA* **11**(5): 837–846.

Sharma S, Rao A, 2009. RNAi screening: Tips and techniques. *Nat Immunol* **10**(8): 799–804.

Silva JM, Marran K, Parker JS, Silva J, Golding M, Schlabach MR, Elledge SJ, Hannon GJ, Chang K, 2008. Profiling essential genes in human mammary cells by multiplex RNAi screening. *Science* **319**(5863): 617–620.

Simpson KJ, Davis GM, Boag PR, 2012. Comparative high-throughput RNAi screening methodologies in *C. elegans* and mammalian cells. *N Biotechnol* **29**(4): 459–470.

Sledz CA, Holko M, de Veer MJ, Silverman RH, Williams BR, 2003. Activation of the interferon system by short-interfering RNAs. *Nat Cell Biol* **5**(9): 834–839.

Sledz CA, Williams BR 2004a. RNA interference and double-stranded-RNA-activated pathways. *Biochem Soc Trans* **32**(Pt 6): 952–956.

Sledz CA, Williams BRG 2004b. RNA interference and double-stranded-RNA-activated pathways. *Biochem Soc Trans* **32**: 952–956.

Sleno L, Emili A, 2008. Proteomic methods for drug target discovery. *Curr Opin Chem Biol* **12**(1): 46–54.

Snijder B, Sacher R, Ramo P, Liberali P, Mench K, Wolfrum N, Burleigh L et al. 2012. Single-cell analysis of population context advances RNAi screening at multiple levels. *Mol Syst Biol* **8**: 579.

Sonnichsen B, Koski LB, Walsh A, Marschall P, Neumann B, Brehm M, Alleaume AM et al. 2005. Full-genome RNAi profiling of early embryogenesis in *Caenorhabditis elegans*. *Nature* **434**(7032): 462–469.

St. Onge RP, Mani R, Oh J, Proctor M, Fung E, Davis RW, Nislow C, Roth FP, Giaever G, 2007. Systematic pathway analysis using high-resolution fitness profiling of combinatorial gene deletions. *Nat Genet* **39**(2): 199–206.

Stein RA, 2010. Transitioning toward three-dimensional cell culture. *Genet Eng Biotechnol News*, 30, 1, 18, 20–21.

Stelling J, Sauer U, Szallasi Z, Doyle FJ, 3rd, Doyle J, 2004. Robustness of cellular functions. *Cell* **118**(6): 675–685.

Stielow B, Sapetschnig A, Kruger I, Kunert N, Brehm A, Boutros M, Suske G, 2008. Identification of SUMO-dependent chromatin-associated transcriptional repression components by a genome-wide RNAi screen. *Mol Cell* **29**(6): 742–754.

Swami M, 2010. Small RNAs: Pseudogenes act as microRNA decoys. *Nat Rev Cancer* **10**(8): 535.

Tai AW, Benita Y, Peng LF, Kim SS, Sakamoto N, Xavier RJ, Chung RT, 2009. A functional genomic screen identifies cellular cofactors of hepatitis C virus replication. *Cell Host Microbe* **5**(3): 298–307.

Terenius O, Papanicolaou A, Garbutt JS, Eleftherianos I, Huvenne H, Kanginakudru S, Albrechtsen M et al. 2010. RNA interference in Lepidoptera: An overview of successful and unsuccessful studies and implications for experimental design. *J Insect Physiol* **57**(2): 231–245.

Terstappen GC, Schlupen C, Raggiaschi R, Gaviraghi G, 2007. Target deconvolution strategies in drug discovery. *Nat Rev Drug Discov* **6**(11): 891–903.

Thierbach R, Steinberg P, 2009. Automated soft agar assay for the high-throughput screening of anticancer compounds. *Anal Biochem* **387**(2): 318–320.

Torarinsson E, Sawera M, Havgaard JH, Fredholm M, Gorodkin, J. 2006. Thousands of corresponding human and mouse genomic regions unalignable in primary sequence contain common RNA structure. *Genome Res* **16**(7): 885–889.

Tyner JW, Deininger MW, Loriaux MM, Chang BH, Gotlib JR, Willis SG, Erickson H et al. 2009. RNAi screen for rapid therapeutic target identification in leukemia patients. *Proc Natl Acad Sci USA* **106**(21): 8695–8700.

Vogel CL, Cobleigh MA, Tripathy D, Gutheil JC, Harris LN, Fehrenbacher L, Slamon DJ et al. 2002. Efficacy and safety of trastuzumab as a single agent in first-line treatment of HER2-overexpressing metastatic breast cancer. *J Clin Oncol* **20**(3): 719–726.

Westbrook TF, Martin ES, Schlabach MR, Leng Y, Liang AC, Feng B, Zhao JJ et al. 2005a. A genetic screen for candidate tumor suppressors identifies REST. *Cell* **121**(6): 837–848.

Westbrook TF, Stegmeier F, Elledge SJ (2005b) Dissecting cancer pathways and vulnerabilities with RNAi. *Cold Spring Harb Symp Quant Biol* **70**: 435–444.

Whitehead KA, Langer R, Anderson DG, 2009. Knocking down barriers: Advances in siRNA delivery. *Nat Rev Drug Discov* **8**(2): 129–138.

Whitehurst AW, Bodemann BO, Cardenas J, Ferguson D, Girard L, Peyton M, Minna JD et al. 2007. Synthetic lethal screen identification of chemosensitizer loci in cancer cells. *Nature* **446**(7137): 815–819.

Williams SE, Beronja S, Pasolli HA, Fuchs E, 2011. Asymmetric cell divisions promote Notch-dependent epidermal differentiation. *Nature* **470**(7334): 353–358.

Wishart DS, Knox C, Guo AC, Cheng D, Shrivastava S, Tzur D, Gautam B, Hassanali M, 2008. DrugBank: A knowledgebase for drugs, drug actions and drug targets. *Nucleic Acids Res* **36**(Database issue): D901–D906.

Wishart DS, Knox C, Guo AC, Shrivastava S, Hassanali M, Stothard P, Chang Z, Woolsey J, 2006. DrugBank: A comprehensive resource for in silico drug discovery and exploration. *Nucleic Acids Res* **34**(Database issue): D668–D672.

Woodcock J, 2007. The prospects for "personalized medicine" in drug development and drug therapy. *Clin Pharmacol Ther* **81**(2): 164–169.

Xue W, Krasnitz A, Lucito R, Sordella R, Vanaelst L, Cordon-Cardo C, Singer S et al. 2008. DLC1 is a chromosome 8p tumor suppressor whose loss promotes hepatocellular carcinoma. *Genes Dev* **22**(11): 1439–1444.

Yildirim MA, Goh KI, Cusick ME, Barabasi AL, Vidal M, 2007. Drug-target network. *Nat Biotechnol* **25**(10): 1119–1126.

Yokokura T, Dresnek D, Huseinovic N, Lisi S, Abdelwahid E, Bangs P, White K, 2004. Dissection of DIAP1 functional domains via a mutant replacement strategy. *J Biol Chem* **279**(50): 52603–52612.

Zambrowicz BP, Sands AT, 2003. Knockouts model the 100 best-selling drugs—Will they model the next 100? *Nat Rev Drug Discov* **2**(1): 38–51.

Zamore PD, Haley B, 2005. Ribo-gnome: The big world of small RNAs. *Science* **309**(5740): 1519–1524.

Zender L, Xue W, Zuber J, Semighini CP, Krasnitz A, Ma B, Zender P et al. 2008. An oncogenomics-based *in vivo* RNAi screen identifies tumor suppressors in liver cancer. *Cell* **135**(5): 852–864.

Zhang JH, Chung TD, Oldenburg KR, 1999. A simple statistical parameter for use in evaluation and validation of high throughput screening assays. *J Biomol Screen* **4**(2): 67–73.

Zhao HF, L'Abbe D, Jolicoeur N, Wu M, Li Z, Yu Z, Shen SH, 2005. High-throughput screening of effective siRNAs from RNAi libraries delivered via bacterial invasion. *Nat Methods* **2**(12): 967–973.

Zheng CJ, Han LY, Yap CW, Ji ZL, Cao ZW, Chen YZ, 2006. Therapeutic targets: Progress of their exploration and investigation of their characteristics. *Pharmacol Rev* **58**(2): 259–279.

Zhou H, Xu M, Huang Q, Gates AT, Zhang XD, Castle JC, Stec E et al. 2008. Genome-scale RNAi screen for host factors required for HIV replication. *Cell Host Microbe* **4**(5): 495–504.

Zhu F, Han B, Kumar P, Liu X, Ma X, Wei X, Huang L et al. 2010. Update of TTD: Therapeutic target database. *Nucleic Acids Res* **38**(Database issue): D787–D791.

3

Current Advances in Epigenetics

Ewan Hunter and Alexandre Akoulitchev

CONTENTS

3.1 Introduction to Epigenetics

It has been over 70 years since Conrad Waddington has coined the terms "epigenetics" and "epigenetic landscape" [1,2], setting off a race toward an understanding of the fundamental mechanism that mediates between genetic risks and the environment and which is ultimately responsible for "the interaction … with the environment" and brings the phenotype into being. The progress made in molecular biology today gives us some of the earliest insights into the molecular mechanisms behind the epigenetic phenomenon. The sign of big changes to come in biology is the fact that we have moved a long way from the first studies demonstrating relevance of epigenetics for early organism development to the multitude of evidence of epigenetic contributions into onset, development, and manifestation of many diseases [3,4]. New approaches in personalized medicine are seen today in light of the individual epigenetic state of the patients. Biomarker readouts of epigenetic differences and deregulations help to improve early diagnosis, prognosis, and prediction of response to treatment.

In an exemplary case, an extensive study of identical monozygous twins demonstrated a clear difference in epigenetic profiles between the twins, despite them having a common genotype. These epigenetic differences, when measured at different stages of life and development, were clearly accumulated with time [5]. A closer look showed that the accumulation of various epigenetic markers took place both globally, across the genome, and at specific loci [5]. Today, we can correlate some of these epigenetic differences with susceptibilities to specific diseases and phenotypic discordances. Studies of phenotypes originated from the same genotype of monozygous twins have revealed individual susceptibility to a remarkable spectrum of disorders: from rheumatoid arthritis (RA), Crohn's disease, stroke, breast and prostate cancers, multiple sclerosis (MS), type 2 diabetes (T2DM), hypertension, bipolar disorder, dementia, and autism [6,7].

In order to discuss the latest developments, it is helpful to briefly review the major regulatory aspects of epigenetic machinery and its dynamics. This will be followed by a closer look at the epigenetic advances in the context of personalized medicine.

3.2 Regulatory Components of Epigenetic Machinery

Any regulation of an epigenetic nature should be viewed as part of a fundamental biological mechanism responsible for the controlled, predetermined, and heritable access to genetic information. This is not a trivial matter, and in the context of individual differences observed among the patients this aspect becomes of critical importance in the context of a personalized approach to diagnosis and treatment.

Epigenetics is frequently described as a phenomenon of heritable changes in gene expression in the absence of changes in the DNA sequence. Today, it represents one of the most exciting and fastest-expanding fields of biology. Historically, studies of human diseases often have focused on genetic mechanisms. However, with a better understanding of the epigenetic control over timing and the magnitude of individual gene responses, one appreciates the role of epigenetics and the importance of epigenetic status in modulation of disease phenotypes, from one individual to another. Today, human disorders are thought to be driven by combinations of genetic and epigenetic abnormalities. It is the epigenetic component that proves most relevant to all aspects of personalized medicine.

Biochemically, the full set of genetic information is present in every individual cell, where it is encoded within sets of DNA molecules comprising in total approximately 2 m length, all packaged within less than 6–10 µm nuclei [8,9]. The packaging of genomic DNA into chromatin, a biochemical entity that simultaneously ensures storage, replication, and functional access to genetic information, is based on the building blocks of nucleosomes. The x-ray structure of the nucleosome has identified a histone octamer core particle containing two copies each of histones H2A, H2B, H3, and H4, with about 146 bases of DNA wrapped around it [8–10]. Each histone octamer is linked together with the help of histone H1, forming a highly condensed and, at the same time, highly dynamic chromatin entity [11,12]. The dynamic aspect of chromatin is an important regulatory aspect of chromatin and gene expression, importance of which is hard not to overestimate.

Regulatory markers monitored for the assessment of the epigenetic status of the loci and their chromatin dynamics include DNA methylation, core histones posttranscriptional modifications, such as acetylation, methylation, phosphorylation, and ubiquitination. Addition and removal of these epigenetic markers, as well as changes in rates of their turnover, are under the control of specific enzymes and nonhistone adaptor molecules—readers, erasers, modifiers, all remodel and modify chromatin dynamics structure with measurable effects on gene expression [13]. At the higher level of chromatin organization, long-range chromosomal interactions and specialized noncoding RNAs (ncRNAs) involved in epigenetic posttranscriptional modulation of gene expression constitute a highly valuable new class of epigenetic biomarkers.

Historically, in the early days of epigenetics, its primary focus was on developmental biology [3]. Now the focus has shifted toward chromosomal and molecular biology mechanisms modulating gene expression in the broader context of the life cycle [4]. Interestingly, the developmental component of epigenetics is now considered a very important component of the developmental origins of age-related diseases, marked by time-dependent accumulation of differences in epigenetic profiles of individual patients [14]. In fact, every day brings reports on newly discovered epigenetic aberrations specific to one or other disease [15–17]. As a fundamental consequence of this phenomenon, treatment of many diseases could be influenced by accumulated epigenetic variations [18–20].

Since the advances from human genome project and a low tally of about 23,000 discovered genes, the challenges of "personalized genomics" brought forth the problem of missing heritability. As acknowledged by one of the heads of the human genome project, Dr. Francis Collins: for many complex disease phenotypes, available genetic data offered a very limited basis for explanation and stratification [21,22]. Latest evidence points at epigenetics as the fundamental biological mechanism responsible for a large proportion of heritable complex disease phenotypes and their manifestation. According to latest assessments, a significant proportion of complex disease phenotypes are driven by defects in epigenetic regulation [23]. Even for fairly straightforward causal genetic defects, epigenetics profiles account for important phenotypical differences in the onset and progression of the disease.

One of the main functions of the epigenetic mechanisms is to act as a functional intermediary between the heritable genomic information [24] and the stresses imposed by the environment. Personalized epigenetic approach to therapeutic and preventive measures relies on understanding of epigenetic mechanisms and on reliable monitoring of changes through epigenetic-based biomarkers. This can help determine the choice of targeted therapies and offer molecular diagnostic tests that will help doctors identify those patients who can benefit from particular therapies.

3.2.1 Epigenetic Patterns and Signatures

The organs and tissues of the human body are formed by over 200 types of the specialized cells of the same genetic background. The distinct functional differences displayed by each cell type are very much due to the strict epigenetic controls imposed across the majority of the genome, so that only a small subset of genes is expressed and actively regulated in each cell type. The epigenetic state, with all the hallmarks of its regulations, is certainly subject to changes in response to various stages in development [14,25], age [26,27], chemicals in the environment [28–32], nutrients [33], and stress [34].

Normally, the patterns of epigenetic marks are inherited by a cell so that the daughter cells develop and mature according to a program that is similar to that of their parent cells. Because the epigenome of the whole organism reflects all cellular epigenetic states of all the cells, screening for specific epigenetic marks as an evidence of pathology present somewhere within the organism could be very informative, although a data-intensive process. These epigenetic marks, directly related to the specific deregulation events, include DNA methylation and posttranslational modifications of core histones at the microlevel of epigenetic organizations, and regulatory ncRNAs and chromosome conformation signatures at the macrolevel.

3.2.2 DNA Modifications

The most famous and long-studied epigenetic modification—methylation of cytosine—is a modification of eukaryotic DNA in which a methyl group is enzymatically transferred from *S-adenosylmethionine* (SAM) to the 5-position of cytosine. The methyl group is situated in the major groove of the DNA and inhibits transcription *in vitro* by interfering with the binding of transcription factors. The pattern of genomic methylation reflects two distinct processes— de novo methylation by enzymes Dnmt3a and Dnmt3b and maintenance methylation by Dnmt1.

De novo methylation is the enzymatic transfer of the methyl group to unmethylated cytosines of CpG nucleotides (nt), and is first observed in early embryo. Maintenance methylation converts a CpG, in which only one strand of DNA is methylated, into a symmetrically methylated form.

The significance of DNA methylation was first noted in the 1980s, when high-density methylation at "CpG" islands in the genome of vertebrates was first described [35]. Interestingly, up to 35% of disease-related mutations are located within those CpG islands, occurring at a frequency 42-fold higher than that predicted from random mutation [36].

Originally, DNA methylation was thought to prevent damage from transposable proviruses by suppressing their capacity to disrupt gene structure and function. This was thought to be an ancestral function of methylation in invertebrates. In this context, vertebrates might have retained this function and adapted it as DNA methylation at CpG residues to suppress endogenous promoters [37,38]. Similarly high methylation patterns were later described for large, repetitive genomic regions, such as ribosomal DNA, satellite sequences, centromeric repeats, parasitic elements, and endogenous retroviruses [39,40].

How are the markings of DNA methylation related to gene expression? As an early insight into epigenetic regulation, it was reported that gene silencing involved coordinated controls of DNA methylation and chromatin acetylation [41,42]. Furthermore, histone deacetylases (HDACs) were found to cooperate with histone methylases, establishing a "histone code" that resulted in self-propagating heterochromatin assembly [43–45]. One of the histone modification marks that emerged from those early studies was a conserved lysine residue, lysine 9 of histone 3 (H3K9), which was often methylated in heterochromatic regions of yeast and humans [45]. The heterochromatin conformation of chromatin was also associated with deacetylation marks and was generally considered to reflect a closed, nontranscribed state. One of the explanations for this connection pointed out that deacetylation of lysine ε-amino groups might allow greater interaction between positively charged N-terminal histone tails and the negatively charged DNA phosphate backbone [46]. Methylation of CpG islands was reported as part of the gene silencing in such processes as x-inactivation, imprinting, and cancer [40].

With the help of molecular biology a series of comprehensive studies analyzed the patterns of methylation, their generation and maintenance, as well as transmission to the next cellular generation. A recent study has demonstrated that the human genome contains nearly 28 million CpG sites of which about 60% of the cytosines are methylated [47]. Oxidation of 5-methylcytosine (5mC) by the Tet family of enzymes converts the standard methylation mark into 5-hydroxymethylcytosine (5hmC), which is often considered as an intermediate of 5mC demethylation process [48,49]. Although first discovered in 1952 [50], it is only in 2009 that its abundant presence has been confirmed in neuronal tissues and embryonic stem cells [48,51].

Latest reports with regard to 5hmC indicate that it is a valid epigenetic biomarker reflecting a specific regulatory role in gene expression. For example, reduction of 5hmC levels in embryonic stem cells has been linked to the loss of pluripotency [52]. Exposure to phenobarbital, a nongenotoxic carcinogen, induced well-defined changes in 5hmC genome wide [53].

The use of the bisulfate sequencing technique is the standard analysis of 5mC but it appears not to discriminate 5mC from 5hmC [54]. In a number of studies, significant efforts have now been made to discriminate between 5mC and 5hmC with further improvement in clinical stratifications.

From the early studies in 1980s, when *in vitro* DNA methylation of promoters by purified DNA methylases was shown to suppress reconstituted transcription, DNA methylation has evolved into a biomarker with a rather complex relationship with gene transcription. Most genes that have CpG-rich promoters lack methylation in the corresponding CpG-rich region even when the genes are silent (i.e., the globin genes in nonerythroid cells). In cell lines and tumors, DNA methylation at CpG-rich promoters is often associated with transcriptional silencing; in oocytes and preimplantation embryos, one finds evidence for thousands of heavily methylated CpG islands. Also, to make things even more complicated, the inactive X chromosome in all female mammals is hypermethylated at only a subset of gene-rich regions and, unexpectedly, is generally hypomethylated relative to its active counterpart [55,56].

3.2.3 Histone Code

Alteration of chromatin structure at the nucleosomal level influences the cellular phenotype by recruiting activating or repressing chromatin protein complexes, generating unique regulatory microenvironment and an additional layer of complexity to epigenetic regulation [13].

One of the striking features of the core histones is the diversity of post-translational modifications they possess [57,58]. Another common feature of many modified residues is that they protrude from the nucleosome core and are accessible to the factors that attach, recognize, or remove them—the so-called modifiers, readers, and erasers.

Over 50 different modifications are known to occur on four main histones. Among them are modifications for histone H3: H3R2me2, K4me3, K9Ac, K9me3, S10P, K14Ac, R17me2, K18Ac, K23Ac, R26me2, K27me3, S28P, K36me3, K79me3; modifications for histone H4: H4S1P, R3me2, K5Ac, K8Ac, K12Ac, K16Ac, K20me3; modifications for histone H2A: H2AS1P, K5Ac, K9Ac, K119Ub; and modifications for histone H2B: H2BK5Ac, K12Ac, K15Ac, K20Ac, K123Ub. Multiple effort has been made in the analysis of acetylation, methylation, and phosphorylation at several of these sites [57,59,60].

On the basis of the early observations that distinct histone modifications correlated with specific transcriptional states, it was proposed that histone modifications dictated specific functional modulation of transcription, that is, carried the "histone code" [59]. For example, it was suggested that specific marks of acetylation, methylation, phosphorylation, and ubiquitination were involved in activation, whereas deacetylation, methylation, ubiquitination, sumoylation, deamination, and proline isomerization were involved in repression.

Today, it is clear that for many occasions the functional role of a histone modification could be defined only in the context of other modifications as well as in the context of the preceding epigenetic state (epigenetic memory) reflecting the complex nature of the epigenetic regulatory system.

3.2.4 Chromosome Conformation Signatures

A powerful alternative to the described epigenetic markers is offered from the macrolevel of epigenetic regulation. Chromosome conformation signatures reflect the regulatory aspects of three-dimensional organization of chromatin, juxtaposition of distant regulatory sites, and regulated expression in the controlled microenvironment of genes. These biomarkers are associated with the regulatory aspects of chromatin conformation and epigenetics of gene expression [61–64]. The information encoded in the primary genome sequence is highly organized spatially and topologically within the cellular nucleus to ensure the efficient access and accurate control of gene expression that is crucial to development and homeostasis [63,64]. At the macrolevel, the chromatin generated via DNA–nucleosome interactions is organized into higher-order loop structures that define specific boundaries that limit accessibility and transcriptional responsiveness of individual genes or gene clusters and creates autonomous microenvironments with defined sensitivity, robustness, and timing of gene expression. These regulatory long-range interactions, that is, chromatin conformation signatures, can occur both within (*cis-*) and between genes or chromosomes (*trans-*). While chromatin conformation signatures may change in response to gene expression, their reorganization appears to be one of the earliest events in the cascade of changes associated with switches in the modes of gene expression, preceding both other epigenetic modifications events (methylation, acetylation, etc.), transcription factor binding and transcription of mRNA itself [65]. Importantly, in terms of their potential use as biomarkers, a key feature of chromatin conformation signatures is their stability: a conformation signature remains the same until a physiological signal induces a switch into alternative topological arrangement. This macroevent offers stable binary targets for the detection amongst a population of cells for a particular chromosome conformation signature which would be either present or not in any of the cells.

The spatial organization of the genome can be determined using technologies based on chromatin conformation capture and related techniques [61] which detects juxtaposition of distant DNA sites brought into close proximity by the topological organization of the chromatin. In these procedures, chromatin is first fixed using a cross-linking agent to capture intra-chromatin associations, digested with restriction enzymes to generate intermediates consistent of cross-linked chromatin fragments, re-ligated under conditions favoring intramolecular ligation of cross-linked fragments. These fragments contain sequence tags from juxtaposed distant sites, which are then analyzed with PCR or any other sequence-based readout platforms to confirm the presence of particular chromatin conformations.

The potential advantages of chromosome conformation biomarkers have been clearly demonstrated in a wide spectrum of disease applications. For example, chromosome conformation signatures allow the monitoring of how activated oncogenes mediate alterations in epigenetic status [66], cancer-specific chromosomal alterations [67], gene-specific deregulation in hepatocellular carcinoma (HCC) [68], regulation of p53 and its targets [69,70], deregulation of c-Myc in colorectal cancer (CRC) [71], and deregulation of BRCA1 [72,73].

Beyond oncology, high-order epigenetic chromatin regulation has been described for INFγ-induced JAK/STAT-mediated transcriptional activation of classical HLA genes [65], autoimmune diseases (RA, Lupus, MS) [74], cytokine regulation [75–77], diabetes [78], induced pluripotent stem cells [79], senescence [80,81], memory T-cell response [82], transgenerational epigenetic inheritance [83], single-nucleotide polymorphism (SNP) interlink between coronary artery disease (CAD) and T2DM [84], and metabolic disorders [85].

3.2.5 Noncoding RNA

Chromatin dynamic organization, its sustainability, and resetting involve a number of factors. Regulatory ncRNAs, in many varieties, lately have become the main focus of interest in the mechanisms of epigenetic posttranscriptional gene regulation [86,87]. This is not surprising as coding exons of genes account for only 1.5% of the genome, whereas most of the rest of genome transcribes ncRNAs.

Today, several classes of ncRNAs are recognized for their role in the regulation of gene expression. A class of small ncRNAs called microRNAs (miRNAs) [88,89] has been shown to be linked to epigenetic and genetic defects as a common hallmark of cancers and many other diseases [90–93]. Other ncRNAs, such as transcribed ultraconserved regions (T-UCRs), small nucleolar RNAs (snoRNAs), PIWI-interacting RNAs (piRNAs), large intergenic noncoding RNAs (lincRNAs), and the heterogeneous group of long noncoding RNAs (lncRNAs), also contribute to the development of many different human disorders [94]. The discovery that many genomic sequences are transcribed in a developmental and tissue-regulated fashion [95,96] has brought attention to the regulatory roles all of the different types of ncRNAs detected in human cells.

The most widely studied class of ncRNAs are miRNAs, which are small ncRNAs of ~22 nt that can mediate posttranscriptional gene silencing by controlling the translation of mRNA into proteins. miRNAs are estimated to regulate the translation of more than 60% of protein-coding genes [88,89]. They are involved in regulating many processes including proliferation, differentiation, apoptosis, and regulation of other ncRNAs in cancer and other types of diseases. While some miRNAs regulate specific individual targets, others can function as master regulators of a process, regulating the expression levels of hundreds of genes simultaneously and often, cooperatively [88,89]. miRNAs called epiRNAs influence target gene expression by directly regulating epigenetic processes [97]. Multiple studies have shown that tumor-derived miRNAs can be detected in blood in a stable form, responsible for horizontal transfer of miRNA and synchronization between living cells [98]. miRNAs act as good markers for early detection and as prognosis, as well as predictors for response to therapy [99].

piRNAs are ncRNAs of 24–30 nt in length, which are, unlike miRNA, dicer-independent and bind the PIWI subfamily of Argonaute family proteins that are involved in maintaining genome stability in germ line cells [100,101]. They are transcribed from regions in the genome that contain transcribed transposable elements and other repetitive elements. The complex that is formed by piRNAs and PIWI proteins suppresses transposable element expression and mobilization. Not surprisingly, piRNAs and PIWI proteins have also been linked to DNA methylation [100,102] and heterochromatin-mediated gene silencing [103]. Consistently with this, a single piRNA was recently reported to mediate locus-specific methylation of an imprinted region [104].

lncRNAs are a heterogeneous group of noncoding transcripts more than 200 nt long that are involved in many biological processes. This class of ncRNA makes up the largest portion of the mammalian noncoding transcriptome [94]. Various mechanisms of transcriptional regulation of gene expression by lncRNAs have been proposed. Among these, lncRNAs are known to mediate epigenetic modifications of DNA by recruiting chromatin remodeling complexes to specific loci [105,106]. At the human HOX loci, there is sequential temporal and spatial expression of hundreds of lncRNAs, which regulate chromatin accessibility in a process that involves histone modification enzymes and RNA polymerase [107]. lncRNAs are essential in many physiological processes, such as X-chromosome inactivation in mammals, in which the X-inactivation-specific transcript (XIST) lncRNA (17 kb) recruits the polycomb complex to silence the X chromosome from which it is transcribed [26]. *TSIX*, another lncRNA, is transcribed from the opposite strand to *XIST* and regulates *XIST* levels during X-chromosome inactivation [105]. As another example, many lncRNAs are expressed by imprinted loci, at which they have a central functional role [94].

Another class of lncRNAs are lincRNAs, which are transcribed from intergenic regions. These transcripts are identified by searching for chromatin signatures that are associated with active transcription in the regions across which transcriptional elongation takes place [108]. Key roles for lincRNAs in certain biological processes are starting to emerge. A specialized type of lncRNA, known as telomeric repeat-containing RNAs (TERRAs), is transcribed from telomeres. TERRAs help to maintain the integrity of telomeric heterochromatin by regulating telomerase activity [108].

Finally, it is important to mention a study that suggested a functional link between antisense transcription in organization of gene expression and the epigenetic status of the chromatin for transcribed genes, including possible implications in the formation of conditional long-range chromosome interactions, that is, chromosome conformation signatures, described separately in this chapter [109].

3.3 Aberrant Epigenetic Signatures

Since the discovery of DNA structure and with the advancement of the human genome project, the study of human disease has focused on genetic mechanisms and heritable mutations responsible for the aberrant regulation in pathological cases. Considerable evidence is now pointing to the fact that the disruption of epigenetic networks and the differences in epigenetic profiles are a significant and often critical step, in the onset of major diseases in individual patients. While the first examples of epigenetic applications came from the field of oncology, deregulations of epigenetic mechanisms have been now described as causative in neurological, autoimmune, cardiovascular, metabolic, and nutritional disorders [15,33,110–112]. The epigenetic markers of deregulation clearly involve DNA methylation, histone modifications, and changes in ncRNA profiles and chromosome conformation signatures. Systemic epigenetic deregulations are also evidenced through specific signatures observed for epigenetic biomarkers in peripheral blood from patients with various cancers, inflammatory diseases, and other disorders [113–116].

3.3.1 DNA Methylation

Aberrant patterns in DNA methylation became the first examples of cancer-specific deregulation. Global hypomethylation was noted in some of the first studies of cancer cells [7,117]. Hypomethylation is typically observed at the intergenic regions, marked by genomic instability and chromosomal rearrangements. At the same time, promoters of genes involved in cancer-related pathways showed a degree of hypermethylation, largely linked with transcriptional silencing of tumor suppressor phenotypes [118–120]. An extensive study of 600 primary tumor samples representing 15 tumor types revealed hypermethylation of promoters for 12 preselected genes of interest [119]. Further studies have focused on epigenetic deregulations of various other genes whose primary functional importance includes tumor suppression, metastasis, DNA repair, apoptosis, hormone response, cell cycle regulation, Ras, and Wnt signaling [119–122].

Genome-wide methylation technologies have demonstrated that in normal cells the repetitive portion of the genome is heavily methylated and most CpG islands are unmethylated, while in cancer cells one could observe widespread loss of intergenic DNA methylation with gain of methylation at many gene-associated CpG islands [123]. Within individual tumors, up to 10% of CpG islands are aberrantly hypomethylated, and CpG islands normally methylated become transcriptionally active. At the same time, promoter-associated CpG islands are not the only islands affected by aberrant DNA methylation, as the CpG islands located within 3' ends of genes and in intergenic regions also start to exhibit hypermethylation in cancer cells. Analysis of genes with methylated 3' CpG islands showed increased expression, suggesting a new function for DNA methylation in this location. These alterations in methylations are part of epigenetic regulation, with little understanding of its role on gene expression and cellular functions currently.

Interestingly, in a genome-wide study of differential DNA methylation specific for colon cancer, most alterations were observed not in the promoter regions or CpG islands as such, but in adjacent regions within 2 kb, named "CpG island shores" [124]. Methylation at those sites is best conserved for stratification of tissue types. One of the conclusions from this observation is that epigenetic changes and alterations in cancer take place at the sites normally involved in tissue differentiation. It may even be a predominant mechanism by which epigenetic deregulation can cause the onset of cancer.

DNA methylation is the most extensively studied mechanism of epigenetic gene regulation. Increasing evidence indicates that DNA methylation is labile in response to nutritional and environmental influences. Alterations in DNA methylation profiles can lead to changes in gene expression, resulting in diverse phenotypes with the potential for increased disease risk. The primary methyl donor for DNA methylation is SAM, a species generated in the cyclical cellular process called one-carbon metabolism. One-carbon metabolism is catalyzed by several enzymes in the presence of dietary micronutrients, including folate, choline, betaine, and other B-vitamins. For this reason, nutritional status, particularly micronutrient intake, has been a focal point when investigating epigenetic mechanisms. Although animal evidence linking nutrition and DNA methylation is fairly extensive, epidemiological evidence remains today less comprehensive [125].

In a fundamental study of epigenetic polymorphism, Amos Tanay identified distinct modes of highly controlled methylation loci against loci open to stochastic components of polymorphic methylation [126]. Interestingly, in a related analysis, control over polymorphic stochasticity has been linked with epigenetic regulation imposed through chromosomal domain compartmentalization, monitored through the chromosome conformation signatures [127].

3.3.2 Histone Modifications

Another fundamental aspect of epigenetic machinery is aberrant chromatin packaging and remodeling, with regulatory effects on genes involved in cell differentiation, proliferation, and survival. A specific group of chromatin modifier enzymes is influencing these process by catalyzing modifications of histones, particularly histone acetylation, deacetylation, methylation, and demethylation. Deregulation of epigenetic modifiers has been characterized in many malignancies and plays a crucial role in certain other disorders [15,33,110]. It is now widely accepted that DNA methylation, histone modifications, and nucleosome remodeling are functionally interlinked and contribute to epigenetic deregulations observed in cancer and other disease indications [128].

Aberrant histone modifications observed during the onset and progression of carcinogenesis include, for example, a pattern of global loss of monoacetylation at H4-Lys16 (H4K16ac), as well as loss of trimethylation of H4-Lys20 (H4K20me3) [129], these changes appear early and accumulate with the progression of tumorigenesis. Parallel studies revealed a global decrease in H4K20me2/3, H3K9me2, and H4 acetylation, particularly at H4K16, in premalignant lesions and also become more pronounced through tumorigenesis [123]. The loss of H4K16ac and H4K20me2/3 takes place in the repetitive part of the genome, which is also affected by changes in DNA methylation. Loss of DNA methylation at the sites of changes in H3K9me2 and H4K20me3 marks deregulation of transcriptional repression and may promote tumorigenesis through derepression of exogenous repetitive elements, such as transposons, or miRNA, impaired DNA damage response, and chromosomal instability. Normally, a euchromatin, or an open chromatin structure, is marked by hyperacetylation of histones H3 and H4 and di- and trimethylation of histone H3 at lysine 4 (H3K4me2/3) and constitutes a permissive region for transcription. Repressed regions exhibit heterochromatin, or a compact chromatin structure, that lacks H3/H4 acetylation and H3K4 methylation, and is enriched instead in repressive modifications, di- and trimethylation of H3K9 (H3K9me2/3), trimethylation of H3K27 (H3K27me3), and trimethylation of H4K20 (H4K20me3).

In an instructive example of epigenetic carcinogenesis, nongenotoxic exposure to carcinogen phenobarbital leads to the development of liver cancer. Epigenetic signatures developed in response to this carcinogen revealed a dynamic change from 5mC to 5hmC at the subset of the promoters of transcriptionally upregulated genes, paralleled by the changes in histone marks H3K4me2, H3K27me3, and H3K36me3 [53].

3.3.3 Chromosome Conformation Signatures

As part of the epigenetic regulatory context, chromatin adopts a nonrandom three-dimensional topology. The organization of genes into structural hubs and domains becomes an important part of their transcriptional status. An unbiased high-resolution mapping of intra- and interchromosome interactions upon overexpression of oncogene ERG demonstrated association with global, reproducible, and functionally coherent changes in chromosome conformation signature organization [66]. In another study, in the context of somatic copy-number alterations in cancer, analysis of three-dimensional genome architecture [130] suggested that the distribution of chromosomal alterations in cancer was spatially related to three-dimensional genomic architecture and that somatic evolution of cancer cells involved somatic copy number alterations based on their three-dimensional genome architecture [67].

A study of gene deregulation in HCC revealed how the three-dimensional context of chromosome conformation signatures contributed to the regulation of gene clusters [76]. Influence of interactions between transcriptional regulatory elements was observed as a result of tumor necrosis factor alpha (TNFα) signaling on a set of long-range interactions between enhancer and promoter in the human tumor necrosis factor (TNF)/lymphotoxin (LT) gene locus. The cytokine genes *LTα, TNF,* and *LTβ* are differentially regulated by NF-κB signaling in both inflammatory and oncogenic responses. In the *TNF/LT* locus, there are at least four CTCF-enriched sites with enhancer-blocking activities and a TNF-responsive TE2 enhancer. One of the CTCF-enriched sites is located between the early-inducible *LTα/TNF* promoters and the late-inducible *LTβ* promoter. After TNF stimulation, the CTCF insulators mediated specific long-range interactions, that is, conditional chromosome conformation signatures, between the enhancer and the *LTα/TNF* promoters, followed by interaction with the *LTβ* promoter. These results provided a striking example of conditional spatiotemporal control of enhancer–promoter associations in the *TNF/LT* gene cluster, all achieved and monitored through the regulatory entity of chromosome conformation signatures [68]. In a separate study of TNFα and NF-κB, by using primary human endothelial cells, using variants of chromosome conformation capture (3C), and fluorescence *in situ* hybridization to detect single nascent transcripts, it was shown that TNFα-induced responsive genes change their localization and congregate at discrete sites—"NF-κB factories." Interestingly, some of those sites further specialized in transcribing miRNAs targeted downregulated mRNAs. Many of the signaling pathways may share the same property of rearranging the localization of responding genes and leaving a clear mark of changed, conditional chromosome conformation signatures [76].

p53 is a tumor suppressor protein critical for genome integrity. As a transcription factor, p53 regulates the expression of genes involved in cellular responses to stress, including cell cycle arrest and apoptosis. Although its control at the protein level is well-known, the transcriptional regulation of the *TP53* gene is still unclear. A study reported detailed analysis of the organization of the *TP53* gene domain in several breast cancer and control cell lines. In the control breast epithelial cell line, HB2, the *TP53* gene is positioned within a relatively small DNA domain, encompassing 50 kb. Interestingly, the chromosome conformation signature structure was found to be radically different in the studied breast cancer cell lines, MCF7, T47D, MDA-MB-231, and BT474, in which the domain size was increased and *TP53* transcription was decreased. In this example, organization of the three-dimensional structure of the *TP53* locus correlated directly with the transcriptional status of *TP53* and neighboring genes [69].

Evidence for gene-specific mechanisms affecting expression of three important p53 target genes reveals a series of conditional chromosome conformation interactions. The apoptotic gene *PUMA* is regulated through long-range interactions between intragenic chromatin boundaries, recognized by insulator factors, such as CTCF. Further analysis of PUMA locus revealed distinct histone modification H3K27me3 territories that correlated with binding of the insulator factors. Another interesting epigenetic biomarker discovered for the regulation of *PUMA* locus was an evolutionary-conserved lncRNA [70].

Genome-wide association studies have mapped many SNPs that are linked to cancer risk, but the mechanism by which most of these SNPs promote cancer remains undefined. The rs6983267 SNP at 8q24 has been associated with several cancers, yet this SNP is 335 kb away from the nearest gene, c-MYC. It now has been shown that the beta-catenin-TCF4 transcription factor complex binds preferentially to the cancer risk-associated rs6983267(G) allele in colon cancer cells. The rs6983267 SNP bears epigenetic modifications specific of active enhancers—H3K4me2, H3-Ac, and H4-Ac, but it also forms a 335-kb chromatin loop to interact directly with the c-MYC promoter. Thus, this suggests that cancer risk is a direct consequence of elevated c-MYC expression from increased distal enhancer activity. The findings of these studies support a general mechanism by which intergenic SNPs that can promote cancer through the regulation of distal genes by utilizing or altering preexisting large chromatin loops [71].

The 85-kb breast cancer-associated gene BRCA1 is an established tumor suppressor gene, widely implicated in breast and ovarian cancers. Analysis of chromosome conformation signatures in human cells as well as in mouse mammary tissue demonstrated first evidence for conditional long-range interactions imposed on BRCA1 between the promoter, introns, and terminator region. Interestingly, association between the BRCA1 promoter and terminator regions changed upon estrogen stimulation and during lactational development. The BRCA1 terminator region is able to suppress estrogen-induced transcription. Significantly, BRCA1 promoter and terminator interactions vary in different breast cancer cell lines, indicating that defects in BRCA1 chromatin structure may contribute to deregulated expression of BRCA1 as seen in breast tumors [72]. In a separate study, it was shown that cancer-predisposing mutations of BRCA1 display an allele-specific effect on chromosome conformation signature profile: 5′ mutations that result in gross truncation of the protein and abolish the chromatin unfolding activity, whereas those in the 3′ region of the gene markedly enhance this activity [73].

High-order epigenetic chromatin regulation has been described for a wide range of clinical indications extending beyond oncological applications. In transcriptional activation of the major histocompatibility complex (MHC) by IFNγ, a key step in cell-mediated immunity, the entire MHC locus first loops out from the chromosome territory by forming a specific conditional chromosome conformation signature at an early stage of induction. As part of transcriptional activation of *HLA* class II genes, JAK/STAT signaling triggers chromatin remodeling and the decondensation of the entire *MHC* locus. The onset of chromatin remodeling coincides with the binding of activated STAT1 and the chromatin remodeling enzyme BRG1 at sites within the MHC, and is followed by RNA-polymerase recruitment and histone hyperacetylation. This study strongly suggested that the higher-order chromatin reorganization and remodeling of the MHC locus were essential early epigenetic step necessary for transcriptional activation of classical *HLA* genes [65].

The chromosome 16p13 region has been associated with several autoimmune diseases, including type 1 diabetes (T1DM) and MS. CLEC16A has been reported as the most likely candidate gene in this region, since it contains the most disease-associated SNPs. However, it appears that it is the intron 19 of CLEC16A, containing the most autoimmune disease-associated SNPs, which acts as a regulatory sequence, affecting the expression of a neighboring gene, DEXI. The CLEC16A alleles that are protective from T1DM and MS are associated with increased expression of DEXI, and no other genes in the region. 3C analysis demonstrated the presence of chromosome conformation signature with a physical proximity between the DEXI promoter region and intron 19 of CLEC16A, separated by >150 kb. Also, a 20 kb fragment of intron 19 of CLEC16A, containing SNPs associated with T1DM and MS, was shown to interact with the promoter region of DEXI but not with other potential causal genes in the region. These data indicate that although the causal variants in the 16p13 region lie within CLEC16A, DEXI is an unappreciated autoimmune disease candidate gene. It also illustrates the power of the chromosome conformation signature approach in understanding the causal relationship underlying the disease [74].

Until recently, the cytokine-mediated signaling toward the polarization and differentiation of a T-helper cell lineage lacked clear understanding into the mechanisms of the transcriptional regulation of cytokine receptor genes. Significant progress was made with the discovery of a new mechanism for the transcriptional regulation of the interferon gamma receptor 1 gene via long-range intrachromosomal interactions with the *IFNγ* locus mediated by the protein CTCF. These interactions sustained the mono-allelic expression of the differentially methylated IFNγ R1 gene and were implicated in selective blocking of active transcription. These findings suggest that regulatory elements for a cytokine gene locus can also positively regulate the transcription of its receptor [75].

Insulin (INS) synthesis and secretion from pancreatic β-cells are tightly regulated; their deregulation causes diabetes. Mapping of the *INS*-associated loci in human pancreatic islets showed that the *INS* gene physically interacted with the *SYT8* gene located over 300 kb away, by forming a conditional chromosome conformation signature. This interaction was elevated by glucose and accompanied by an increase in *SYT8* expression. Furthermore,

SYT8 knockdown decreases INS secretion in islets. These results revealed a nonredundant role for *SYT8* in INS secretion and indicated that the *INS* promoter acted from a distance to stimulate *SYT8* transcription. Together this suggested a function for the INS promoter in coordinating INS transcription and secretion through long-range regulation of *SYT8* expression in human islets [78].

Embryonic stem cells and induced pluripotent stem cells use a complex network of genetic and epigenetic pathways to maintain a delicate balance between self-renewal and multilineage differentiation. Recently developed high-throughput molecular tools greatly facilitated the study of epigenetic regulation in pluripotent stem cells. Increasing evidence suggests the existence of extensive crosstalk among epigenetic pathways that modify DNA, histones, and nucleosomes. Novel methods of mapping higher-order chromatin structure and chromatin–nuclear matrix interactions also provide the first insight into the three-dimensional organization of the genome and a framework in which existing genomic data of epigenetic regulation can be integrated to discover new rules of gene regulation [79]. It is well-known that somatic cells can be reset to oncogene-induced senescent (OIS) cells or induced pluripotent stem cells by expressing specified factors [118]. The *INK4/ARF* locus encodes *p15INK4b*, *ARF,* and *p16INK4a* genes in human chromosome 9p21, the products of which are known as common key reprogramming regulators. Compared with growing fibroblasts, the CCCTC-binding factor CTCF is remarkably upregulated in iPS cells with silencing of the three genes in the locus and is reversely downregulated in OIS cells with high expression of *p15INK4b* and *p16INK4a* genes. There are at least three CTCF-enriched sites in the *INK4/ARF* locus, which possess chromatin loop-forming activities, recognized as chromosome conformation signatures. These CTCF-enriched sites and the *p16INK4a* promoter associate to form compact chromatin loops in growing fibroblasts, while CTCF depletion disrupts the loop structure. Interestingly, the loose chromatin structure is found in OIS cells. In addition, the *INK4/ARF* locus has an intermediate type of chromatin compaction in iPS cells. These results suggest that senescent cells have distinct higher-order chromatin signature in the *INK4/ARF* locus [80]. Indeed, higher-order chromatin structure modulates differential expression of the human INK4b-ARF-INK4a locus during progenitor cell differentiation, cellular ageing, and senescence of cancer cells. Indeed, INK4b and INK4a, but not ARF, are upregulated following the differentiation of hematopoietic progenitor cells, in ageing fibroblasts and in senescing malignant rhabdoid tumor cells. The expression pattern of the locus is reflected by its organization in space. In the repressed state, the PRC-binding regions are in close proximity, while the intervening chromatin harboring ARF loops out. Downregulation of polycomb PcG silencer EZH2 causes release of the approximately 35 kb repressive chromatin loops and induction of both INK4a and INK4b, whereas ARF expression remains unaltered. PcG silencers bind and coordinately regulate INK4b and INK4a, but not ARF, during a variety of physiological processes. Developmentally regulated EZH2 levels are one of the factors that can determine the higher-order chromatin structure and expression pattern of the INK4b-ARF-INK4a locus, coupling human progenitor cell differentiation to proliferation control. The analysis revealed long-range control via chromosome conformation signatures [81].

The identification of pathogen-specific memory lymphocytes that arise after an infection provided a cellular basis for immunological memory. But the molecular mechanisms of immunological memory remain only partially understood. The emerging evidence suggests that epigenetic changes have a key role in controlling the distinct transcriptional profiles of memory lymphocytes and thus in shaping their function. The recent progress in assessing the differential gene expression and chromatin modifications in memory CD4(+) and CD8(+) T cells have made interesting contributions to the current understanding of the molecular basis of memory T-cell function [82].

In another example of genome-wide association studies, an SNP in the 9p21 gene desert was associated with CAD and T2DM. Despite evidence for a role of the associated interval in neighboring gene regulation, the biological underpinnings of these genetic associations with CAD or T2DM have not yet been explained. By using chromosome conformation signature analysis, it was shown that in human vascular endothelial cells the enhancer interval containing the CAD locus physically interacts with the CDKN2A/B locus, the MTAP gene, and an interval downstream of IFNA21. In human vascular endothelial cells, IFNγ activation strongly affects the structure of the chromatin and the transcriptional regulation in the 9p21 locus, including STAT1-binding, long-range enhancer interactions, and altered expression of neighboring genes. This study established a link between CAD genetic susceptibility and the response to inflammatory signaling in a vascular cell type and demonstrated the utility of high-order chromatin organization [84].

Chromatin interactions play important roles in transcription regulation. To better understand the underlying evolutionary and functional constraints of these interactions, a study implemented a systems approach to examine RNA polymerase-II-associated chromatin interactions in human cells. The authors found that 40% of the total genomic elements involved in chromatin interactions converged to a giant, scale-free-like, hierarchical network organized into chromatin communities. The communities were enriched with specific functions and were synthetic through evolution. Disease-associated SNPs from genome-wide association studies were enriched among the nodes with fewer interactions, implying their selection against deleterious interactions by limiting the total number of interactions, a model that we further reconciled using somatic and germ line cancer mutation data. The hubs lacked disease-associated SNPs, constituted a nonrandomly interconnected core of key cellular functions, and exhibited lethality in mouse mutants, supporting an evolutionary selection that favored the nonrandom spatial clustering of the least-evolving key genomic domains against random genetic or transcriptional errors in the genome. Altogether, the analyses revealed a systems-level evolutionary framework that shapes functionally compart-mentalized and error-tolerant transcriptional regulation of human genome in three dimensions [131]. This is similar to the findings mentioned early for TNFα induction in endothelial cells, of NFκB "factory," and reinforces the concept of three-dimensional regulatory hubs is a common phenomenon.

3.3.4 Noncoding RNA

ncRNAs has been most thoroughly studied in tumorigenesis, in particular with respect to miRNAs [90–93]. In human cancer, miRNA expression profiles clearly differ between normal tissues, tumors, and tumor types. miRNAs can be attributed properties of an oncogene or a tumor suppressors and can have critical functions in tumorigenesis [90–93]. Deregulation of miRNAs in cancer can occur through epigenetic changes, for example, through promoter CpG island hypermethylation in the case of the miR-200 family [132], and genetic alterations, which can affect the production of the primary miRNA transcript, their processing to mature miRNAs, and/or interactions with mRNA targets. One of the first associations to be observed between miRNAs and cancer development was deregulation of miR-15 and miR-16 in most B-cell chronic lymphocytic leukemias (CLL) as a result of chromosome 13q14 deletion [133]. Interestingly, miRNAs are frequently located in fragile regions of the chromosomes that are involved in ovarian, breast carcinomas, and melanomas and epigenetically carry distinct markers [133,134].

piRNAs have been found to be involved in tumorigenesis in testicular tissue and a range of other tumor types [135–138], although their specific functions in tumorigenesis are unknown. PIWI proteins have also been implicated in cancer development; for example, PIWIL1 and PIWIL2 are overexpressed in a variety of somatic tumors [139–142]. Furthermore, studies in human cancer cell models have linked PIWIL1 overexpression to cell cycle arrest [142] and PIWIL2 overexpression to antiapoptotic signaling and cell proliferation [143]. The mechanisms that underlie the putative oncogenic effects of piRNAs and PIWIs are largely unknown, although several pathways seem feasible. PIWI proteins are associated with epigenetic properties of stem cell self-renewal [144] and are reexpressed in precancerous stem cells that have the potential for malignant differentiation [145]. In some cancers, PIWIL2 overexpression has been suggested to lead to cells becoming resistant to cisplatin, which might arise because of increased chromatin condensation that prevents the normal process of DNA repair [146]. Strikingly, PIWI-associated RNAs were also found to be aberrantly expressed in human somatic tumors [147], implying that the PIWI pathway has a more profound function outside germ line cells than was originally thought.

lncRNAs originated from T-UCR are also altered in human tumorigenesis and that different types of human cancer can be distinguished according to their specific aberrant T-UCR expression profiles [148]. T-UCR expression signatures have been described for CLL, CRC, and HCC. Both downregulation and upregulation of different T-UCRs are seen when comparing expression in tumors and in normal tissues. Like miRNAs, T-UCRs that are differentially expressed in a specific cancer tend to be located in cancer-associated genomic regions (CARGs) that are associated with that type of cancer: for example, fragile sites, HOX gene clusters, minimal regions of loss of heterozygosity, and minimal regions of amplification [148,149]. So far, the aberrant regulation of T-UCR expression in cancer has been found to occur in two main ways: by altered interactions with miRNAs [148] and by hypermethylation of CpG island promoters [150]. Many T-UCRs show significant complementarity to specific miRNAs, which suggests that the T-UCRs could act as miRNA targets [151,152]. Experimental results support this hypothesis, and further link miRNAs with epigenetic mode of regulation. For instance, transfection of miR-155 into leukemia cells significantly reduces expression of the T-UCR uc.160+ [148]. As occurs in coding genes, DNA hypermethylation of a CpG island that is located in the promoter can also downregulate T-UCR expression [150]. This has been shown for several T-UCRs in a manner that is specific to cancer type.

Among various other examples of the involvement of lncRNAs in cancer, the role of *HOTAIR* in human neoplasia is the most well understood [106]. In epithelial cancer cells, *HOTAIR* overexpression causes polycomb to be retargeted across the genome. The invasiveness of these cells and propensity to metastasize is also increased in these cells, both changes of which are dependent on the polycomb protein PRC2. By contrast, cancer invasiveness is decreased when *HOTAIR* expression is lost—an effect that is increased in cells with higher than usual levels of PRC2 activity. As such, *HOTAIR* might have an active role in modulating the cancer epigenome and mediating cell transformation. A similar function has been postulated for some other lincRNAs, such as lincRNA-p21, which functions as a repressor in p53-dependent transcriptional responses [153]. The p15 antisense lncRNA, *p15AS*, which was first identified in human leukemia, has also been shown to induce the silencing of the p15 tumor suppressor gene locus by inducing the formation of heterochromatin [154].

Just as in cancer, aberrant miRNA expression patterns are observed in neurodegenerative, inflammatory, and cardiovascular diseases. Many miRNAs are essential for the correct function of the nervous system, which has the broadest spectrum of miRNA expression of all human tissues. Around 70% of miRNAs are expressed in the brain, and many of them are specific to neurons [155]. They are involved in neurodevelopment, dendritic spine formation and neurite outgrowth, and their deregulation has been described in almost all neurological diseases studied. Disruption of miRNA processing has been shown to cause hallmarks of ataxia in Purkinje cells [156]; MS in oligodendrocyte cells [157]; Parkinson's disease in dopaminergic cells [158]; and Alzheimer's disease in α-calcium/calmodulin-dependent protein kinase type II (αCaMKII)-expressing neurons [159]. Specific miRNAs have been linked to particular neurological diseases. For example, miR-206 deficiency accelerates amyotrophic lateral sclerosis [160], miR-9 leads to defects in spinal motor neuron disease [161], and miR-19, miR-101, and miR-130 levels, which modify the penetrance of spinocerebellar ataxia type 1 by the coregulation of ataxin 1 levels [162]. In Alzheimer's disease, abnormally expressed miRNAs have consistently been reported as downregulating the expression of the enzyme β-secretase 1 (BACE1), which leads to the production of β-amyloid peptide [159,163,164]. miRNAs are also known to control the inflammatory process that leads to the development of MS [165,166]. Finally, miRNAs regulate α-synuclein expression [167] and E2F1 and dopamine production [168]; factors underlying Parkinson's disease.

Several lines of evidence suggest key roles for miRNAs in cardiovascular disorders. The most abundant miRNA in cardiac myocytes is miR-1, which is involved in heart development [169]. This miRNA has been linked with the development of arrhythmias as it downregulates expression of the ion channel genes [170]. Myocardial tissue from heart failure patients has a distinct miRNA expression profile as compared to a healthy myocardium [171]. miRNAs also have a role in vascular disease. Here, the formation of the atheroma plaque and the physiological phenotype of vascular smooth muscle cells depend on the correct expression of several miRNAs, such as miR-10a, miR-145, miR-143, and miR-126 [172–174]. As with heart failure, miRNA expression signature distinguishes the vascular lesion from healthy tissue [175]. Finally, SNPs that affect miRNA-binding sites, including those for miR-1, have been associated with unrestricted muscular growth [176] and hypertension [177], which increases the risk of cardiovascular disease.

Several monogenic disorders have been found to have aberrant miRNA expression profiles in tissue types that are relevant to the pathophysiology of the disease, and this list is rapidly increasing. In addition, specific miRNA defects have been shown to underlie particular diseases; for example, miR-145 and miR-146a deletions are involved in the 5q syndrome phenotype [178]. As well as genetic mutations, alterations of epigenetic marks cause deregulation of miRNA expression. Recent disease studies have found disrupted expression of miRNAs that are transcribed from CpG islands, at which the expression of the miRNA is regulated by DNA methyltransferases (DNMTs). First examples for such deregulation were described in immunodeficiency, centromere instability, and facial anomalies syndrome (mutations in the gene that encodes DNMT3B107), and in Rett's syndrome (mutations in the methyl CpG-binding protein 2 [MECP2] gene) [179,180]. Deregulation of miRNAs in ICF syndrome has also been associated with an aberrant histone modification profile [181].

Other types of ncRNA have been implicated in nonneoplastic disease. For example, in Alzheimer's disease, a conserved noncoding antisense transcript drives rapid feed-forward regulation of BACE1 [182]. In addition, enrichment for T-UCR loci is seen in chromosomally imbalanced regions that are associated with pathology in neurodevelopmental disorders [183]. snoRNAs have been found to have an important role in imprinting disorders, specifically those with a neurodevelopmental component such as Prader–Willi and Angelman syndromes [184]. These disorders are caused by several genetic and epigenetic mechanisms involving the 15q11–q13 imprinted locus [185,186].

Contribution of ncRNAs to the onset and progression of human disorders is one of the most exciting problems today, with a direct link to better understanding of epigenetic regulation of disease phenotypes. One of the challenges is to identify novel functional ncRNAs that are encoded in the human genome. The project of encyclopedia of DNA elements [187] aims to identify all functional elements in the human genome. Methods based on second-generation sequencing, such as RNA sequencing, provide a more detailed picture of the whole human ncRNA transcriptome. Effective bioinformatics tools for identifying potentially functional ncRNAs are critically important. Because ncRNAs fold into complex secondary structures that are crucial to function, sequence-based alignments alone might not be enough to identify ncRNAs. Pattern recognition algorithms provide invaluable help in identifying functional classes of RNA secondary structures present in ncRNA. A number of algorithms that use different approaches have been developed to identify potentially functional ncRNAs (e.g., RNAfold, RNAalifold, Pfold, EvoFold, RNAz, QRNA, CMFinder, and FOLDALIGN). Low expression levels of some of ncRNAs by no means diminish their functional importance; however they make their detection and characterization a highly challenging task. Restricted spatiotemporal expression of many ncRNAs, and the binding of transcription factors to noncoding loci could also be used as evidence of functionality beyond nonspecific "noise" [188].

Finally, expectations in the therapeutic arena have been raised as a result of the recognition of ncRNA roles in human diseases. Molecules based on ncRNAs broaden the universe of potential "druggable" targets, and important genes that are not considered to be viable conventional drug targets can now be readily inhibited by siRNAs or miRNAs. The first clinical trials using ncRNA-based molecules are underway.

3.4 Diseases and Biomarkers

Human diseases are driven by combinations of genetic and epigenetic abnormalities. Very often, like in the case of cancer or autoimmune disease, these disorders bear hallmarks of heterogeneous disorders, with shared features that define clinical diagnosis, and with distinct differences in genetic and epigenetic make up to grant distinct prognostic and predictive characteristics for the individual patient. A fundamental difference in properties of epigenetic deregulation, when compared with genetic inheritable make-up, is that it could be in principle reversed through the turnover and resting of the epigenetic marks, such as DNA methylation, histone modifications, ncRNA, and chromosome conformation signatures.

Signatures of epigenetic deregulation can be detected in peripheral blood even within a few hours of environmental exposure. The field now faces the demand for thorough, systematic, and rationalized approaches to establish the relation of epigenetic changes to clinical outcomes, by using reliable designs and tools [189]. In disease epidemiology, the epigenetic approach aims to address the questions about disease risk and prognosis using the epigenetic variability. As early examples, rare "epimutations" were detected in peripheral blood and reported for the genes MLH1, MSH2, and IGF2 from cancer patients [190].

A very interesting biological effect evident in cells damaged by ionizing radiation (IR) is the radiation-induced bystander effect (BE). IR can affect neighboring cells in proximity, giving rise to a BE. IR effects can also span several generations and influence the progeny of exposed parents, leading to transgeneration effects. Bystander and transgeneration IR effects are linked to the phenomenon of the IR-induced genome instability that manifests itself as chromosome aberrations, gene mutations, late cell death, and aneuploidy. Evidence suggests that the IR-induced genome instability, bystander, and transgeneration effect are epigenetically mediated. The epigenetic changes encompass chromatin remodeling, small RNA regulation, and DNA methylation. Studies demonstrated that IR exposure alters epigenetic parameters in the directly exposed tissues and in the distant bystander tissues [191,192]. A similar epigenetic effect of BE is seen in somatic organs (liver, kidney, and heart) when patients or animals undergo a stroke [193].

In HCC [194], over 30 tumor suppressors and other cancer-related genes have been found consistently hypermethylated. Those also included genes implicated in cell-cycle regulation, apoptosis, DNA repair, cell adhesion, and invasion. On the other hand, expression of CD147 was shown to be directly correlated with hypomethylation and risk of recurrence. A set of methylated biomarkers on *SPINT2, SRD5A2, AFP,* and *PIVKA-II* genes showed promising potential for early detection of HCC. Moreover, in tumor tissues, expression of HDACs 1–3 was highly correlated with tumor grade. Multiple studies showed that tumor-derived miRNAs can be detected in blood in highly stable form and miRNA deregulation was an early event in liver carcinogenesis. For example, miR-122, -192, -21, -223, 26a, -27a, and -801 provided high diagnostic accuracy in detecting early-stage HCC [99,194].

Another example concerns endometrial cancer, the seventh most common cancer in women worldwide. Analysis of epigenetic deregulations identified aberrant DNA hypermethylation associated with endometrial cancer in a number of genes, including *SPRY2*. This gene encodes an antagonist regulator of receptor tyrosine kinase in the fibroblast growth factor (FGF) and RAS–MAPK pathways and is a tumor suppressor gene involved in cell proliferation, differentiation, and angiogenesis. Parts of FGF and RAS–MAPK pathways are changed in endometrial cancer and expression of *SPRY2* is known to be reduced in several types of cancer. In direct link with DNA methylation are several miRNAs consistently associated with the changes in their mode of expression—miR-124, -126, -137, and -491. miR-152 is found to be downregulated at high frequency not only in endometrial cancer, but also in acute lymphomic leukemia, digestive system cancers, and cholangiocellular cancer. Interestingly, one of the known targets of miR-152 is *MET* that encodes a cell-surface receptor and is a known cancer gene [195].

Myeloid hematological malignancies are among the epigenetically best-characterized neoplasms. The comparatively low number of recurring balanced and unbalanced chromosomal abnormalities as well as common genetic mutations has enabled researchers to relate epigenetic states to these defects. A number of distinct mutations have been recognized as interfering with the epigenetic state. While clinical and pathological diagnosis of AML has never been a problem, determining minimal residual disease (MRD) as a sign of early relapse remains a challenge, largely dependent on epigenetic insight. A study of promoter methylation of ERα and *CDKN2B* was found to correlate well with high relapse risk in AML. Latest advances suggest that these biomarkers may be utilized not only on bone marrow samples but also in the peripheral blood. Methylation analysis on samples from patients with myelodysplastic syndromes (MDS), a group of clonal bone marrow disorders, demonstrated strong cooperation between chromosomal deletions and epigenetic silencing. For chronic myeloid leukemia (CML), a common trend is strong hypermethylation on a number of promoters, except for *CDKN2B* which, unlike the AML and MDS cases, remains unmethylated [196].

CpG hypermethylation is a common feature in ovarian cancer, including common immunosuppressors *BRCA1*, *p16*, *MLH1*, putative immunosuppressors *OPCML*, *RASSF1A*, imprinted genes *ARHI*, *PEG3*, and proapoptotic genes *LOT1*, *DAPK*, *PAR-4*. Interestingly, *BRCA1* has been shown to be hypermethylated in sporadic, but never in hereditary types of ovarian cancers. *BRCA1* methylation is strongly associated with the loss of BRCA1 RNA and protein. Comparing methylation status of *SFRP1, 2, 4, 5, SOX1, PAX1,* and *LMX1A* between benign, borderline, and malignant ovarian tumors showed that methylation rates were highest in ovarian cancer and decreased in patients with borderline malignancy and nonmalignant tissue. In addition to redistribution of DNA methylation patterns, changes in histone modifications in ovarian carcinogenesis were observed on aberrantly expressed class III beta-tubulin, surviving, *PAGE4*, and *Claudin 3*. Altered histone modifications of the promoter loci were found in silenced *GATA4* and *GATA6* transcription factors in ovarian cancer cell lines. As part of the epigenetic posttranscriptional gene downregulation, miRNA-200a, -200b, -200c, and -141 were shown to be overexpressed in ovarian cancer. At the same time, miR-21, -203, and -205 were among the most downregulated. miRNA signatures of ovarian cancer could be helpful to distinguish the tumors based on their histological subtype: miR-200b and miR-141 are upregulated in endometrioid and serous subtypes. Nineteen miRNAs are downregulated in all three histotypes, miR-145 is downregulated in both serous and clear cell carcinoma, while miR-222 is downregulated in both endometrioid and clear cell carcinoma [197].

In early diagnosis of ovarian cancer, despite late presentation of symptoms, specific methylated DNA markers were reported in the serum, plasma, and peritoneal fluid of ovarian cancer patients. Tumor-specific methylation pattern of six tumor suppressor genes—*BRCA1, RASSF1A, APC, p14, p16, DAPK*—was detected in the serum of ovarian cancer patients with 82% sensitivity. Detection of specific epigenetic markers in the blood of patients appears to be a promising approach for early detection of ovarian cancer.

Tumor stage, residual disease after surgery, histological type, and tumor grade are all the most important clinical–pathological factors most relevant to diagnosis and treatment of ovarian cancer. Today, individual methylated genes with possible prognostic value include *HOXA11*, linked with postsurgical residual tumor and overall poor prognosis, *FBXO32*, associated with a progression-free survival, and *IGFBP-3*, associated with disease progression and death. A panel of predictive biomarkers *SFRP1, SFRP2, SOX1, LMX1A* showed good correlation with recurrence and overall survival. In terms of miRNA, a lower ratio of miR-221 and miR-222 was reported to be a significant predictor for worse survival in high-grade, advanced stage sporadic ovarian carcinoma [197].

Variations in methylation patterns can occur within the same tumor type. In addition to providing prognostic information, these patterns can be associated with response to therapy. A major impediment for survival is the development of chemoresistance. One well-documented example is the use of *MLH1* methylation status as a biomarker. Silencing of MLH1 by methylation has been linked with platinum resistance. In a recent study, demethylation agent cytidine analog 5-axzacytidine (azacitidine, 5-aza-CR; Celgene, NJ, USA) demethylates MLH1 and enhanced response to platinum in patients with platinum resistant ovarian cancer [198]. With regard to miR-NAs, over 27 miRNAs, including tumor suppressor Let-7i, have been linked today with chemotherapy responses [197,199].

Chemoresistance in CRC also turns out to be largely an epigenetic issue. CRC is the second leading cause of cancer-related deaths in the world. Despite many therapeutic opportunities, prognosis remains dismal for patients with metastatic disease, and a significant portion of early-stage patients develop recurrence after chemotherapy. Emerging evidence indicates that epigenetics mechanisms are responsible for chemoresistance to three commonly used agents in CRC: 5-fluorouracil, irinotecan, and oxaliplatin. It is therefore considered that epigenetic biomarkers may help stratify CRC patients and reverse epigenetic modifications through specific drugs: histone-deacetylase and DNA-methyl-transferase inhibitors. Early preclinical studies suggest that these drugs may reverse chemoresistance in colorectal tumors [200].

Glioblastoma, medulloblastoma, and ependymoma represent molecularly and clinically diverse forms of adult and pediatric brain tumors, arising from both genetic and epigenetic causation. Glioblastoma shows extensive pattern of CpG methylation, analyzed on over 27,000 CpG sites [201], with significant prognostic value for survival rates. Analysis of ncRNA shows upregulation of miR-26a involved in development and proliferation of GBM, silencing of miR-128, a glioma proliferation inhibitor and silencing of miR-451, an inhibitor of invasion. For medulloblastoma, an interesting example of a link with genetic and epigenetic synergy identified DNA hypermethylation on chromosome 17p11.2, a region frequently deleted in 30–50% of all medulloblastomas. Downregulation of miR-126b, 324-5p, 326 in medulloblastoma results in increased proliferation of tumor cells. Interestingly, miR-17–92, implicated previously in leukemia and lung adenocarcinomas, has been identified as overexpressed in medulloblastoma as well. Ependymoma, despite its heterogeneity across CNS, demonstrated examples of specific promoter methylation, primarily upon locations within known regions of chromosomal loss specific for ependymoma. One of the examples is *RASSF1A* hypermethylated with the incidence of 86% and present universally in all histological subtypes [202].

Emerging data suggest that these epigenetic modifications also impact on the development of cardiovascular disease and heart failure [203–205]. A large population of CpG islands within gene promoters has significant hypomethylation at end-stage cardyomyopathic hearts and convergent methylation pattern in genes relevant to myocyte apoptosis, fibrosis, and altered contractility. In addition, genome-wide analysis showed distinct pattern of enrichment in H3K36me3. A number of miRNAs altered by environmental stress have been directly implicated in cardiovascular diseases and associated epigenetic changes. Those include miR-222, induced in response to air and metal pollutants and linked to angiogenesis, miR-146a, induced by exposure to aluminum and linked to cardiac hypertrophy, miR-199a, associated with exposure to alcohol and with prevention of hypoxia injury [189].

Osteoarthritis (OA) is a complex multifactorial disease with a strong genetic component. Several studies have suggested or identified epigenetic events that may play a role in OA progression and the gene expression changes observed in diseased cartilage. Metalloproteinase expression in normal cartilage is relatively low, but is elevated in OA leading to extracellular matrix degradation. A number of metalloproteinase promoters show decreased methylation, which underlies the disease-associated change in expression. This includes *MMP3, MMP9, MMP13*, and *ADAMTS4*. A region of the *IL1B* promoter is demethylated in human articular chondrocytes correlating with an increase in *IL1B* expression. In terms of histone modifications, chondrocytes display induced histone H3K4 di- and tri-methylation around the *COX2* and *NOS* promoters. On the part of ncRNA, miR-140 has been extensively studied as one of the originally defined cartilage-restricted miRNAs, with direct target of *ADAMTS4*. Latest screens identified miR-9, -98, -146 as potential biomarker candidates, with miR-146 directly modulating *MMP13* expression. Latest screens in dedifferentiating articular chondrocytes, cartilage, chondrosarcoma, and osteochondroma have identified novel and unique miRNA profiles. Interestingly, some of these miRNAs have also been found in plasma, able to reenter recipient cells and opening up possibility of exogenous regulation of gene expression via systemic synchronization [206,207].

In RA, the epigenetic data are currently very limited. However, some interesting stratifying epigenetic patterns have already started to emerge. Analysis of T-cell DNA methylation has revealed global hypomethylation in RA patients [208]. Hypomethylation, as a general trend, has also been observed in RA fibroblast-like synoviocytes (FLS) [209]. According to one study, FLS derived from RA patients showed differences in methylation in as many as 1859 loci genome wide [210]. In a gene-targeted approach, analysis of *IL6* in peripheral blood mononuclear cells identified a motif hypomethylated in RA patients [211]. On the ncRNA side of epigenetic regulation, increased expression of miR-115 and -203 has been observed in RA FLS [212,213]. These and other epigenetic alterations may prove useful markers for disease progression and response to treatment. Correct study design, choice of panels of epigenetic markers, and scope and resolution of coverage in longitudinal cohorts would be an essential prerequisite for distinguishing causal from consequence at the level of epigenetic readouts [214]. In a recent study, 354 anti-citrullinated protein antibody-associated RA cases and 337 controls, and two clusters within the MHC region were identified, whose differential methylation potentially mediates genetic risk for RA. To reduce confounding factors that have hampered previous epigenome-wide studies, the authors corrected for cellular heterogeneity by estimating and adjusting for cell-type proportions in our blood-derived DNA samples and used mediation analysis to filter out associations likely to be a consequence of disease. Four CpGs showed an association between genotype and variance of methylation. In an independent cohort of 12 RA cases and 12 controls, the methylation analysis was only done on the monocyte cell fractions separated from blood by using cytometry. This identified that the DNA methylation differences were seen in monocytes. This shows that monitoring epigenetic causes of disease peripherally is viable and that the blood is a conduit of epigenetic epitype [215].

Diabetes mellitus is a chronic metabolic disease due to insufficient INS response to elevated blood glucose levels, caused by autoimmune destruction of INS-producing pancreatic beta cells in T1DM or by impaired sensitivity to INS of INS-responsive tissues such as liver and skeletal muscle, together with insufficient β-cell compensation in T2DM. Classical genetic studies established a link between T1DM, a common childhood autoimmune disease and genes that encode MHC antigens, and several immune-related determinants. Emerging data indicate a role for epigenetic mechanisms of metabolic memory, including Set7-mediated histone methylation. Relevance for histone lysine methylation to diabetic deregulation in gene expression was indicated by the constitutive demethylation of H3K9 at two candidate genes in peripheral blood monocytes derived from T1DM and T2DM patients

[216,217]. Genome-wide epigenetic studies of human pancreatic islets, based on high-throughput sequencing characterized mono-, di-, and tri-methylation profiles of histone 3 (H3K4me1, me2, me3, H3K27me3, H3K79me2) and the binding sites for epigenetic regulator CTCF, implicated in formation of chromosome conformation signatures [218,219]. Epigenetic mechanisms were shown to be involved in β-cell differentiation and proliferation. Analysis of the human INS locus in pancreatic islets demonstrated not only a role for regulatory long-range interactions with adjacent genes over the distance of 300 kb, as mentioned earlier, but also demonstrated distinct kinetics in epigenetic changes on the INS promoter distinguishing a scenario for impaired glucose response. The existence of a regulatory network between the INS gene and other distant genes, like SYT8, through long-range chromosomal interactions, suggests that such networks of chromosome conformation signatures have general importance for INS biology and diabetes [78,220–222].

In a related area of research, insights into the role of epigenetics in nutrition revealed that maternal dietary fat, folic acid, protein, and total energy intakes induced altered epigenetic regulation of specific genes in the offspring which were often associated with altered tissue function. Passage of induced phenotypic and epigenetic traits between generations involves intergenerational modifications in the interaction between maternal phenotype and environment. The methylation of specific CpG loci in fetal tissues is associated with differential future risk of T2DM, and variation in adiposity and height. Methylation of specific CpGs in adult blood also marks differential risk of T2DM and breast cancer [223]. The mechanism by which the maternal nutritional environment induces changes is beginning to be understood and involves the altered epigenetic regulation of specific genes. The demonstration of a role for altered epigenetic regulation of genes in the developmental induction of a disease opens the possibility that interventions—either through nutrition or specific drugs—may modify long-term risks and reduce the prevalence of epigenetically driven diseases [223].

In early attempts to treat epigenetic diseases, a number of clinical trials have tested hemoglobinopathies, myelodysplastic, leukemic, and fragile X syndromes with demethylating agents [23,60,224–227], histone deacetylating (HDAC) agents, or combined manipulation of cytosine methylation and histone acetylation. Agents used in these trials included 5-azacytidine, 2-deoxy-5-azacytidine, as well as newer demethylating agents (antisense oligonucleotide MG98, which suppresses DNMT1), histone deacetylase inhibitors (HDACs) such as sodium butyrate, sodium phenyl butyrate, trichostatin, suberoylanilide hydroxamic acid (SAHA) [228], and depsipeptide [226].

In cancer, the use of epigenetic targets has already shown itself as a valuable approach [229]. Epigenetic drugs can be used therapeutically as part of a synergistic combination with other therapeutic treatments such as chemotherapy, immunotherapy, or radiotherapy. HDAC inhibitors have been shown to induce enhanced sensitivity to IR treatment. Various combinations of demethylating agents and HDAC inhibitors are being studied for

reactivation of tumor suppressor genes, DNA repair, increase in cellular che-
mosensitivity, alleviation of resistance to other drugs, and increased efficacy
of existing therapies.

3.5 Epigenetic Analysis

Epigenetic biomarkers—DNA methylation, posttranslational modifications of histones, ncRNAs, and chromosome conformation signatures—are
important regulatory markers that functionally control chromatin architecture, modes of gene expression, and cellular phenotypes. The mechanisms
underlying the deposition of these marks, their propagation during cell replication, and alteration in their distribution are subject to some of the most
exciting biological research.

Epigenetic methodologies have until recently been small-scale, focused
on low-throughput analysis of single genes, many of them based on using
polymerase chain reaction (PCR) as the final quantitative readout step. Many
of the new techniques now employ tiling genome array-hybridization techniques, high-throughput sequencing, making it possible to analyze the epigenome on a large scale.

DNA methylation analysis is based primarily on the use of methylation sensitive and insensitive restriction endonucleases, affinity enrichment steps against
5mC and 5hmC, and methyl-binding protein affinities for proteins like MBD2.
After enrichment, tiling arrays or high-throughput DNA sequencing methods
are often employed.

Chromatin modifications are analyzed with the chromatin immuno-
precipitation [230] or advanced sequencing techniques that combine ChiP
[230], with real-time PCR as a final readout. ChiP paired with hybridization
to genomic tiling array or deep sequencing (ChiP-seq) is also increasingly
common.

ncRNAs analysis depends on either miRNA microarrays or high-throughput sequencing. Chromosome conformation signatures are still largely identified and monitored on the basis of low-throughput research techniques
[61], with only one industrial methodology offering high-throughput platform *EpiSwitch*™, which combines the advantages of bioinformatics, tiling
microarray, and new generation sequencing for the discovery and monitoring of epigenetic biomarkers [231].

A number of alternative platforms available today, including arrays and
PCR profiling [74], serial analysis of chromatin occupancy (SACO), and
genome-wide mapping technique (GMAT) have generated precise maps of
epigenetic marks in different cell types [232,233]. Epigenomic maps have
improved our understanding of chromatin organization and epigenetic differences in regulation in health and disease. The Alliance for the Human

Epigenome and Disease (AHEAD) project has recommended an international effort to characterize the human epigenetic changes that accompany normal development, adult cell renewal and disease, and epigenetic variation that accompanies a healthy state. The Encyclopedia of DNA Elements Consortium [187] is an international collaboration of research groups funded by the National Human Genome Research Institute (NHGRI). The goal of ENCODE is to build a comprehensive parts list of functional elements in the human genome, including elements that act at the protein and RNA levels, and regulatory elements that control cells and circumstances in which a gene is active.

Successful use of epigenetic biomarkers and biomarker panels is intricately linked to their biological properties. High turnover for some of the histone modification markers and histone variants, close link of 5mC levels to metabolic rates, nutritional status, and stochastic component at the sites of high polymorphism, low copy numbers, and short half-life for some of ncRNAs— all constitute serious challenges in designing robust and reproducible biomarker applications for routine use in clinical practice. Interestingly, chromosome conformation signatures and some of the ncRNA offer a more robust and consistent source of targets, associated with established epigenetic status, which could be monitored in a binary way for presence or absence of specific chromosome conformation signatures/ncRNA. Such readout is in striking contrast to the continuum readout of varying levels of DNA methylation, histone modifications, and most of the ncRNAs. Against the continuum readout for most of the biomarkers, data analysis, which includes stratification classifies for biomarker panels, benefits significantly from the binary modes of phenotypical differences.

Substantial contributions have already been made toward understanding the importance of epigenetics to human disease [233]. Ever-growing numbers of reported epigenetic alterations in disease offer a chance to increase sensitivity and specificity of future diagnostics and therapies. Challenges—modern clinical management strategies require to combine and integrate data from genomic, transcriptomic, and epigenomic data sets to determine profiles predicting disease outcome in terms of patient prognosis and treatment response. The integration of data and the comparison of epigenetic profiles from normal and diseased tissues allow the development of predictive models for disease outcomes using epigenetic biomarkers and signatures. As we advance from studying alterations at single loci, groups of disease-specific biomarkers will soon be able to diagnose and to predict disease prognosis more accurately than is possible at present.

For certain diseases, especially cancers, combinations of epigenetic biomarkers already have achieved good sensitivities in the detection of cancer cells and in the prediction of tumor progression, when performed on primary tissue [234]. However, before being of clinical value, noninvasive detection of biomarkers in biological fluids has to be improved to the levels of high sensitivity and specificity. High-throughput epigenetic screening approaches and the identification of biomarkers are now achievable for increasing number of clinical indications. Because of the high costs of high-resolution techniques, these approaches are only applicable to biomarker identification *per se*, while for clinical assays, limited biomarker panels will still be the methods of choice because of the costs.

The key to successful therapy lies in leveraging of patient's altered epigenetic profiles with combinations of conventional treatments and novel drugs under predictive models, which aim at low-dose, customized, and high-impact treatments.

Acknowledgments

The authors are grateful for the important discussions and comments from Professor Jane Mellor, Biochemistry Department, University of Oxford; Professor Colin Goding, Ludwig Institute for Cancer Research, University of Oxford; Dr. Dmitry Pshezhetskiy, Imperial College, Hammersmith Hospital, London; Christian Hoyer Millar, Oxford BioDynamics and Chronos Therapeutics Limited.

References

1. Goldberg, A.D., Allis, C.D., and E. Bernstein, Epigenetics: A landscape takes shape. *Cell*, 2007. **128**: 635–8.
2. Slack, J.M., Conrad Hal Waddington: The last Renaissance biologist? *Nat Rev Genet*, 2002. **3**(11): 889–95.
3. Holliday, R., Epigenetics: A historical overview. *Epigenetics*, 2006. **1**(2): 76–80.
4. Bird, A., Perceptions of epigenetics. *Nature*, 2007. **447**(7143): 396–8.
5. Fraga, M.F. et al., Epigenetic differences arise during the lifetime of monozygotic twins. *Proc Natl Acad Sci USA*, 2005. **102**(30): 10604–9.
6. Poulsen, P. et al., The epigenetic basis of twin discordance in age-related diseases. *Pediatr Res*, 2007. **61**(5 Pt 2): 38R–42R.
7. Feinberg, A.P. and B. Vogelstein, Hypomethylation distinguishes genes of some human cancers from their normal counterparts. *Nature*, 1983. **301**(5895): 89–92.
8. Kornberg, R.D. and Y. Lorch, Twenty-five years of the nucleosome, fundamental particle of the eukaryote chromosome. *Cell*, 1999. **98**(3): 285–94.
9. Luger, K. et al., Crystal structure of the nucleosome core particle at 2.8 A resolution. *Nature*, 1997. **389**(6648): 251–60.
10. Cheung, P., C.D. Allis, and P. Sassone-Corsi, Signaling to chromatin through histone modifications. *Cell*, 2000. **103**(2): 263–71.
11. Kornberg, R.D. and Y. Lorch, Chromatin-modifying and -remodeling complexes. *Curr Opin Genet Dev*, 1999. **9**(2): 148–51.

12. Mellor, J., Dynamic nucleosomes and gene transcription. *Trends Genet*, 2006. **22**(6): 320–9.
13. Saha, A., J. Wittmeyer, and B.R. Cairns, Mechanisms for nucleosome movement by ATP-dependent chromatin remodeling complexes. *Results Probl Cell Differ*, 2006. **41**: 127–48.
14. Hanson, M.A. and P.D. Gluckman, Developmental origins of health and disease: New insights. *Basic Clin Pharmacol Toxicol*, 2008. **102**(2): 90–3.
15. Portela, A. and M. Esteller, Epigenetic modifications and human disease. *Nat Biotechnol*, 2010. **28**(10): 1057–68.
16. Johnstone, S.E. and S.B. Baylin, Stress and the epigenetic landscape: A link to the pathobiology of human diseases? *Nat Rev Genet*, 2010. **11**(11): 806–12.
17. Halfmann, R. and S. Lindquist, Epigenetics in the extreme: Prions and the inheritance of environmentally acquired traits. *Science*, 2010. **330**(6004): 629–32.
18. Gomez, A. and M. Ingelman-Sundberg, Epigenetic and microRNA-dependent control of cytochrome P450 expression: A gap between DNA and protein. *Pharmacogenomics*, 2009. **10**(7): 1067–76.
19. Gomez, A. and M. Ingelman-Sundberg, Pharmacoepigenetics: Its role in interindividual differences in drug response. *Clin Pharmacol Ther*, 2009. **85**(4): 426–30.
20. Brockmoller, J. and M.V. Tzvetkov, Pharmacogenetics: Data, concepts and tools to improve drug discovery and drug treatment. *Eur J Clin Pharmacol*, 2008. **64**(2): 133–57.
21. Manolio, T.A. et al., Finding the missing heritability of complex diseases. *Nature*, 2009. **461**(7265): 747–53.
22. Khoury, M.J., J. Evans, W. Burke, A reality check for personalized medicine. *Nature*, 2010. **464**: 680.
23. Egger, G. et al., Epigenetics in human disease and prospects for epigenetic therapy. *Nature*, 2004. **429**(6990): 457–63.
24. Feinberg, A.P. et al., Personalized epigenomic signatures that are stable over time and covary with body mass index. *Sci Transl Med*, 2010. **2**(49): 49ra67.
25. He, F. and P.K. Todd, Epigenetics in nucleotide repeat expansion disorders. *Semin Neurol*, 2011. **31**(5): 470–83.
26. Murrell, A., V.K. Rakyan, and S. Beck, From genome to epigenome. *Hum Mol Genet*, 2005. **14**(1): R3–10.
27. Gilbert, S.F., Ageing and cancer as diseases of epigenesis. *J Biosci*, 2009. **34**(4): 601–4.
28. Dolinoy, D.C., D. Huang, and R.L. Jirtle, Maternal nutrient supplementation counteracts bisphenol A-induced DNA hypomethylation in early development. *Proc Natl Acad Sci USA*, 2007. **104**(32): 13056–61.
29. Liu, Y. et al., Aberrant promoter methylation of p16 and MGMT genes in lung tumors from smoking and never-smoking lung cancer patients. *Neoplasia*, 2006. **8**(1): 46–51.
30. Schuebel, K.E. et al., Comparing the DNA hypermethylome with gene mutations in human colorectal cancer. *PLoS Genet*, 2007. **3**(9): 1709–23.
31. Kim, D.H. et al., p16(INK4a) and histology-specific methylation of CpG islands by exposure to tobacco smoke in non-small cell lung cancer. *Cancer Res*, 2001. **61**(8): 3419–24.
32. Tessema, M. et al., Promoter methylation of genes in and around the candidate lung cancer susceptibility locus 6q23-25. *Cancer Res*, 2008. **68**(6): 1707–14.
33. Duthie, S.J., Epigenetic modifications and human pathologies: Cancer and CVD. *Proc Nutr Soc*, 2011. **70**(1): 47–56.

34. Heijmans, B.T. et al., Persistent epigenetic differences associated with prenatal exposure to famine in humans. *Proc Natl Acad Sci USA*, 2008. **105**(44): 17046–9.
35. Gardiner-Garden, M. and M. Frommer, CpG islands in vertebrate genomes. *J Mol Biol*, 1987. **196**(2): 261–82.
36. Cooper, D.N. and H. Youssoufian, The CpG dinucleotide and human genetic disease. *Hum Genet*, 1988. **78**(2): 151–5.
37. Bird, A.P., CpG-rich islands and the function of DNA methylation. *Nature*, 1986. **321**(6067): 209–13.
38. Bird, A.P., Functions for DNA methylation in vertebrates. *Cold Spring Harb Symp Quant Biol*, 1993. **58**: 281–5.
39. Yoder, J.A., C.P. Walsh, and T.H. Bestor, Cytosine methylation and the ecology of intragenomic parasites. *Trends Genet*, 1997. **13**(8): 335–40.
40. Cross, S.H. and A.P. Bird, CpG islands and genes. *Curr Opin Genet Dev*, 1995. **5**(3): 309–14.
41. Nan, X. et al., Transcriptional repression by the methyl-CpG-binding protein MeCP2 involves a histone deacetylase complex. *Nature*, 1998. **393**(6683): 386–9.
42. Jones, P.L. et al., Methylated DNA and MeCP2 recruit histone deacetylase to repress transcription. *Nat Genet*, 1998. **19**(2): 187–91.
43. Ng, H.H. et al., MBD2 is a transcriptional repressor belonging to the MeCP1 histone deacetylase complex. *Nat Genet*, 1999. **23**(1): 58–61.
44. Tamaru, H. and E.U. Selker, A histone H3 methyltransferase controls DNA methylation in *Neurospora crassa*. *Nature*, 2001. **414**(6861): 277–83.
45. Nakayama, J. et al., Role of histone H3 lysine 9 methylation in epigenetic control of heterochromatin assembly. *Science*, 2001. **292**(5514): 110–3.
46. Bestor, T.H., Gene silencing. Methylation meets acetylation. *Nature*, 1998. **393**(6683): 311–2.
47. Edwards, J.R. et al., Chromatin and sequence features that define the fine and gross structure of genomic methylation patterns. *Genome Res*, 2010. **20**(7): 972–80.
48. Tahiliani, M. et al., Conversion of 5-methylcytosine to 5-hydroxymethylcytosine in mammalian DNA by MLL partner TET1. *Science*, 2009. **324**(5929): 930–5.
49. Ito, S. et al., Role of Tet proteins in 5mC to 5hmC conversion, ES-cell self-renewal and inner cell mass specification. *Nature*, 2010. **466**(7310): 1129–33.
50. Warren, R.A., Modified bases in bacteriophage DNAs. *Annu Rev Microbiol*, 1980. **34**: 137–58.
51. Kriaucionis, S. and N. Heintz, The nuclear DNA base 5-hydroxymethylcytosine is present in Purkinje neurons and the brain. *Science*, 2009. **324**(5929): 929–30.
52. Freudenberg, J.M. et al., Acute depletion of Tet1-dependent 5-hydroxymethylcytosine levels impairs LIF/Stat3 signaling and results in loss of embryonic stem cell identity. *Nucleic Acids Res*, 2012. **40**(8): 3364–77.
53. Thomson, J.P. et al., Non-genotoxic carcinogen exposure induces defined changes in the 5-hydroxymethylome. *Genome Biol*, 2012. **13**(10): R93.
54. Jin, S.G., S. Kadam, and G.P. Pfeifer, Examination of the specificity of DNA methylation profiling techniques towards 5-methylcytosine and 5-hydroxymethylcytosine. *Nucleic Acids Res*, 2010. **38**(11): e125.
55. Esteller, M., Cancer epigenomics: DNA methylomes and histone-modification maps. *Nat Rev Genet*, 2007. **8**(4): 286–98.
56. Esteller, M., Epigenetics in cancer. *N Engl J Med*, 2008. **358**(11): 1148–59.
57. Kouzarides, T., Chromatin modifications and their function. *Cell*, 2007. **128**(4): 693–705.

58. Cosgrove, M.S. and C. Wolberger, How does the histone code work? *Biochem Cell Biol*, 2005. **83**(4): 468–76.

59. Strahl, B.D. and C.D. Allis, The language of covalent histone modifications. *Nature*, 2000. **403**(6765): 41–5.

60. Spannhoff, A. et al., The emerging therapeutic potential of histone methyltransferase and demethylase inhibitors. *Chem Med Chem*, 2009. **4**(10): 1568–82.

61. Jennifer, L., X.Q.D.W., Crutchley M.A. Ferraiuolo, and J.E. Dostie, Chromatin conformation signatures—Ideal human disease biomarkers? *Biomarkers Med*, 2010. **4**(4): 611–29.

62. Ling, J.Q. and A.R. Hoffman, Epigenetics of long-range chromatin interactions. *Pediatr Res*, 2007. **61**(5 Pt 2): 11R–16R.

63. Deng, W. and G.A. Blobel, Do chromatin loops provide epigenetic gene expression states? *Curr Opin Genet Dev*, 2010. **20**(5): 548–54.

64. Kadauke, S. and G.A. Blobel, Chromatin loops in gene regulation. *Biochim Biophys Acta*, 2009. **1789**(1): 17–25.

65. Christova, R. et al., P-STAT1 mediates higher-order chromatin remodelling of the human MHC in response to IFNgamma. *J Cell Sci*, 2007. **120**(Pt 18): 3262–70.

66. Rickman, D.S. et al., Oncogene-mediated alterations in chromatin conformation. *Proc Natl Acad Sci USA*, 2012. **109**(23): 9083–8.

67. Fudenberg, G. et al., High order chromatin architecture shapes the landscape of chromosomal alterations in cancer. *Nat Biotechnol*, 2011. **29**(12): 1109–13.

68. Watanabe, T. et al., Higher-order chromatin regulation and differential gene expression in the human tumor necrosis factor/lymphotoxin locus in hepatocellular carcinoma cells. *Mol Cell Biol*, 2012. **32**(8): 1529–41.

69. Goes, A.C. et al., Loop domain organization of the p53 locus in normal and breast cancer cells correlates with the transcriptional status of the TP53 and the neighboring genes. *J Cell Biochem*, 2011. **112**(8): 2072–81.

70. Gomes, N.P. and J.M. Espinosa, Disparate chromatin landscapes and kinetics of inactivation impact differential regulation of p53 target genes. *Cell Cycle*, 2010. **9**(17): 3428–37.

71. Wright, J.B., S.J. Brown, and M.D. Cole, Upregulation of c-MYC in *cis* through a large chromatin loop linked to a cancer risk-associated single-nucleotide polymorphism in colorectal cancer cells. *Mol Cell Biol*, 2010. **30**(6): 1411–20.

72. Tan-Wong, S.M. et al., Dynamic interactions between the promoter and terminator regions of the mammalian BRCA1 gene. *Proc Natl Acad Sci USA*, 2008. **105**(13): 5160–5.

73. Ye, Q. et al., BRCA1-induced large-scale chromatin unfolding and allele-specific effects of cancer-predisposing mutations. *J Cell Biol*, 2001. **155**(6): 911–21.

74. Davison, L.J. et al., Long-range DNA looping and gene expression analyses identify DEXI as an autoimmune disease candidate gene. *Hum Mol Genet*, 2012. **21**(2): 322–33.

75. Deligianni, C. and C.G. Spilianakis, Long-range genomic interactions epigenetically regulate the expression of a cytokine receptor. *EMBO Rep*, 2012. **13**(9): 819–26.

76. Papantonis, A. et al., TNFalpha signals through specialized factories where responsive coding and miRNA genes are transcribed. *EMBO J*, 2012. **31**(23): 4404–14.

77. Emily Rowell, M.M. and C.B. Wilson, Long-range regulation of cytokine gene expression. *Curr Opin Immunol*, 2008. **20**(3): 272–80.

78. Xu, Z. et al., Mapping of INS promoter interactions reveals its role in long-range regulation of SYT8 transcription. *Nat Struct Mol Biol*, 2011. **18**(3): 372–8.
79. Li, M., G.H. Liu, and J.C. Izpisua Belmonte, Navigating the epigenetic landscape of pluripotent stem cells. *Nat Rev Mol Cell Biol*, 2012. **13**(8): 524–35.
80. Akiyuki Hirosue, K.I., K. Tokunaga, T. Watanabe, N. Saitoh, M. Nakamoto, T. Chandra, M. Narita, M. Shinohara, and M. Nakao, Quantitative assessment of higher-order chromatin structure of the INK4/ARF locus in human senescent cells. *Aging Cell*, 2012. **11**: 553–6.
81. Kheradmand Kia, S. et al., EZH2-dependent chromatin looping controls INK4a and INK4b, but not ARF, during human progenitor cell differentiation and cellular senescence. *Epigenet Chromatin*, 2009. **2**(1): 16.
82. Weng, N.P., Y. Araki, and K. Subedi, The molecular basis of the memory T cell response: Differential gene expression and its epigenetic regulation. *Nat Rev Immunol*, 2012. **12**(4): 306–15.
83. Daxinger, L. and E. Whitelaw, Understanding transgenerational epigenetic inheritance via the gametes in mammals. *Nat Rev Genet*, 2012. **13**(3): 153–62.
84. Harismendy, O. et al., 9p21 DNA variants associated with coronary artery disease impair interferon-gamma signalling response. *Nature*, 2011. **470**(7333): 264–8.
85. Katada, S., A. Imhof, and P. Sassone-Corsi, Connecting threads: Epigenetics and metabolism. *Cell*, 2012. **148**(1–2): 24–8.
86. Harries, L.W., Long non-coding RNAs and human disease. *Biochem Soc Trans*, 2012. **40**(4): 902–6.
87. Esteller, M., Non-coding RNAs in human disease. *Nat Rev Genet*, 2011. **12**(12): 861–74.
88. He, L. and G.J. Hannon, MicroRNAs: Small RNAs with a big role in gene regulation. *Nat Rev Genet*, 2004. **5**(7): 522–31.
89. Mendell, J.T., MicroRNAs: Critical regulators of development, cellular physiology and malignancy. *Cell Cycle*, 2005. **4**(9): 1179–84.
90. Esquela-Kerscher, A. and F.J. Slack, Oncomirs—MicroRNAs with a role in cancer. *Nat Rev Cancer*, 2006. **6**(4): 259–69.
91. Hammond, S.M., MicroRNAs as tumor suppressors. *Nat Genet*, 2007. **39**(5): 582–3.
92. Croce, C.M., Causes and consequences of microRNA dysregulation in cancer. *Nat Rev Genet*, 2009. **10**(10): 704–14.
93. Nicoloso, M.S. et al., MicroRNAs—The micro steering wheel of tumour metastases. *Nat Rev Cancer*, 2009. **9**(4): 293–302.
94. Mercer, T.R., M.E. Dinger, and J.S. Mattick, Long non-coding RNAs: Insights into functions. *Nat Rev Genet*, 2009. **10**(3): 155–9.
95. Carninci, P. et al., The transcriptional landscape of the mammalian genome. *Science*, 2005. **309**(5740): 1559–63.
96. Kapranov, P. et al., RNA maps reveal new RNA classes and a possible function for pervasive transcription. *Science*, 2007. **316**(5830): 1484–8.
97. Valeri, N. et al., Epigenetics, miRNAs, and human cancer: A new chapter in human gene regulation. *Mamm Genome*, 2009. **20**(9–10): 573–80.
98. Kosaka, N. and T. Ochiya, Unraveling the mystery of cancer by secretory microRNA: Horizontal microRNA transfer between living cells. *Front Genet*, 2011. **2**: 97.
99. Liu, W.R. et al., Epigenetics of hepatocellular carcinoma: A new horizon. *Chin Med J (Engl)*, 2012. **125**(13): 2349–60.

100. Aravin, A.A. et al., Developmentally regulated piRNA clusters implicate MILI in transposon control. *Science*, 2007. **316**(5825): 744–7.

101. Brennecke, J. et al., Discrete small RNA-generating loci as master regulators of transposon activity in Drosophila. *Cell*, 2007. **128**(6): 1089–103.

102. Kuramochi-Miyagawa, S. et al., MVH in piRNA processing and gene silencing of retrotransposons. *Genes Dev*, 2010. **24**(9): 887–92.

103. Pal-Bhadra, M. et al., Heterochromatic silencing and HP1 localization in Drosophila are dependent on the RNAi machinery. *Science*, 2004. **303**(5658): 669–72.

104. Watanabe, T. et al., Role for piRNAs and noncoding RNA in de novo DNA methylation of the imprinted mouse Rasgrf1 locus. *Science*, 2011. **332**(6031): 848–52.

105. Navarro, P. et al., Tsix-mediated epigenetic switch of a CTCF-flanked region of the Xist promoter determines the Xist transcription program. *Genes Dev*, 2006. **20**(20): 2787–92.

106. Gupta, R.A. et al., Long non-coding RNA HOTAIR reprograms chromatin state to promote cancer metastasis. *Nature*, 2010. **464**(7291): 1071–6.

107. Rinn, J.L. et al., Functional demarcation of active and silent chromatin domains in human HOX loci by noncoding RNAs. *Cell*, 2007. **129**(7): 1311–23.

108. Guttman, M. et al., Chromatin signature reveals over a thousand highly conserved large non-coding RNAs in mammals. *Nature*, 2009. **458**(7235): 223–7.

109. Murray, S.C. et al., A pre-initiation complex at the 3′-end of genes drives antisense transcription independent of divergent sense transcription. *Nucleic Acids Res*, 2012. **40**(6): 2432–44.

110. Lillycrop, K.A. and G.C. Burdge, Epigenetic changes in early life and future risk of obesity. *Int J Obes (Lond)*, 2011. **35**(1): 72–83.

111. Cox, G.F. et al., Intracytoplasmic sperm injection may increase the risk of imprinting defects. *Am J Hum Genet*, 2002. **71**(1): 162–4.

112. DeBaun, M.R., E.L. Niemitz, and A.P. Feinberg, Association of in vitro fertilization with Beckwith-Wiedemann syndrome and epigenetic alterations of LIT1 and H19. *Am J Hum Genet*, 2003. **72**(1): 156–60.

113. Samantarrai, D. et al., Genomic and epigenomic cross-talks in the regulatory landscape of miRNAs in breast cancer. *Mol Cancer Res*, 2013. **11**(4): 315–28.

114. Lorincz, A.T., The promise and the problems of epigenetics biomarkers in cancer. *Expert Opin Med Diagn*, 2011. **5**(5): 375–9.

115. Wong, I.H., Methylation profiling of human cancers in blood: Molecular monitoring and prognostication (review). *Int J Oncol*, 2001. **19**(6): 1319–24.

116. Xu, X. et al., DNA methylation in peripheral blood measured by LUMA is associated with breast cancer in a population-based study. *FASEB J*, 2012. **26**(6): 2657–66.

117. Feinberg, A.P. et al., Reduced genomic 5-methylcytosine content in human colonic neoplasia. *Cancer Res*, 1988. **48**(5): 1159–61.

118. Baylin, S.B. et al., DNA methylation patterns of the calcitonin gene in human lung cancers and lymphomas. *Cancer Res*, 1986. **46**(6): 2917–22.

119. Esteller, M. et al., A gene hypermethylation profile of human cancer. *Cancer Res*, 2001. **61**(8): 3225–9.

120. Jacinto, F.V. and M. Esteller, Mutator pathways unleashed by epigenetic silencing in human cancer. *Mutagenesis*, 2007. **22**(4): 247–53.

121. Jones, P.A. and S.B. Baylin, The fundamental role of epigenetic events in cancer. *Nat Rev Genet*, 2002. **3**(6): 415–28.

122. Cheung, H.H. et al., DNA methylation of cancer genome. *Birth Defects Res C Embryo Today*, 2009. **87**(4): 335–50.
123. McCabe, M.T., J.C. Brandes, and P.M. Vertino, Cancer DNA methylation: Molecular mechanisms and clinical implications. *Clin Cancer Res*, 2009. **15**(12): 3927–37.
124. Irizarry, R.A. et al., The human colon cancer methylome shows similar hypo- and hypermethylation at conserved tissue-specific CpG island shores. *Nat Genet*, 2009. **41**(2): 178–86.
125. Anderson, O.S., K.E. Sant, and D.C. Dolinoy, Nutrition and epigenetics: An interplay of dietary methyl donors, one-carbon metabolism and DNA methylation. *J Nutr Biochem*, 2012. **23**(8): 853–9.
126. Landan, G. et al., Epigenetic polymorphism and the stochastic formation of differentially methylated regions in normal and cancerous tissues. *Nat Genet*, 2012. **44**(11): 1207–14.
127. Tanay, A. and G. Cavalli, Chromosomal domains: Epigenetic contexts and functional implications of genomic compartmentalization. *Curr Opin Genet Dev*, 2013. **23**(2):197–203.
128. Jones, P.A. and S.B. Baylin, The epigenomics of cancer. *Cell*, 2007. **128**(4): 683–92.
129. Fraga, M.F. et al., Loss of acetylation at Lys16 and trimethylation at Lys20 of histone H4 is a common hallmark of human cancer. *Nat Genet*, 2005. **37**(4): 391–400.
130. Zaenker, K.S., E. Mihich, and E. Liu, Personalized cancer medicine 2011: Toward individualized cancer treatments. *XV International Fritz Bender Symposium, February 21–23, 2011 at Matrix, Biopolis, Singapore. Transl Oncol*, 2011. **4**(4): 199–202.
131. Sandhu, K.S. et al., Large-scale functional organization of long-range chromatin interaction networks. *Cell Rep*, 2012. **2**(5): 1207–19.
132. Davalos, V. et al., Dynamic epigenetic regulation of the microRNA-200 family mediates epithelial and mesenchymal transitions in human tumorigenesis. *Oncogene*, 2012. **31**(16): 2062–74.
133. Calin, G.A. et al., Frequent deletions and down-regulation of micro-RNA genes miR15 and miR16 at 13q14 in chronic lymphocytic leukemia. *Proc Natl Acad Sci USA*, 2002. **99**(24): 15524–9.
134. Zhang, L. et al., MicroRNAs exhibit high frequency genomic alterations in human cancer. *Proc Natl Acad Sci USA*, 2006. **103**(24): 9136–41.
135. Lu, Y. et al., Identification of piRNAs in Hela cells by massive parallel sequencing. *BMB Rep*, 2010. **43**(9): 635–41.
136. Park, C.W. et al., Mature microRNAs identified in highly purified nuclei from HCT116 colon cancer cells. *RNA Biol*, 2010. **7**(5): 606–14.
137. Cichocki, F. et al., Cutting edge: KIR antisense transcripts are processed into a 28-base PIWI-like RNA in human NK cells. *J Immunol*, 2010. **185**(4): 2009–12.
138. Yan, Z. et al., Widespread expression of piRNA-like molecules in somatic tissues. *Nucleic Acids Res*, 2011. **39**(15): 6596–607.
139. Taubert, H. et al., Expression of the stem cell self-renewal gene Hiwi and risk of tumour-related death in patients with soft-tissue sarcoma. *Oncogene*, 2007. **26**(7): 1098–100.
140. Sun, G. et al., Clinical significance of Hiwi gene expression in gliomas. *Brain Res*, 2011. **1373**: 183–8.

141. Lee, J.H. et al., Stem-cell protein Piwil2 is widely expressed in tumors and inhibits apoptosis through activation of Stat3/Bcl-XL pathway. *Hum Mol Genet*, 2006. **15**(2): 201–11.

142. Liu, X. et al., Expression of hiwi gene in human gastric cancer was associated with proliferation of cancer cells. *Int J Cancer*, 2006. **118**(8): 1922–9.

143. Lee, T.I. et al., Control of developmental regulators by Polycomb in human embryonic stem cells. *Cell*, 2006. **125**(2): 301–13.

144. Sharma, A.K. et al., Human CD34(+) stem cells express the hiwi gene, a human homologue of the Drosophila gene piwi. *Blood*, 2001. **97**(2): 426–34.

145. Chen, L. et al., Precancerous stem cells have the potential for both benign and malignant differentiation. *PLoS One*, 2007. **2**(3): e293.

146. Wang, Q.E. et al., Stem cell protein Piwil2 modulates chromatin modifications upon cisplatin treatment. *Mutat Res*, 2011. **708**(1–2): 59–68.

147. Cheng, J. et al., piRNA, the new non-coding RNA, is aberrantly expressed in human cancer cells. *Clin Chim Acta*, 2011. **412**(17–18): 1621–5.

148. Calin, G.A. et al., Ultraconserved regions encoding ncRNAs are altered in human leukemias and carcinomas. *Cancer Cell*, 2007. **12**(3): 215–29.

149. Rossi, S. et al., Cancer-associated genomic regions (CAGRs) and noncoding RNAs: Bioinformatics and therapeutic implications. *Mamm Genome*, 2008. **19**(7–8): 526–40.

150. Lujambio, A. et al., CpG island hypermethylation-associated silencing of non-coding RNAs transcribed from ultraconserved regions in human cancer. *Oncogene*, 2010. **29**(48): 6390–401.

151. Bejerano, G. et al., A distal enhancer and an ultraconserved exon are derived from a novel retroposon. *Nature*, 2006. **441**(7089): 87–90.

152. Scaruffi, P. et al., Transcribed-ultra conserved region expression is associated with outcome in high-risk neuroblastoma. *BMC Cancer*, 2009. **9**: 441.

153. Huarte, M. et al., A large intergenic noncoding RNA induced by p53 mediates global gene repression in the p53 response. *Cell*, 2010. **142**(3): 409–19.

154. Yu, W. et al., Epigenetic silencing of tumour suppressor gene p15 by its antisense RNA. *Nature*, 2008. **451**(7175): 202–6.

155. Cao, X. et al., Noncoding RNAs in the mammalian central nervous system. *Annu Rev Neurosci*, 2006. **29**: 77–103.

156. Schaefer, A. et al., Cerebellar neurodegeneration in the absence of microRNAs. *J Exp Med*, 2007. **204**(7): 1553–8.

157. Shin, D. et al., Dicer ablation in oligodendrocytes provokes neuronal impairment in mice. *Ann Neurol*, 2009. **66**(6): 843–57.

158. Kim, J. et al., A MicroRNA feedback circuit in midbrain dopamine neurons. *Science*, 2007. **317**(5842): 1220–4.

159. Hebert, S.S. et al., Genetic ablation of Dicer in adult forebrain neurons results in abnormal tau hyperphosphorylation and neurodegeneration. *Hum Mol Genet*, 2010. **19**(20): 3959–69.

160. Williams, A.H. et al., MicroRNA-206 delays ALS progression and promotes regeneration of neuromuscular synapses in mice. *Science*, 2009. **326**(5959): 1549–54.

161. Haramati, S. et al., miRNA malfunction causes spinal motor neuron disease. *Proc Natl Acad Sci USA*, 2010. **107**(29): 13111–6.

162. Lee, Y. et al., miR-19, miR-101 and miR-130 co-regulate ATXN1 levels to potentially modulate SCA1 pathogenesis. *Nat Neurosci*, 2008. **11**(10): 1137–9.

163. Wang, W.X. et al., The expression of microRNA miR-107 decreases early in Alzheimer's disease and may accelerate disease progression through regulation of beta-site amyloid precursor protein-cleaving enzyme 1. *J Neurosci*, 2008. **28**(5): 1213–23.
164. Boissonneault, V. et al., MicroRNA-298 and microRNA-328 regulate expression of mouse beta-amyloid precursor protein-converting enzyme 1. *J Biol Chem*, 2009. **284**(4): 1971–81.
165. De Santis, G. et al., Altered miRNA expression in T regulatory cells in course of multiple sclerosis. *J Neuroimmunol*, 2010. **226**(1–2): 165–71.
166. Cox, M.B. et al., MicroRNAs miR-17 and miR-20a inhibit T cell activation genes and are under-expressed in MS whole blood. *PLoS One*, 2010. **5**(8): e12132.
167. Junn, E. et al., Repression of alpha-synuclein expression and toxicity by microRNA-7. *Proc Natl Acad Sci USA*, 2009. **106**(31): 13052–7.
168. Gehrke, S. et al., Pathogenic LRRK2 negatively regulates microRNA-mediated translational repression. *Nature*, 2010. **466**(7306): 637–41.
169. Zhao, Y. et al., Dysregulation of cardiogenesis, cardiac conduction, and cell cycle in mice lacking miRNA-1-2. *Cell*, 2007. **129**(2): 303–17.
170. Yang, B. et al., The muscle-specific microRNA miR-1 regulates cardiac arrhythmogenic potential by targeting GJA1 and KCNJ2. *Nat Med*, 2007. **13**(4): 486–91.
171. van Rooij, E. et al., A signature pattern of stress-responsive microRNAs that can evoke cardiac hypertrophy and heart failure. *Proc Natl Acad Sci USA*, 2006. **103**(48): 18255–60.
172. Fang, Y. et al., MicroRNA-10a regulation of proinflammatory phenotype in athero-susceptible endothelium in vivo and in vitro. *Proc Natl Acad Sci USA*, 2010. **107**(30): 13450–5.
173. Cordes, K.R. et al., miR-145 and miR-143 regulate smooth muscle cell fate and plasticity. *Nature*, 2009. **460**(7256): 705–10.
174. Nicoli, S. et al., MicroRNA-mediated integration of haemodynamics and Vegf signalling during angiogenesis. *Nature*, 2010. **464**(7292): 1196–200.
175. Ji, R. et al., MicroRNA expression signature and antisense-mediated depletion reveal an essential role of MicroRNA in vascular neointimal lesion formation. *Circ Res*, 2007. **100**(11): 1579–88.
176. Clop, A. et al., A mutation creating a potential illegitimate microRNA target site in the myostatin gene affects muscularity in sheep. *Nat Genet*, 2006. **38**(7): 813–8.
177. Sethupathy, P. et al., Human microRNA-155 on chromosome 21 differentially interacts with its polymorphic target in the AGTR1 3′ untranslated region: a mechanism for functional single-nucleotide polymorphisms related to phenotypes. *Am J Hum Genet*, 2007. **81**(2): 405–13.
178. Starczynowski, D.T. et al., Identification of miR-145 and miR-146a as mediators of the 5q- syndrome phenotype. *Nat Med*, 2010. **16**(1): 49–58.
179. Urdinguio, R.G. et al., Disrupted microRNA expression caused by Mecp2 loss in a mouse model of Rett syndrome. *Epigenetics*, 2010. **5**(7): 656–63.
180. Wu, H. et al., Genome-wide analysis reveals methyl-CpG-binding protein 2-dependent regulation of microRNAs in a mouse model of Rett syndrome. *Proc Natl Acad Sci USA*, 2010. **107**(42): 18161–6.
181. Gatto, S. et al., Epigenetic alteration of microRNAs in DNMT3B-mutated patients of ICF syndrome. *Epigenetics*, 2010. **5**(5): 427–43.

182. Faghihi, M.A. et al., Expression of a noncoding RNA is elevated in Alzheimer's disease and drives rapid feed-forward regulation of beta-secretase. *Nat Med*, 2008. **14**(7): 723–30.
183. Martinez, F. et al., Enrichment of ultraconserved elements among genomic imbalances causing mental delay and congenital anomalies. *BMC Med Genomics*, 2010. **3**: 54.
184. Horsthemke, B. and J. Wagstaff, Mechanisms of imprinting of the Prader-Willi/Angelman region. *Am J Med Genet A*, 2008. **146A**(16): 2041–52.
185. Kishore, S. and S. Stamm, The snoRNA HBII-52 regulates alternative splicing of the serotonin receptor 2C. *Science*, 2006. **311**(5758): 230–2.
186. Sahoo, T. et al., Prader-Willi phenotype caused by paternal deficiency for the HBII-85 C/D box small nucleolar RNA cluster. *Nat Genet*, 2008. **40**(6): 719–21.
187. Consortium, E.P. et al., Identification and analysis of functional elements in 1% of the human genome by the ENCODE pilot project. *Nature*, 2007. **447**(7146): 799–816.
188. Ponjavic, J., C.P. Ponting, and G. Lunter, Functionality or transcriptional noise? Evidence for selection within long noncoding RNAs. *Genome Res*, 2007. **17**(5): 556–65.
189. Baccarelli, A. and S. Ghosh, Environmental exposures, epigenetics and cardiovascular disease. *Curr Opin Clin Nutr Metab Care*, 2012. **15**(4): 323–9.
190. Brennan, K. and J.M. Flanagan, Epigenetic epidemiology for cancer risk: Harnessing germline epigenetic variation. *Methods Mol Biol*, 2012. **863**: 439–65.
191. Baskar, R., Emerging role of radiation induced bystander effects: Cell communications and carcinogenesis. *Genome Integr*, 2010. **1**(1): 13.
192. Kovalchuk, A. et al., Epigenetic bystander-like effects of stroke in somatic organs. *Aging (Albany NY)*, 2012. **4**(3): 224–34.
193. Kovalchuk, O. and J.E. Baulch, Epigenetic changes and nontargeted radiation effects—Is there a link? *Environ Mol Mutagen*, 2008. **49**(1): 16–25.
194. Zhou, J. et al., Plasma microRNA panel to diagnose hepatitis B virus-related hepatocellular carcinoma. *J Clin Oncol*, 2011. **29**(36): 4781–8.
195. Banno, K. et al., Epigenetics and genetics in endometrial cancer: New carcinogenic mechanisms and relationship with clinical practice. *Epigenomics*, 2012. **4**(2): 147–62.
196. Deneberg, S., Epigenetics in myeloid malignancies. *Methods Mol Biol*, 2012. **863**: 119–37.
197. Seeber, L.M. and P.J. van Diest, Epigenetics in ovarian cancer. *Methods Mol Biol*, 2012. **863**: 253–69.
198. Hofstetter, B. et al., Impact of genomic methylation on radiation sensitivity of colorectal carcinoma. *Int J Radiat Oncol Biol Phys*, 2010. **76**(5): 1512–9.
199. Boren, T. et al., MicroRNAs and their target messenger RNAs associated with ovarian cancer response to chemotherapy. *Gynecol Oncol*, 2009. **113**(2): 249–55.
200. Crea, F. et al., Epigenetics and chemoresistance in colorectal cancer: An opportunity for treatment tailoring and novel therapeutic strategies. *Drug Resist Updat*, 2011. **14**(6): 280–96.
201. Noushmehr, H. et al., Identification of a CpG island methylator phenotype that defines a distinct subgroup of glioma. *Cancer Cell*, 2010. **17**(5): 510–22.
202. Dubuc, A.M. et al., The epigenetics of brain tumors. *Methods Mol Biol*, 2012. **863**: 139–53.

203. Lorenzen, J.M., F. Martino, and T. Thum, Epigenetic modifications in cardiovascular disease. *Basic Res Cardiol*, 2012. **107**(2): 245.
204. Zaina, S. and G. Lund, Epigenetics: A tool to understand diet-related cardiovascular risk? *J Nutrigenet Nutrigenomics*, 2011. **4**(5): 261–74.
205. Movassagh, M., A. Vujic, and R. Foo, Genome-wide DNA methylation in human heart failure. *Epigenomics*, 2011. **3**(1): 103–9.
206. Barter, M.J., C. Bui, and D.A. Young, Epigenetic mechanisms in cartilage and osteoarthritis: DNA methylation, histone modifications and microRNAs. *Osteoarthritis Cartilage*, 2012. **20**(5): 339–49.
207. Reynard, L.N. and J. Loughlin, Genetics and epigenetics of osteoarthritis. *Maturitas*, 2012. **71**(3): 200–4.
208. Richardson, B. et al., Evidence for impaired T cell DNA methylation in systemic lupus erythematosus and rheumatoid arthritis. *Arthritis Rheum*, 1990. **33**(11): 1665–73.
209. Karouzakis, E. et al., DNA hypomethylation in rheumatoid arthritis synovial fibroblasts. *Arthritis Rheum*, 2009. **60**(12): 3613–22.
210. Nakano, K. et al., DNA methylome signature in rheumatoid arthritis. *Ann Rheum Dis*, 2013. **72**(1): 110–7.
211. Nile, C.J. et al., Methylation status of a single CpG site in the IL6 promoter is related to IL6 messenger RNA levels and rheumatoid arthritis. *Arthritis Rheum*, 2008. **58**(9): 2686–93.
212. Stanczyk, J. et al., Altered expression of MicroRNA in synovial fibroblasts and synovial tissue in rheumatoid arthritis. *Arthritis Rheum*, 2008. **58**(4): 1001–9.
213. Stanczyk, J. et al., Altered expression of microRNA-203 in rheumatoid arthritis synovial fibroblasts and its role in fibroblast activation. *Arthritis Rheum*, 2011. **63**(2): 373–81.
214. Viatte, S., D. Plant, and S. Raychaudhuri, Genetics and epigenetics of rheumatoid arthritis. *Nat Rev Rheumatol*, 2013. **9**(3): 141–53.
215. Liu, Y. et al., Epigenome-wide association data implicate DNA methylation as an intermediary of genetic risk in rheumatoid arthritis. *Nat Biotechnol*, 2013. **31**(2): 142–7.
216. Miao, F. et al., Genome-wide analysis of histone lysine methylation variations caused by diabetic conditions in human monocytes. *J Biol Chem*, 2007. **282**(18): 13854–63.
217. Jayaraman, S., Epigenetic mechanisms of metabolic memory in diabetes. *Circ Res*, 2012. **110**(8): 1039–41.
218. Gaulton, K.J. et al., A map of open chromatin in human pancreatic islets. *Nat Genet*, 2010. **42**(3): 255–9.
219. Stitzel, M.L. et al., Global epigenomic analysis of primary human pancreatic islets provides insights into type 2 diabetes susceptibility loci. *Cell Metab*, 2010. **12**(5): 443–55.
220. Xu, Z., G.M. Lefevre, and G. Felsenfeld, Chromatin structure, epigenetic mechanisms and long-range interactions in the human insulin locus. *Diabetes Obes Metab*, 2012. **14 Suppl 3**: 1–11.
221. Bramswig, N.C. and K.H. Kaestner, Epigenetics and diabetes treatment: An unrealized promise? *Trends Endocrinol Metab*, 2012. **23**(6): 286–91.
222. Khare, S. and M. Verma, Epigenetics of colon cancer. *Methods Mol Biol*, 2012. **863**: 177–85.

223. Burdge, G.C., S.P. Hoile, and K.A. Lillycrop, Epigenetics: Are there implications for personalised nutrition? *Curr Opin Clin Nutr Metab Care*, 2012. **15**(5): 442–7.
224. Weber, W.W., The promise of epigenetics in personalized medicine. *Mol Interv*, 2010. **10**(6): 363–70.
225. Gilbert, J. et al., The clinical application of targeting cancer through histone acetylation and hypomethylation. *Clin Cancer Res*, 2004. **10**(14): 4589–96.
226. Karberg, S., Switching on epigenetic therapy. *Cell*, 2009. **139**(6): 1029–31.
227. Spannhoff, A., W. Sippl, and M. Jung, Cancer treatment of the future: Inhibitors of histone methyltransferases. *Int J Biochem Cell Biol*, 2009. **41**(1): 4–11.
228. Marks, P.A. and R. Breslow, Dimethyl sulfoxide to vorinostat: Development of this histone deacetylase inhibitor as an anticancer drug. *Nat Biotechnol*, 2007. **25**(1): 84–90.
229. Yoo, C.B. and P.A. Jones, Epigenetic therapy of cancer: Past, present and future. *Nat Rev Drug Discov*, 2006. **5**(1): 37–50.
230. Jones, K.L. et al., The magic nature of (132)Sn explored through the single-particle states of (133)Sn. *Nature*, 2010. **465**(7297): 454–7.
231. Tan, Y.O. et al., A blood-based epigenetic test for early detection of nasopharyngeal carcinoma (NPC), in American Society of Clinical Oncology (ASCO), *J Clin Oncol*, 2013. **31**(suppl, abstr 6063).
232. Schones, D.E. and K. Zhao, Genome-wide approaches to studying chromatin modifications. *Nat Rev Genet*, 2008. **9**(3): 179–91.
233. Jones, P.A., The AACR human epigenome task force and EUNE SAB. Moving AHEAD with an international human epigenome project. *Nature*, 2010. **454**: 711–5.
234. Heyn, H. and M. Esteller, DNA methylation profiling in the clinic: Applications and challenges. *Nat Rev Genet*, 2012. **13**(10): 679–92.

4

Biomarkers and Precision Medicine: The Case of Rare Diseases

Candida Fratazzi and Claudio Carini

CONTENTS

4.1 Introduction

Personalized medicine helps to move the population-based evidence of therapeutic interventions toward individual evidence on how to treat the specific person based on the biological profile, clinical history, and environment. The aim of precision medicine is to offer personalized health care to everyone. Precision medicine is based on the integration of individual information, from genome and cellular phenotype to the interaction with the personal environment leading toward a proactive, preventive, and prospective model of patient care [1–3], contrary to the more traditional reactive approach to the health status of an individual.

Traditionally, precision medicine has been applied to oncology, cardiovascular diseases, and recently to autoimmune diseases.

In recent years, rare disease (RD) has become an important topic raising considerable interest for both translational research and the application of precision medicine to individual patients.

During the past few decades, several efforts have been made to identify appropriate prognostic and predictive factors in many of the rare diseases (RDs). Indeed, although what may be seen as a commonality among RDs in terms of biochemistry or molecular underpinnings, this further defines the biochemical and molecular characteristics thus, making each RD a rather unique entity. RDs are a broad and heterogeneous group of severe and disabling disorders, involving a small number of individuals in specific populations. Thus, the situation today reflects the partial knowledge we have about this conglomerate of diseases, so that why very few "biomarkers" are available in most of these RDs to assist the clinicians to know, which patients *a priori* will suffer from more severe manifestations or will benefit the most from specific therapies.

Eight percent of RDs are estimated to be genetic, mostly monogenic. Knowledge about the genetic causes, mutations, and the underlying pathomechanisms is very important to further address RD translational research and clinical medicine. As previously mentioned, therapeutic options in RD are generally scarce and ineffective. However, the development of new therapies for these diseases aimed at specific molecular targets for RD. This may be useful not only for RD but also for the common diseases that may share such biological targets or pathophysiological pathways.

RDs are now becoming targets for precision medicine approaches, owing to the view that individual susceptibility might now be explained by the subject's genetic background and the epigenetic changes. Based on this paradigm, a massive increase in data generated by different types of novel high-throughput technologies is resulting in a great amount of traditional phenotypes being split into different diseases. Applying omic approaches in a chosen group of RDs should help in understanding the clinical heterogeneity of certain individual RDs as well as in revealing the pathophysiological commonalities between different clinical RDs.

Biomarkers (BMs) are now needed to speed up precision medicine for RDs and monitor diagnosis and responses to therapies. BMs are clearly the drivers in identifying and developing new drugs for RDs.

It is widely recognized that BMs play a critical role in disease diagnosis and treatment. Recent omic technologies such as transcriptomics, proteomics, metabonomics, and others are important in accelerating the rate of BM discovery [4]. Several research initiatives have been investigating BMs for RD, for example, Huntington's disease [8], pulmonary arterial hypertension [5], Hailey–Hailey disease [6,7], hepatoblastoma [8], and multiple osteochondroma [4].

However, it is crucial that the BMs used in the clinic get validated. The approach of validating a BM has to be addressed clearly. The major challenge for BM validation is the high degree of variability of BM levels across the population and the considerable molecular heterogeneity of individual RDs [9]. The main challenge in BMs identification for precision medicine in RDs is that they may be common to other diseases and partly specific for RDs. A better understanding of RDs will increase our awareness of RDs, improving the clinical and molecular diagnosis, which will result in early application of the available therapeutic intervention. RDs, which are often disregarded by the pharma companies, can instead be considered a benchmark for testing models that will help us in understanding other more common diseases [10].

Specific requirements are needed for selecting a BM: (1) it should be technically feasible; (2) easy to measure; (3) useful, with a consistent relative magnitude between treated and untreated subjects; (4) clinically reliable, precise, and accurate; (5) classifiable as a strong predictive or prognostic. In recruiting patients with lysosomal disorders for clinical trials, the use of BMs is a double-edged sword: whereas biomarkers may meet all of the above criteria, they must be clearly related to the disease burden in the vast majority of patients and also be capable of detecting at both ends of the spectrum, from very mild-to-severe patients, and equally reactive to specific therapy within the same range. If all these prerequisites cannot be met, then the use of the BM may be unjustified clinically. The purpose of this chapter is to review the literature and practice of BMs in lysosomal storage diseases and use current practices to discuss guidelines for the use of BMs in upcoming clinical trials.

4.2 Identification of Specific Lysosomal Storage Diseases

The more rare a disease is, the more likely it is that BMs are unavailable. In terms of some of the lysosomal diseases, of which there are more than 50 separate diseases, there are actually no universally recognized BMs other than specific protein (enzyme) or substrate markers. Thus, for four mucoploysaccharidoses disorders (MPS I, MPS II, MPS III, and MPS VI) and Pompe disease, Gaucher disease, and Fabry disease, there are protein markers, either enzymes or macrophage BMs; and for seven diseases (MPS I, MPS II, MPS IIIA, MPS IIIB, MPS IVA, MPS VII, and Fabry disease), there are substrate markers [10]. Urinary heparan sulfates can be used to differentiate MPS IIIC (Sanfilippo C syndrome) and MPS II (Hunter disease) [11], keratin sulfate to identify MPS IV and possibly other MPS disorders [12] and antibodies against gangliosides, that is, anti-G_{M2} and anti-G_{M3} based on animal modeling. Monoclonal and/or polyclonal antibodies have been generated against diseases' enzymes. Immunohistochemical techniques, which can also be used to identify proteins [13], may prove to have considerable potential as predictive markers if teamed with other techniques such as mass spectrometry or various forms of chromatography.

In the first decade of the 2000s, Chamoles [14] has developed assays to identify various enzymes whose deficiencies implicated a lysosomal disorder: α-L-iduronidase (MPS I), α-galactosidase (Fabry disease), β-D-galactosidase (G_{M1} gangliosidosis), and others were developed [15–20]. This multiplex assay led to the identification of enzymes for Fabry, Gaucher, Hurler,

Krabbe, Niemann-Pick A/B, and Pompe diseases [21], raising the need to utilize simple and reliable diagnostic markers for patient's identification, given the fact that new specific therapies were of imminent development. The methodological advancement highlights the importance of using an easily obtainable patient sample that can be shipped worldwide without special precautions. For the majority of the above enzymes, the filter paper system is reliable; however, in Pompe disease, for example, measured α-glucosidase activity may be a composite of other activities, making this specific assay less reliable. However, in cases where inhibition of nonspecific (substrate) activities cannot be totally suppressed, other assays such as immune-capture need to be used [22].

There have also been evidences for the use of diagnostic BMs from amniotic fluid in lysosomal disorders, with the express purpose of distinguishing normal from affected and even correlation with specific storage material in some of the disorders [23,24]. Within the past few years, the list of diseases that can be profiled on the basis of various proteins, oligosaccharides, and glycolipids include six MPS disorders and at least eight other diseases.

Of note is a urinary measure of oligosaccharides (glycosaminoglycan derivatives) which has met the criteria of sensitivity and specificity in identifying individuals with MPS disorders and, based on unique profiles, can differentiate among (all but MPS IIIB and MPS IIIC) subtypes [24].

Generally, to be useful, a BM has to show correlation with clinical disease expression, that is, predictive or prognostic value must be proven. A urinary diagnostic test that may be an appropriate marker of both disease progression and response to therapy is urinary globotriaosylceramide (Gb_3) in Fabry disease [21], although residual enzyme activity in the blood is a poorer marker of disease status. Similarly, in Gaucher disease, the most common lysosomal storage disorder, which has a range of clinical expression from virtually asymptomatic octogenarians to lethal neonatal forms, residual activity is a poor predictor of disease severity. Therefore, in other diseases, a combination of analyses of enzyme activity with genotype or molecular phenotypes has been recommended, for example, in MPS II (Hunter disease), to improve predictability. In summary, within the past few decades, various specific assays have been developed that identify patients with enzyme deficiencies and can even quantify residual enzyme activity (relative to normal controls), based on the kinetics model of Conzelmann and Sandhoff [25] of a correlation between lipid accumulation and deficient enzyme activity [26], but residual activity is not always correlated with clinical status. Alternatively, improper or "derailed" processing of the enzyme may be indicative of disease severity since these enzymes undergo trafficking from endosome to Golgi to lysosome. This thinking has been applied in estimates of lysosomal-associated membrane proteins (LAMP-1 and LAMP-2) with the expectation of uncovering a processing defect common to all lysosomal disorders that would also be predictive of disease severity [27], but this was not proven. It has also been suggested that mutant enzyme variants may be retained in the endoplasmic reticulum and that this may be one of the factors that determine disease severity [28].

Accumulation of lipid in the endosomes or lysosomes was shown to characterize variants of Type C Niemann–Pick disease because of the presence of cholesterol [29], thereby making this a good marker, but again, this was true only for a highly specific variant of this rare disorder. It should be noted that one ramification from these and similar findings is that response to therapy, even if the modality is identical for more than one lysosomal disease, may not be uniquely or sensitively monitored using nondisease-specific markers.

4.3 Identification of Clinical Markers

Clinical markers with a predictive or prognostic value would be attractive if quantifiable and if assessment was noninvasive. It was hoped that the use of animal models would be illustrative of human conditions. In a recent study of murine MPS I, Braunlin et al. [30] demonstrated that "murine MPS I is not identical to human MPS I" [31] and each has unique clinical features. Nonetheless, a more recent study by Randall et al. 2006 [32] in murine MPS I, employing proteomic analysis of heparin cofactor II-thrombin (HCII-T), showed highly elevated serum levels in mice and in human patients that were correlated with disease severity and responsive to therapy [33]. HCII-T may therefore indeed meet the requirements of a good BM for MPS I, given that it implicates a specific pathophysiology. A second good example in the MPSs is the use of accumulation of a disaccharide (HNS-UA), a marker of heparin sulfate storage in disease-specific sites of MPS IIIA [33], because the rate of accumulation is commensurate with disease severity at these sites and is appropriately reactive to disease-specific therapy.

Along these lines, therefore, it is commendable to find disease-specific parameters that lend themselves to quantification and test correlation with clinical severity and responsiveness to therapy. Biopsies and bone marrow aspirations or repeat radiological workups to stage severity should not be condoned if there is a better option, even, some might say, if that option does not exactly meet our criteria of a "good" BM. In Gaucher disease, because of concern about Gaucher-related skeletal involvement as associated with considerable morbidity, one study showed a reduction in osteoblast and osteoclast bone markers [34], but there was no correlation with incidence of bone pathology [35]. BMs in this sense might therefore be misleading. Another example in Fabry disease showed no correlation between plasma concentrations of endothelial markers or homocysteine with response to therapy, although endothelial and leukocyte activation is a good measure of renal and cardiovascular involvement in Fabry disease [31].

4.4 Inflammatory Markers as Secondary BMs

Among the most prevalent hypothetical constructs used in lysosomal storage disorders is that of inflammation as a mediator, either as a causative or consequent effect, of lipid storage material. A pathway common to all MPS disorders (originally to describe MPS VI and MPS VII) has been developed based on inflammatory reactivity of connective tissues correlated with metalloproteinases in chondrocytes [36], but it is not a qualitative measure of severity or responsiveness to therapy. In G_{M1} gangliosidosis, assessment of inflammatory cerebrospinal fluid markers showed correlation with clinical course but were not responsive to therapeutic interventions because it is known that neuronal apoptosis and abnormalities in the central nervous system are secondary to storage [37]. However, in a mouse model of gangliosidoses that showed disease progression with increased inflammatory cells in the microglia, the difference in G_{M1} (Sandhoff disease) and G_{M2} gangliosidosis (Tay–Sachs and late-onset Tay–Sachs disease) models was the timing of the onset of clinical signs [38], which is not always taken into consideration. Thus, while inflammation may be postulated to be either a primary or secondary index of disease activity, not all markers meet the criteria of sensitivity or clinical relevance. Similarly, in an early study of Gaucher disease using macrophage-derived inflammatory markers, there were some cytokines that correlated with disease severity and clinical parameters, but the results were equivocal in many markers [39]. In a knockout mouse model of Types A and B of Niemann–Pick disease, the macrophage inflammatory cytokine MIP-1α was elevated in disease-specific sites and declined with therapy [40], but this marker cannot be disease specific. On a global level, however, mouse models for the various lysosomal disorders have recently shown a connection between lipid storage in the endosome or lysosome and invariant natural killer T (iNKT) cell function, indicative of thymic involvement; however, these findings would conflict with the theory of elaboration of inflammatory markers in lysosomal storage disorders [41].

4.5 Macrophage Surrogate BMs

Of the many avenues attempted in the various common and less common lysosomal storage diseases, none has provided a satisfactory BM. This is a distinct disadvantage when the alternative may be invasive procedures. A class of BMs has been incorporated into the evaluation initially of Gaucher disease, but now also of Fabry disease and Type B Niemann–Pick disease, which are surrogate in the sense that they measure the plasma levels of macrophage lipid or chemokines. Examples of this class are chitotriosidase and C–C chemokine ligand 18 (CCL 18; also called pulmonary and activation-regulated chemokine, PARC), which can be measured in plasma and in urine. Chitotriosidase in Gaucher disease [42] was considered a specific marker of disease severity and then as a measure of response to therapy [43]. Among the methodological issues with using chitotriosidase is that it is genetically deficient in 6% of all individuals and genotyping should be performed. The surrogate marker CCL18/PARC was then introduced [43] because it had the advantage of being present in all individuals, yet it is not nearly as elevated in patients with Gaucher disease relative to healthy individuals. An advantage of CCL18/PARC over chitotriosidase assays is the less difficult assay of CCL18/PARC. In male patients with Fabry disease, the chitotriosidase levels were found to be significantly elevated but were not correlated with disease severity, although in some cases they may have normalized with therapy [44]. In two siblings with Type B Niemann–Pick disease, there were elevated levels of both markers, which were not commensurate with clinical severity [43]. Recently, the urinary levels of chitotriosidase and CCL 18/PARC have been measured in Gaucher disease, but they do not appear to correlate with the plasma levels, although there was correlation after exposure to treatment [45]. Interestingly, despite the popularity of chitotriosidase as a putative BM and its indirect relationship to disease-specific parameters, it has nonetheless led to its use in testing other nonspecific markers [46]. This, of course, should not be the intention of BMs (i.e., that they correlate with each other) because then one would get caught up in loops of correlation, not one of which is directly related to a disease-specific parameter.

4.6 BMs and Clinical Trials

Initiation of clinical trials is a costly and time-consuming commitment which has as a goal decreased the time to market of a novel modality that will be a gold standard. This is definitely the case in RDs, where the availability of a single therapeutic option that is safe and effective may be the only hope of affected individuals. If a pharmaceutical company undertakes commitment to a clinical trial in a rare disorder, the candidate modality must have tremendous promise to survive rigorous examination of the preclinical stages. By the time a putative therapy achieves Phase II or Phase III status, the patients too will be highly motivated to see a successful treatment brought to market. Thus, on the one hand, there is an incentive for the company and for the patients to get the treatment into the market but, on the other, there is awareness that in clinical trials of patients, many hopeful candidate therapies do not meet their primary outcome measures, resulting in dismissal of that option.

Choosing outcome measures for clinical trials is both a science and an art in RDs because of the paucity of candidate patients. The current practice is to have primary and secondary endpoints. In the past, BMs have been seen as adjuncts in assessing clinical efficacy of therapy. However, recently, the popularity of BMs has increased and they are being recognized by the regulatory agencies, especially since they have been regarded as crucial for the registration of some oncological drugs. In RDs, however, one must be cautious in applying BMs merely because they are more convenient to assess compared to disease-specific clinical endpoints.

It should be said that BMs are not all equal in their capacity to be of predictive or prognostic value. This has to be taken into consideration in establishing whether to include a BM as an outcome measure. Similarly, there is a difference between markers that measure disease-specific events and those that substitute clinical endpoints (as is the case for surrogate markers). In making clinical decisions, one should create a good balance between putatively related markers and clinically relevant parameters that correlate well with disease severity.

4.7 Conclusions

BMs are a means to better prediction and follow-up, especially from the perspective of regulatory issues involving diagnostics and novel therapeutic options. This is even more cogent in cases where ancillary or additive therapies are considered to "fine-tune" previously achieved therapeutic achievements.

References

1. Snydeman R, Yoediono Z, 2006. Prospective care: A personalized preventive approach to medicine. *Pharmacogenomics* 7:5–9.
2. Snydeman R, Langheier J, 2006. Prospective health care: The second transformation of medicine. *Genome Biol.* 7:104.
3. Snydeman R, 2009. The role of genomics in enabling prospective health care. In *Genomic and Personalized Medicine* (Vol. 1). Willard HF and Ginsburg GD (eds.) Academic Press, Elsevier Inc, San Diego, USA, 378–385.
4. Zuntini M, Salvatore M, Pedrini E et al., 2010. MicroRNA profiling of multiple osteochondromas: Identification of disease-specific and normal cartilage signature. *Clin. Genet.* 78:507–516.
5. Heresi GA, Dweik RA, 2010. Biomarkers in pulmonary hypertension. *Pulmonary Vasc. Res. Inst. Rev.* 2:12–16.

6. Manca S, Magrelli A, Cialfi S et al. Oxidative stress activation of miR-125b is part of the molecular switch for Hailey–Hailey disease manifestations. *Exp. Dermatol.* 11:932–937.

7. Cialfi S, Oliviero C, Ceccarelli S et al., 2010. Complex multipathways alterations and oxidative stress are associated with Hailey–Hailey disease. *Br. J. Dermatol.* 162:518–526.

8. Magrelli A, Azzalin G, Salvatore M et al., 2009. Altered micro RNA expression patterns in hepatoblastoma patients. *Transl Onc.* 2:157–163.

9. Zhang XW, Li L, Wei D, Yap YL, Chen F, 2007. Moving cancer diagnostics from bench to bedside. *Trends Biotechnol.* 2:166–173.

10. Parkinson-Lawrence E, Fuller M, Hopwood JJ, Meikle PJ, Brooks DA, 2006. Immunochemistry of lysosomal storage disorders. *Clin Chem* 52:1660–1668.

11. Toma L, Dietrich CP, Nader HB, 1996. Differences in the nonreducing ends of heparan sulfates excreted by patients with mucopolysaccharidoses revealed by bacterial heparitinases: A new tool for structural studies and differential diagnosis of Sanfilippo's and Hunter's syndromes. *Lab Invest* 75:771–781.

12. Tomatsu S, Okamura K, Maeda H, Taketani T, Castrillon SV, Gutierrez MA, Nishioka T et al. 2005. Keratan sulphate levels in mucopolysaccharidoses and mucolipidoses. *J Inherit Metab Dis* 28:187–202.

13. Walkley SU, 2004. Secondary accumulation of gangliosides in lysosomal storage disorders. *Semin Cell Dev Biol* 15:433–444.

14. Chamoles NA, Blanco M, Gaggioli D, Cosentini C, 2002. Tay-Sachs and Sandhoff diseases: Enzymatic diagnosis in dried blood spots on filter papers retrospective diagnosis in new born screening cards. *Clin. Chim. Acta* 318:133–137.

15. Chamoles NA, Blanco M, Gaggioli D, 2001. Diagnosis of alpha-L-iduronidase deficiency in dried blood spots on filter paper: The possibility of newborn diagnosis. *Clin Chem* 47:780–781.

16. Chamoles NA, Blanco M, Gaggioli D, 2001. Fabry disease: Enzymatic diagnosis in dried blood spots on filter paper. *Clin Chim Acta* 308(1–2):195–196.

17. Chamoles NA, Blanco MB, Iorcansky S, Gaggioli D, Specola N, Casentini C, 2001. Retrospective diagnosis of GM1 gangliosidosis by use of a newborn-screening card. *Clin Chem* 47:2068.

18. Chamoles NA, Blanco MB, Gaggioli D, Casentini C, 2001. Hurler-like phenotype: Enzymatic diagnosis in dried blood spots on filter paper. *Clin Chem* 47:2098–2102.

19. Chamoles NA, Blanco M, Gaggioli D, Casentini C, 2002. Gaucher and Niemann–Pick diseases—Enzymatic diagnosis in dried blood spots on filter paper: Retrospective diagnoses in newborn-screening cards. *Clin Chim Acta* 317: 191–197.

20. Chamoles NA, Niizawa G, Blanco M, Gaggioli D, Casentini C, 2004. Glycogen storage disease type II: Enzymatic screening in dried blood spots on filter paper. *Clin Chim Acta* 347:97–102.

21. Whitfield PD, Calvin J, Hogg S, O'Driscoll E, Halsall D, Burling K, Maguire G et al. 2005. Monitoring enzyme replacement therapy in Fabry disease—Role of urine globotriaosylceramide. *J Inherit Metab Dis* 28:21–33.

22. Fuller M, Lovejoy M, Hopwood JJ, Meikle PJ, 2005. Immunoquantification of beta-glucosidase: Diagnosis and prediction of severity in Gaucher disease. *Clin Chem* 51:2200–2202.

23. Ramsay SL, Maire I, Bindloss C, Fuller M, Whitfield PD, Piraud M, Hopwood JJ, Meikle PJ, 2004. Determination of oligosaccharides and glycolipids in amniotic fluid by electrospray ionisation tandem mass spectrometry: In utero indicators of lysosomal storage diseases. *Mol Genet Metab* 83:231–238.

24. Fuller M, Rozaklis T, Ramsay SL, Hopwood JJ, Meikle PJ, 2004. Disease-specific markers for the mucopolysaccharidoses. *Pediatr Res* 56:733–738.

25. Conzelmann E, Sandhoff K, 1991. Biochemical basis of late-onset neurolipidoses. *Dev Neurosci* 13:197–204.

26. Schueler UH, Kolter T, Kaneski CR, Zirzow G, Sandhoff K, Brady RO, 2004. Correlation between enzyme activity and substrate storage in a cell culture model system for Gaucher disease. *J Inherit Metab Dis* 27:649–658.

27. Zimmer KP, le Coutre P, Aerts HM, Harzer K, Fukuda M, O'Brien JS, Naim HY, 1999. Intracellular transport of acid beta-glucosidase and lysosome-associated membrane proteins is affected in Gaucher's disease (G202R mutation). *J Pathol* 188:407–414.

28. Ron I, Horowitz M, 2005. ER retention and degradation as the molecular basis underlying Gaucher disease heterogeneity. *Hum Mol Genet* 14:2387–2398.

29. Sun X, Marks DL, Park WD, Wheatley CL, Puri V, O'Brien JF, Kraft DL et al. 2001. Niemann–Pick C variant detection by altered sphingolipid trafficking and correlation with mutations within a specific domain of NPC1. *Am J Hum Genet* 68(6):1361–1372.

30. Braunlin E, Mackey-Bojack S, Panoskaltsis-Mortari A, Berry JM, McElmurry RT, Riddle M, Sun LY, Clarke LA, Tolar J, Blazar BR, 2006. Cardiac functional and histopathologic findings in humans and mice with mucopolysaccharidosis type I: Implications for assessment of therapeutic interventions in hurler syndrome. *Pediatr Res* 59:27–32.

31. Demuth K, Germain DP, 2002. Endothelial markers and homocysteine in patients with classic Fabry disease. *Acta Paediatr Suppl* 91:57–61.

32. Randall DR, Sinclair GB, Colobong KE, Hetty E, Clarke LA, 2006. Heparin cofactor II-thrombin complex in MPS I: A biomarker of MPS disease. *Mol Genet Metab* 88:235–243.

33. King B, Savas P, Fuller M, Hopwood J, Hemsley K, 2006. Validation of a heparan sulfate-derived disaccharide as a marker of accumulation in murine mucopolysaccharidosis type IIIA. *Mol Genet Metab* 87:107–112.

34. Drugan C, Jebeleanu G, Grigorescu-Sido P, Caillaud C, Craciun AM, 2002. Biochemical markers of bone turnover as tools in the evaluation of skeletal involvement in patients with type 1 Gaucher disease. *Blood Cells Mol Dis* 28:13–20.

35. Ciana G, Addobbati R, Tamaro G, Leopaldi A, Nevyjel M, Ronfani L, Vidoni L, Pittis MG, Bembi B, 2005. Gaucher disease and bone: Laboratory and skeletal mineral density variations during a long period of enzyme replacement therapy. *J Inherit Metab Dis* 28:723–732.

36. Simonaro CM, D'Angelo M, Haskins ME, Schuchman EH, 2005. Joint and bone disease in mucopolysaccharidoses VI and VII: Identification of new therapeutic targets and biomarkers using animal models. *Pediatr Res* 57:701–707.

37. Satoh H, Yamato O, Asano T, Yonemura M, Yamauchi T, Hasegawa D, Orima H, Arai T, Yamasaki M, Maede Y, 2007. Cerebrospinal fluid biomarkers showing neurodegeneration in dogs with GM1 gangliosidosis: Possible use for assessment of a therapeutic regimen. *Brain Res* 1133:200–208.

38. Jeyakumar M, Thomas R, Elliot-Smith E, Smith DA, van der Spoel AC, d'Azzo A, Perry VH, Butters TD, Dwek RA, Platt FM, 2003. Central nervous system inflammation is a hallmark of pathogenesis in mouse models of GM1 and GM2 gangliosidosis. *Brain* 126:974–987.
39. Hollak CE, Evers L, Aerts JM, van Oers MH, 1997. Elevated levels of M-CSF, sCD14 and IL8 in type 1 Gaucher disease. *Blood Cells Mol Dis* 123:201–212.
40. Dhami R, Passini MA, Schuchman EH, 2006. Identification of novel biomarkers for Niemann–Pick disease using gene expression analysis of acid sphingomyelinase knockout mice. *Mol Ther* 13:556–564.
41. Gadola SD, Silk JD, Jeans A, Illarionov PA, Salio M, Besra GS, Dwek R, Butters TD, Platt FM, Cerundolo V, 2006. Impaired selection of invariant natural killer T cells in diverse mouse models of glycosphingolipid lysosomal storage diseases. *J Exp Med* 203:2293–2303.
42. Hollak CE, van Weely S, van Oers MH, Aerts JM, 1994. Marked elevation of plasma chitotriosidase activity. A novel hallmark of Gaucher disease. *J Clin Invest* 93:1288–1292.
43. Czartoryska B, Tylki-Szymanska A, Gorska D, 1998. Serum chitotriosidase activity in Gaucher patients on enzyme replacement therapy (ERT). *Clin Biochem* 31:417–420.
44. Boot RG, Verhoek M, de Fost M, Hollak CE, Maas M, Bleijlevens B, van Breemen MJ et al. 2004. Marked elevation of the chemokine CCL18/PARC in Gaucher disease: A novel surrogate marker for assessing therapeutic intervention. *Blood* 103:33–39.
45. Vedder AC, Cox-Brinkman J, Hollak CE, Linthorst GE, Groener JE, Helmond MT, Scheij S, Aerts JM, 2006. Plasma chitotriosidase in male Fabry patients: A marker for monitoring lipid-laden macrophages and their correction by enzyme replacement therapy. *Mol Genet Metab* 89:239–244.
46. Brinkman J, Wijburg FA, Hollak CE, Groener JE, Verhoek M, Scheij S, Aten J, Boot RG, Aerts JM, 2005. Plasma chitotriosidase and CCL18: Early biochemical surrogate markers in type B Niemann–Pick disease. *J Inherit Metab Dis* 28:13–20.

5

Biomarker-Informed Adaptive Design

Jing Wang, Mark Chang, and Sandeep Menon

CONTENTS

5.1 Introduction

Personalized medicine aims to deliver the right drug to the right patient. In addition to discovering the right drug, finding the right dose, and identifying the right patient, it's also desirable to shorten the time of drug development in order to bring the drug to the patient faster. Different clinical trial designs have been proposed for this purpose. One such design is a seamless phase II/III drop-the-losers (or pick-the-winner) design, which has the potential to terminate the inferior treatment groups (i.e., the "losers") early if no efficacy is shown. It minimizes "white space" between phase II and phase III of the studies, and efficiently uses all the patient data both in the learning and confirming phases.

Statistical methods exist for controlling the type I error rate and constructing estimators for the drop-the-losers design. Stallard and Todd [1], Kelly et al. [2], and Stallard and Friede [3] proposed approaches for sequential trials; Bauer and Kieser [4] considered the method of combining p-values from different stages; Sampson and Sill [5] developed a uniformly most powerful conditionally unbiased test (UMPCU) for normally distributed data; Chang et al. [6] suggested the contrast test with a p-value combination method.

All methods considered above are for trials where the same endpoint is used for both the interim and final analyses of the study. However, the benefits of such a design or method could be limited if it takes very long to obtain the primary endpoint measurements at the interim. For example, in oncology trials, it usually takes 12–24 months to observe overall survival—the most commonly used and preferred regulatory primary endpoint. The long time needed to reach the interim analyses can present potential operational challenges [7] and may delay bringing a drug to the market.

Considerable interest has been drawn toward the short-term endpoint ("biomarker")-informed adaptive seamless phase II/III designs. These designs incorporate biomarker information at the interim stages of the study. The decision(s) on interim adaptation can be made based upon the biomarker only or on the available joint information of the biomarker and the primary endpoint.

Todd and Stallard [8] presented a group sequential design for which the interim treatment selection is based upon a biomarker. Stallard [9] considered a design that uses both the available biomarker and primary endpoint information for treatment selection. He proposed a method for the adjustment of the usual group sequential boundaries to maintain strong control of the familywise type I error rate. Friede et al. [10] brought together combination tests for adaptive designs and the closure principle for multiple testing, which allowed them to achieve control of the familywise type I error rate in the strong sense. Shun et al. [11] presented a "Two-Stage Winner Design" with normal interim and final endpoint, where the unconditional distribution of the final test statistic was derived for the design with two active treatment arms. They also proposed a normal approximation approach for the final distribution. Liu and Pledger [12], Li et al. [13], and Li et al. [14] considered cases where more than one treatment can be selected at the interim. Scala and Glimm [15] discussed application of the design when the endpoints are time-to-event data. Jenkins et al. [16] proposed a design with time-to-event endpoints that allows subgroup selection based upon biomarker at the interim, and methodology was presented which controls the type I error rate.

Biomarker-informed adaptive designs could be very helpful for the development of personalized medicine, if the biomarker used at the interim is a good indicator of the primary endpoint.

5.2 Motivations and Concepts

To conduct a drug trial that uses biomarker-informed adaptive procedures, statistical simulations are suggested to be performed first in order to understand the operating characteristics, including sample size for a target power, of the design. The conventional approach uses the one-level (individual level only) correlation model, together with historical knowledge, to describe the relationship between the biomarker and the primary endpoint. This approach can easily wrongly estimate the power of a biomarker-informed design if there is no well-established knowledge about how the biomarker and the primary endpoint are correlated. When the rank order of mean responses of the biomarker for each treatment group is assumed to be the same as that of the primary endpoint based on historical observations, the power of the design is very possible to be overestimated by the conventional model, as the uncertainty of the historical knowledge has been ignored. In this case, the sample size suggested by simulation may lead to an underpowered trial.

The approval rate for NDAs (new drug applications) submitted to the FDA recently is about 40% [17]. This fact indicates that there are trials that are underpowered. It is desirable to propose approaches that lead to a reasonable assessment of clinical trial designs.

Wang et al. [18] have proposed a two-level correlation model to assess the performance of biomarker-informed adaptive designs. This model considers not only the individual level correlation between the biomarker and the primary endpoint, but also accounts for the variability of the estimated mean level correlation (or "mean level association"). The uncertainty due to a small sample size of historical data about the relationship between the biomarker and primary endpoint is considered in the model. This chapter is to describe this two-level correlation model and to assess the performance of biomarker-informed adaptive designs using this model.

The new model is illustrated in the context of a two-stage winner design with three active treatment arms and a control arm. We assume both biomarker and primary endpoint are normally distributed, the distribution of the final test statistic of the design is proposed, and the type I error rate control issue is discussed. The new approach is shown to provide a more reasonable and sensible assessment for the biomarker-informed adaptive designs.

Throughout this chapter, we want to deliver the message that the conventional one-level correlation model is not sufficient for modeling the relationship between the biomarker and primary endpoint in a biomarker-informed adaptive design. The shape of mean level correlation, as well as the uncertainty about the shape, needs to be considered.

5.3 Issues in Conventional One-Level Correlation Model

The conventional one-level correlation model used for describing the relationship of the two endpoints in a biomarker-informed adaptive design considers only the individual level correlation (ρ). If the one-level correlation model is used in statistical simulations for biomarker-informed designs, the means of the two endpoints have to be specified based on the historical knowledge (see Li et al. [14]). In this way, there would not be much difference in power between different values of correlation coefficient ρ between the biomarker and the primary endpoint.

Friede et al. [10] pointed out that the effect of the individual level correlation ρ between the endpoints on power is small if the means of the biomarker in treatment groups are fixed and are different. In their paper, the authors showed (see Figure 2a) how the estimated power of a biomarker-informed design has changed for different estimations of treatment difference in the biomarker. As shown in their figure, there is almost no difference in the power of the design for different values of the correlation coefficient ρ. For example, when the estimated treatment difference in the biomarker is 0.2, the estimated power of their design changes from around 83% to 85% as ρ increases from 0 to 1. Li et al. [14] also mentioned that the influence of ρ on power is really small when compared to other factors. Their paper showed an increase in simulated power from 70.5% to 73.7% as ρ increased from 0.2 to 0.8. We ran simulations for a "two-stage winner design" [11] with a survival primary endpoint. The design was assumed to have five active treatment arms and one control arm, with fixed survival means 2.46, 2.71, 3.67, 3.32, 3, and 2.22 for each treatment arm, respectively, and fixed biomarker log-means 1.6, 1.7, 2, 1.9, 1.8, and 1.5. The critical value for the final test statistic was obtained by simulation with the type I error rate at 0.05 level. Our simulation results (Table 5.1) are consistent with the previous findings.

TABLE 5.1

Power Evaluation for Two-Stage Winner Design Using Conventional One-Level Model

ρ	Censoring Rate	Interim Size	Max Size	Power (%)	Power with Best Treatment (%)
0.3	0.2	72	216	96.48	66.65
0.5	0.2	72	216	96.91	66.29
0.8	0.2	72	216	97.37	67.71

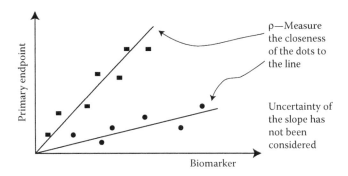

FIGURE 5.1
Illustration of relationship between biomarker and primary endpoint.

We can see from Table 5.1 that if the conventional one-level correlation approach is used, when the correlation between the biomarker and the primary endpoint increases from 0.3 to 0.8, the simulated power of two-stage winner design changes from 96.48% to 97.37%. It is only slightly different. This finding violates the presumption that the biomarker-informed design should have a better performance when the interim endpoint has a stronger correlation with the final endpoint. In addition, the simulation results also suggest that the power is probably overestimated by the one-level correlation model.

Figure 5.1 illustrates different cases where the individual level correlation ρ between the biomarker and the primary endpoint is the same. Two different biomarkers are described in the figure, both of which are correlated with the primary endpoint with correlation coefficient ρ = 0.9. Consider designs that use the two biomarkers at an interim respectively: if the same treatment difference is found on biomarkers at an interim, the power of the two designs might be different, since the treatment difference on the primary endpoint is different due to the different slope. Therefore, it's not sufficient to describe the relationship between the biomarker and the primary endpoint by only considering the individual level correlation ρ. The slope, which is the rate of change of the primary endpoint with respect to the biomarker, should also be incorporated. The conventional one-level correlation model does not incorporate the variability of the slope caused by the uncertainty of historical data, which might easily lead to misestimated power.

5.4 Two-Stage Winner Design with Proposed Model

5.4.1 Two-Stage Winner Design

A two-stage winner design is a special drop-the-losers design, where only a single active treatment will be selected for final evaluation. It combines a phase II and a phase III study, and starts with several active treatment arms and a control arm with a planned interim analysis. At the interim, the inferior treatments will be dropped based on observations of the interim endpoint, and only the most promising one will be carried until the end of the study. The interim endpoint can be different but correlated with the final study primary endpoint. The final comparison of winner treatment with control is performed on the data collected from both stages. This design could potentially shorten the duration of the development, and aid in delivering the personal medicine to the patient at the right time.

For a two-stage winner design, let $\{X_i^{(j)} \mid i = 1,\ldots,n_1\}$ be the measurements of the biomarker obtained at the interim stage, and $\{Y_i^{(j)} \mid i = 1,\ldots,N\}$ be the measurements of primary endpoint obtained at the final stage. n_1 is the interim sample size per group, and N is the maximum sample size for each group, $n_1 < N$; $j = 0,1,2,\ldots,$ M. M is the number of active treatment groups. Let $j = 0$ represent the control group and $j = 1,2,\ldots,$ M the active treatment groups. $\overline{X}_{n_1}^{(j)} = \frac{1}{n_1}\sum X_i^{(j)}$ is the mean of the biomarker measurements for treatment group j and $\overline{Y}_N^{(j)} = (1/N)\sum Y_i^{(j)}$ is the mean of the primary endpoint measurements for treatment group j.

The decision rule of the winner design is if $\overline{X}_{n_1}^{(j)} = \max\left(\overline{X}_{n_1}^{(1)}, \overline{X}_{n_1}^{(2)}, \ldots, \overline{X}_{n_1}^{(M)}\right)$ at interim, carry only the best treatment group j and the control group to the end of the study. The option that more than one treatment group will be kept when the interim outcomes are almost the same is not considered, because either treatment group can be selected in this situation. The final assessment will be based on the primary endpoint Y comparing the selected treatment j group and the control group.

5.4.2 Two-Level Correlation Model for Two-Stage Winner Design

To illustrate the proposed two-level correlation model, we consider a two-stage winner design with three active treatment arms ($M = 3$) and a control arm. For simplicity, we further assume both interim and final endpoints are normally distributed. The two-level correlation approach models the design in the following way:

Assume, u_j^X, $j = 0$, 1, 2, 3, are standardized means of biomarker for treatment group j, and σ_X^2 is the common variance. For a fixed j, assume $\{X_i^{(j)} \mid i = 1,\ldots,n_1\}$ i.i.d. and $(X_i^{(j)}/\sigma_X) \sim N(u_j^X, 1)$.

Assume $\{Y_i^{(j)} \mid i = 1,\ldots,N\}$ i.i.d., denote the true mean level correlation between biomarker and primary endpoint by r_j for treatment group j, assume $(Y_i^{(j)}/\sigma_Y) \mid r_j \sim N(u_j^Y, 1)$, where $u_j^Y = r_j * u_j^X$.

In reality, since the true mean level correlation r_j is unknown, an estimate $\hat{r}_j$ is obtained from historical data to describe the estimated mean level correlation. Assume $\hat{r}_j \sim N(r_j, \sigma_{rj}^2)$, $(Y_i^{(j)}/\sigma_Y) \mid \hat{r}_j \sim N(\hat{r}_j * u_j^X, 1)$. It is easy to show that, under this setting, the unconditional distribution for the primary endpoint is: $(Y_i^{(j)}/\sigma_Y) \sim N\left(u_j^Y, (u_j^X)^2 * \sigma_{rj}^2 + 1\right)$.

The individual level correlation between the biomarker and the primary endpoint is denoted by ρ, where $\rho = Corr(X_i, Y_i)$.

The new variable, r_j, incorporated in the model, and the distribution of its estimate $\hat{r}_j$, accounts for the mean level correlation (or "mean level association") between biomarker and primary endpoint. The uncertainty, due to a small sample size of historical data, about the relationship between the two endpoints should be reflected in the model in this way.

5.4.3 Test Statistic and Its Distribution

Consider the following hypotheses:

$H_0: u_1^Y = u_2^Y = u_3^Y = u_0^Y$

$H_a: u_1^Y > u_0^Y$ or $u_2^Y > u_0^Y$ or $u_3^Y > u_0^Y$

We want to test if there is any treatment that shows significantly better efficacy than the control group.

It is reasonable to assume that $u_1^X = u_2^X = u_3^X = u_0^X$ when $u_1^Y = u_2^Y = u_3^Y = u_0^Y$ and $\rho \neq 0$.

Let the test statistic comparing the primary endpoint of the jth treatment group and the control group be:

$$G_j = \sqrt{\frac{N}{\left[\left(\widehat{u_j^X}\right)^2 * \widehat{\sigma_{rj}^2} + \left(\widehat{u_0^X}\right)^2 * \widehat{\sigma_{r0}^2} + 2\right] * \sigma_Y^2}} \, [\overline{Y_N^{(j)}} - \overline{Y_N^{(0)}}] \quad \text{for} \quad j = 1,2,3$$

G_j is expected to approximately follow the standard normal distribution under H_0 when the sample size is large.

The final test statistic of the study with the given interim selection rule is then:

$$W = G_j, \quad \text{if } \overline{X_{n_1}^{(j)}} = \max\left(\overline{X_{n_1}^{(1)}}, \overline{X_{n_1}^{(2)}}, \overline{X_{n_1}^{(3)}}\right) \quad j = 1,2,3$$

That is, conditional on the interim selection, W takes on the value of the effect from the "winner" treatment group as the final test statistic.

It is well understood that the interim treatment selection will skew the distribution of the final test statistic. In the following, the exact distribution of the final test statistic will be derived. As the test statistic is no longer normally distributed, multidimensional numerical integration is needed for its calculation.

For the very general case under H_a, the distribution of the final test statistic W could be written as

$$F_W(w) = \sum_{j=1}^{3} \Pr(P_{j1} < a_j, P_{j2} > b_j, P_{j3} > c_j) \tag{5.1}$$

where

$$P_{j1} = G_j - \sqrt{\frac{N}{\left[\left(\widehat{u_j^X}\right)^2 * \widehat{\sigma_{rj}^2} + \left(\widehat{u_0^X}\right)^2 * \widehat{\sigma_{r0}^2} + 2\right]}} (u_j^Y - u_0^Y)$$

$$P_{j2} = \frac{\overline{X_{n_1}^{(j)}}}{t} - \frac{\overline{X_{n_1}^{(h)}}}{t} - \left(\frac{u_j^X * \sigma_X}{t} - \frac{u_h^X * \sigma_X}{t}\right)$$

$$P_{j3} = \frac{\overline{X_{n_1}^{(j)}}}{t} - \frac{\overline{X_{n_1}^{(l)}}}{t} - \left(\frac{u_j^X * \sigma_X}{t} - \frac{u_l^X * \sigma_X}{t}\right)$$

$$a_j = w - \sqrt{\frac{N}{\left[\left(\widehat{u_j^X}\right)^2 * \widehat{\sigma_{rj}^2} + \left(\widehat{u_0^X}\right)^2 * \widehat{\sigma_{r0}^2} + 2\right]}} (u_j^Y - u_0^Y)$$

$$b_j = -\left(\frac{u_j^X * \sigma_X}{t} - \frac{u_h^X * \sigma_X}{t}\right)$$

$$c_j = -\left(\frac{u_j^X * \sigma_X}{t} - \frac{u_l^X * \sigma_X}{t}\right)$$

$$t = \sqrt{\frac{\sigma_X^2}{n_1}}$$

$$j \neq h, j \neq l, h \neq l, j, h, l \in \{1, 2, 3\}$$

$(P_{j1} \quad P_{j2} \quad P_{j3})'$ is approximately from a multinormal distribution,

$$\begin{pmatrix} P_{j1} \\ P_{j2} \\ P_{j3} \end{pmatrix} \sim N\left(\begin{pmatrix} 0 \\ 0 \\ 0 \end{pmatrix}, \Sigma_j = \begin{pmatrix} 1 & \gamma_j & \gamma_j \\ \gamma_j & 2 & 1 \\ \gamma_j & 1 & 2 \end{pmatrix}\right)$$

and

$$\gamma_j = \sqrt{\frac{n_1 * \left(\left(\widehat{u_j^X}\right)^2 * \widehat{\sigma_{rj}^2} + 1\right)}{N * \left[\left(\widehat{u_j^X}\right)^2 * \widehat{\sigma_{rj}^2} + \left(\widehat{u_0^X}\right)^2 * \widehat{\sigma_{r0}^2} + 2\right]}} \rho$$

Details of derivations are provided in Appendix A.

5.4.4 Type I Error Rate Control

It is well known that the interim adjustments during a trial might cause inflation of type I error rate. As the two-stage winner design is intended for phase II/III seamless or phase III trials, it's desirable to preserve the type I error rate under a target α level.

Assuming we have the same amount of historical information on the biomarker and the primary endpoint for each treatment group, from Equation 5.1, the distribution of final test statistic W under H_0 is

$$F_0(w) = 3 \int_{-\infty}^{w} \int_{0}^{\infty} \int_{0}^{\infty} f(p_1, p_2, p_3) dp_3 dp_2 dp_1 \tag{5.2}$$

where

$$f(p_1, p_2, p_3) \text{ is the p.d.f of } N\left(\begin{pmatrix} 0 \\ 0 \\ 0 \end{pmatrix}, \Sigma = \begin{pmatrix} 1 & \gamma & \gamma \\ \gamma & 2 & 1 \\ \gamma & 1 & 2 \end{pmatrix}\right)$$

$$\gamma = \sqrt{\frac{n_1}{2N}}\rho$$

$$f(p_1, p_2, p_3) = (2\pi)^{-\frac{3}{2}} |\Sigma|^{-\frac{1}{2}} e^{-\frac{1}{2}\dot{p}'\Sigma^{-1}\dot{p}}$$

$$= (2\pi)^{-\frac{3}{2}}(3 - 2\gamma^2)^{-\frac{1}{2}} e^{-\frac{1}{2}\frac{1}{3-2\gamma^2}\upsilon}$$

$$\upsilon = 3p_1^2 - 2\gamma p_1 p_2 - 2\gamma p_1 p_3 + p_2^2(2 - \gamma^2) + p_2 p_3(2\gamma^2 - 2) + p_3^2(2 - \gamma^2)$$

Let w_α be the upper 100α percent quantile of F_0,

$$w_\alpha = F_W^{-1}(1 - \alpha \mid H_0) = F_0^{-1}(1 - \alpha)$$

The type I error rate is controlled at level α if the 1-sided rejection region is $\Omega = \{W: W > w_\alpha\}$.

The stopping boundary w_α could be easily calculated by numerical integration software. See Table 5.2 for numerical values of $w_{0.025}$ for different values of correlation coefficient ρ when interim information time is 1/2. As expected, the critical value $w_{0.025}$ increases as ρ increases.

R code for the calculation of stopping boundaries can be found in Appendix B.

TABLE 5.2

Critical Value $w_{0.025}$ of Two-Stage Winner Design $((n_1/N) = (1/2))$

ρ	0	0.2	0.5	0.8	1
$w_{0.025}$	1.96	2.041	2.146	2.232	2.279

5.5 Performance Evaluation of Two-Stage Winner Design under Proposed Model

In this section, we show performance evaluation of the two-stage winner design using the proposed two-level model. As illustrated earlier, when the rank order of mean responses of the biomarker is assumed to be the same as that of the primary endpoint, the power of a two-stage winner design could be easily overestimated if the conventional one-level correlation model is used. It will be shown that the new assessment approach is more reasonable, and can help with determining when a two-stage winner design should be used.

As in our earlier study, we consider a two-stage winner design with three active arms and a control arm. Let $\{X_i^{(j)} \mid i = 1,\ldots,n_1\}$ denote the biomarker measurements, and $\{Y_i^{(j)} \mid i = 1,\ldots,N\}$ the primary endpoint measurements; $j = 0, 1, 2, 3$, and $j = 0$ represent the control group and $j = 1, 2, 3$ the three active treatment groups. According to our proposed model, we assume, for a fixed j, $\{X_i^{(j)} \mid i = 1,\ldots,n_1\}$ *i.i.d.*, and $(X_i^{(j)}/\sigma_X) \sim N(u_j^X, 1)$; $\{Y_i^{(j)} \mid i = 1,\ldots,N\}$ *i.i.d.*, and $(Y_i^{(j)}/\sigma_Y) \mid r_j \sim N(u_j^Y, 1)$, where $u_j^Y = r_j * u_j^X$. $\hat{r}_j$ is an estimate of r_j, and it is assumed that $\hat{r}_j \sim N(r_j, \sigma_{r_j}^2)$, $(Y_i^{(j)}/\sigma_Y) \mid \hat{r}_j \sim N(\hat{r}_j * u_j^X, 1)$. The individual level correlation $\rho = Corr(X_i, Y_i)$.

We assume $u_0^X = 1$, $\sigma_X^2 = 1$, $u_0^Y = 1$, $\sigma_Y^2 = 1$—this could always be achieved by scaling—and assume $u_1^Y = 1.1$, $u_2^Y = 1.5$, $u_3^Y = 1.3$. We assume that the biomarker and the primary endpoint are positively related, that is, large values of biomarker measurement correspond to large values of the primary endpoint. We consider the following cases when the means of biomarker and primary endpoint are correlated in linear and in nonlinear ways (see Figure 5.2).

5.5.1 u^X and u^Y Are Linearly Related

If the mean of the biomarker u^X and the mean of primary endpoint u^Y are linearly related, as shown in Figure 5.2, the mean level correlation r_j is same for all treatment groups. Under our assumption here, $r_1 = r_2 = r_3 = r_0 = 1$. Therefore, $u_1^X = 1.1$, $u_2^X = 1.5$, $u_3^X = 1.3$ in this case.

Consider the design with interim sample size $n_1 = 52$ and maximum sample size $N = 104$; and $n_1 = 67$ and $N = 134$, respectively. The two sample sizes will yield 80% and 90% power, respectively, of the corresponding classical design with no interim adaptation.

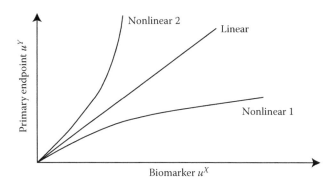

FIGURE 5.2
Mean level correlation shapes.

Tables 5.3 and 5.4 list the simulation results of the two-stage winner design under our setting for the above sample sizes for different values of ρ and σ_r^2. We can see that, when σ_r^2 is fixed, the power of the design for different values of ρ is similar. For example, in Table 5.3, when $\sigma_r^2 = 0.2$, the power of the design is around 78–80%. However, when ρ is fixed, the power of the design has a significant change for different values of σ_r^2. For example, in Table 5.3, for $\rho = 0.5$, the power of the design changes from 87.9% to 78.7% when σ_r^2 increases from 0 to 0.2. The results indicate that the individual level correlation ρ has only a little influence on the performance of the two-stage winner design, while σ_r^2, which measures the uncertainty in the mean level

TABLE 5.3

Power When u^X and u^Y Are Linearly Related ($n_1 = 52$, $N = 104$)

		ρ				
		0	0.2	0.5	0.8	1
σ_r^2	0	88.1%	87.5%	87.9%	88.3%	88.8%
	0.1	85.3%	84.1%	84.0%	83.8%	83.7%
	0.2	80.3%	80.4%	78.7%	79.4%	79.3%

TABLE 5.4

Power When u^X and u^Y Are Linearly Related ($n_1 = 67$, $N = 134$)

		ρ				
		0	0.2	0.5	0.8	1
σ_r^2	0	94.3%	94.5%	94.6%	94.6%	94.8%
	0.1	92.1%	91.9%	91.5%	92.5%	92.4%
	0.2	88.9%	89.2%	88.6%	88.8%	89.6%

correlation estimation, has a significant influence on the design performance. Therefore, it is necessary to consider and incorporate σ_r^2 when evaluating a two-stage winner design. In the conventional one-level correlation model, since σ_r^2 is not considered, the power of the design can be easily overestimated in this case. The simulation results also show that the two-stage winner design is not necessarily always better than the corresponding classical design. In our setting here, only when $\sigma_r^2 < 0.2$ does the two-stage winner design show its advantage in terms of power.

5.5.2 u^X and u^Y Are Not Linearly Related

Cases 1 and 2 in Figure 5.2 show two possible shapes when the mean of biomarker u^X and mean of primary endpoint u^Y are not linearly related.

We assume $u_1^X = 1.2$, $u_2^X = 2.5$, $u_3^X = 1.8$ in case 1 and $u_1^X = 1.05$, $u_2^X = 1.25$, $u_3^X = 1.15$ in case 2.

Simulation results of the two-stage winner design with interim sample size $n_1 = 52$ and maximum sample size $N = 104$ for these two cases are listed in Tables 5.5 and 5.6, respectively. The results agree with the previous findings when u^X and u^Y are linearly related. The individual level correlation ρ does not show large influence on the performance of the design; however, σ_r^2 shows significant influence.

Different from what's been shown when u^X and u^Y are linearly related, under the setting for case 1, the simulation results suggest that the two-stage winner design is a better option than the corresponding classical design only when $\sigma_r^2 < 0.1$; the simulation results also suggest that, under the setting for case 2, the two-stage winner design would never be better than the

TABLE 5.5

Power When u^X and u^Y Are Not Linearly Related—Case 1 ($n_1 = 52$, $N = 104$)

		ρ				
		0	0.2	0.5	0.8	1
σ_r^2	0	94.6%	93.9%	92.7%	91.2%	90.6%
	0.1	86.1%	84.9%	82.6%	80.4%	79.8%

Note: The results are based on 10,000 simulations.

TABLE 5.6

Power When u^X and u^Y Are Not Linearly Related—Case 2 ($n_1 = 52$, $N = 104$)

		ρ				
		0	0.2	0.5	0.8	1
σ_r^2	0	76.5%	76.8%	77.6%	78.6%	79.3%

Note: The results are based on 10,000 simulations.

corresponding classical design. Therefore, the two-stage winner design is not necessarily better than the corresponding classical design. The performance of the two-stage winner design is determined by how u^X and u^Y are related and the uncertainty about the mean level correlation.

Another interesting index for the performance of the two-stage winner design is "power with best treatment," which is the probability that the final hypothesis will be rejected when the best treatment is selected at interim. Tables 5.7 through 5.10 list the "power with best treatment" under the above scenarios associated with Tables 5.3 through 5.6.

TABLE 5.7

Power with Best Treatment When u^X and u^Y Are Linearly Related ($n_1 = 52$, $N = 104$)

		ρ				
		0	0.2	0.5	0.8	1
σ_r^2	0	79.6%	78.0%	78.1%	78.3%	78.1%
	0.1	76.7%	76.1%	75.3%	74.7%	74.7%
	0.2	73.0%	72.9%	71.2%	71.3%	69.8%

Note: The results are based on 10,000 simulations.

TABLE 5.8

Power with Best Treatment When u^X and u^Y Are Linearly Related ($n_1 = 67$, $N = 134$)

		ρ				
		0	0.2	0.5	0.8	1
σ_r^2	0	85.5%	85.7%	84.6%	84.7%	85.2%
	0.1	84.0%	83.8%	82.8%	83.0%	83.3%
	0.2	82.2%	82.1%	81.1%	80.1%	80.6%

Note: The results are based on 10,000 simulations.

TABLE 5.9

Power with Best Treatment When u^X and u^Y Are Not Linearly Related—Case 1 ($n_1 = 52$, $N = 104$)

		ρ				
		0	0.2	0.5	0.8	1
σ_r^2	0	94.7%	93.9%	92.8%	91.5%	90.8%
	0.1	86.2%	84.9%	82.7%	80.3%	79.2%

Note: The results are based on 10,000 simulations.

TABLE 5.10

Power with Best Treatment When u^X and u^Y Are Not Linearly Related—
Case 2 ($n_1 = 52$, $N = 104$)

		ρ				
		0	0.2	0.5	0.8	1
σ_r^2	0	59.7%	60.4%	60.3%	59.7%	60.6%

Note: The results are based on 10,000 simulations.

Notice that the "power with best treatment" is generally lower than the power. However, the difference is affected by the shape of the mean level relationship. When u^X and u^Y are not linearly related, and have a relationship shape similar with the case 1 in Figure 5.2, the difference between "power with best treatment" and the power is small, as can be seen by comparing Tables 5.5 and 5.9. When u^X and u^Y are not linearly related, and have a relationship shape similar to case 2 in Figure 5.2, the difference between the two powers is large. These facts indicate that the probability of choosing the best treatment at interim is affected by the shape of the mean level relationship of the two endpoints used in design.

5.6 Parameter Estimation

In this section, we propose a solution to the question "How to estimate the parameters incorporated in the two-level correlation model using historical data."

It is clear that the two-level correlation model incorporates the following parameters: σ_X, u_j^X, σ_Y, u_j^Y, r_j, σ_{rj}^2, and ρ, $j = 0, 1, 2, \ldots, M$.

Assume there are n_j pairs of historical data for treatment j on biomarker and primary endpoint, $j = 0, 1, 2, \ldots, M$. Let $s_{x_j}^2$ be sample variance of biomarker $X_i^{(j)}$ in treatment group j, $i = 1, 2, \ldots n_j$, and $\overline{x^{(j)}}$ be the observed sample mean of biomarker in treatment group j. Let $s_{y_j}^2$ be sample variance of primary endpoint $Y_i^{(j)}$ in treatment group j, and $\overline{y^{(j)}}$ be the observed sample mean of primary endpoint in treatment group j.

We suggest that the parameters be estimated in the following natural way:

$$\widehat{\sigma_X^2} = \sum (n_j * s_{x_j}^2) \Big/ \sum n_j \quad \widehat{\sigma_X} = \sqrt{\widehat{\sigma_X^2}}$$

$$\widehat{u_j^X} = \overline{x^{(j)}} / \widehat{\sigma_X}$$

$$\widehat{\sigma_Y^2} = \sum (n_j * s_{y_j}^2) \Big/ \sum n_j \quad \widehat{\sigma_Y} = \sqrt{\widehat{\sigma_Y^2}}$$

$$\widehat{u_j^Y} = \overline{y^{(j)}} / \widehat{\sigma_Y}$$

$$\widehat{r_j} = \frac{\widehat{u_j^Y}}{\widehat{u_j^X}}$$

$$\widehat{\sigma_{rj}^2} = \frac{\widehat{\sigma_X^2}}{\widehat{\sigma_Y^2}} \left[\frac{\frac{\widehat{\sigma_Y^2}}{n} + \left(\widehat{u_j^Y}\right)^2}{\frac{\widehat{\sigma_X^2}}{n} + \left(\widehat{u_j^X}\right)^2} \left(\frac{\frac{\widehat{\sigma_Y^2}}{n}}{\frac{\widehat{\sigma_Y^2}}{n} + \left(\widehat{u_j^Y}\right)^2} - 2\frac{\frac{1}{n}\widehat{\rho}\widehat{\sigma_X}\widehat{\sigma_Y}}{\widehat{u_j^X} * \widehat{u_j^Y}} + \frac{\frac{\widehat{\sigma_X^2}}{n}}{\frac{\widehat{\sigma_X^2}}{n} + \left(\widehat{u_j^X}\right)^2} \right) \right] \quad (5.3)$$

$\widehat{\rho} = Corr(X, Y)$, which is the observed correlation coeffient of the pooled sample of $X_i^{(j)}$ and $Y_i^{(j)} \cdot i = 1, 2, \ldots n_j, j = 0, 1, 2, \ldots, M$.

Detailed derivation of Equation 5.3 is provided in Appendix C. An approximation for the variance of ratio was used in the derivation [18].

There are times when a common variance is preferred for $\widehat{r_j}$, that is, $\sigma_{r1}^2 = \cdots = \sigma_{rM}^2 = \sigma_{r0}^2 = \sigma_r^2$ will be assumed. For this case, we suggest:

$$\widehat{\sigma_r^2} = \sum (n_j * \widehat{\sigma_{rj}^2}) \Big/ \sum n_j$$

Table 5.11 lists the simulation results, and compares the true parameter values with their estimators. The three cases in Figure 5.2 were considered here. We assume $\rho = 0.5$, and the simulation results are based on 50 pairs of historical data for each treatment group. The numbers show that the proposed approach provides reasonable estimation for parameters.

5.7 Discussion and Summary

In this new age of personalized medicine, biomarker-informed adaptive designs are very attractive. They have the potential to shorten the time of drug development and to bring the right drug to the right patient earlier, by incorporating a correlated short-term endpoint at the interim stages.

It is strongly suggested that statistical simulations should be performed before a drug trial to understand the operating characteristics of the trial design. The conventional one-level correlation model used in simulations for the biomarker-informed adaptive designs might be inappropriate when the relationship between the biomarker and the primary endpoint is not well known. This model only considers the individual level correlation between the interim and final endpoint of the design. Uncertainty of the mean level correlation between the two endpoints is not considered. Hence, the

TABLE 5.11

Estimation of the Parameters

	Linear		NL 1		NL 2	
	TRUE	EST	TRUE	EST	TRUE	EST
ρ	0.5	0.51	0.5	0.52	0.5	0.50
σ_Y^2	1	1.00	1	1.00	1	1.00
u_0^Y	1	1.01	1	1.00	1	1.00
u_1^Y	1.1	1.11	1.1	1.11	1.1	1.11
u_2^Y	1.5	1.50	1.5	1.50	1.5	1.51
u_3^Y	1.3	1.31	1.3	1.31	1.3	1.31
σ_X^2	1	1.00	1	1.00	1	1.00
u_0^X	1	1.00	1	1.01	1	1.01
u_1^X	1.1	1.11	1.2	1.22	1.05	1.07
u_2^X	1.5	1.51	2.5	2.50	1.25	1.26
u_3^X	1.3	1.30	1.8	1.80	1.15	1.16
r00	1	1.02	1	1.01	1	1.00
r01	1	1.01	0.92	0.92	1.05	1.05
r02	1	1.00	0.6	0.60	1.2	1.21
r03	1	1.01	0.72	0.73	1.13	1.14
σ_r^2	0.014	0.015	0.01	0.0104	0.017	0.019

Note: The results are based on 500 simulations.

simulation results of a biomarker-informed adaptive design using the conventional one-level model can easily misestimate the power.

The new two-level correlation model incorporates correlations at both the individual and the mean level. It's shown that in a biomarker-informed design, the power is much more sensitive to the correlation between the biomarker and the primary endpoint at the mean level than the correlation at the individual level. Simulations using the two-level correlation model for biomarker-informed designs produce more sensible and reasonable results.

The proposed two-level correlation model is illustrated in the context of a two-stage winner design in this chapter. With the derived distribution of the test statistics and stopping boundary information, the type I error rate can be controlled. We considered three cases where the mean level correlations are in different shapes. It is shown that the shape, together with the uncertainty about the shape, should be counted when comparing the biomarker-informed adaptive design with the corresponding classical design. An absolute advantage of the biomarker-informed design is not guaranteed. In addition, it's also shown that the shape of the mean level correlation affects the probability of choosing the best treatment at interim of the design.

Methods were proposed to estimate the parameters. The proposed estimators for the parameters appear to be unbiased by simulations. Hence, based on the prior historical data, we will be able to answer questions such as "which design will provide higher power, the biomarker-informed adaptive design or the classical Dunnett design" and "what should the sample size be in order to get 80% power" by simulations.

In general, when a good portion of the relationship between the biomarker and the primary endpoint is known, the biomarker-informed design is recommended.

5.7.1 Distribution of Final Test Statistic

$$F_W(w) = \Pr(W < w)$$

$$= \sum_{j=1}^{3} \Pr\left(W < w, \overline{X_{m_1}^{(j)}} = \max\left(\overline{X_{m_1}^{(1)}}, \overline{X_{m_1}^{(2)}}, \overline{X_{m_1}^{(3)}}\right)\right)$$

$$= \sum_{j=1}^{3} \Pr\left(G_j < w \mid \overline{X_{m_1}^{(j)}} = \max\left(\overline{X_{m_1}^{(1)}}, \overline{X_{m_1}^{(2)}}, \overline{X_{m_1}^{(3)}}\right)\right) \Pr\left(\overline{X_{m_1}^{(j)}} = \max\left(\overline{X_{m_1}^{(1)}}, \overline{X_{m_1}^{(2)}}, \overline{X_{m_1}^{(3)}}\right)\right)$$

$$= \sum_{j=1}^{3} \Pr\left(G_j < w, \overline{X_{m_1}^{(j)}} = \max\left(\overline{X_{m_1}^{(1)}}, \overline{X_{m_1}^{(2)}}, \overline{X_{m_1}^{(3)}}\right)\right)$$

$$= \sum_{j=1}^{3} \Pr\left(G_j < w, \overline{X_{m_1}^{(j)}} - \overline{X_{m_1}^{(h)}} > 0, \overline{X_{m_1}^{(j)}} - \overline{X_{m_1}^{(l)}} > 0\right)$$

$$= \sum_{j=1}^{3} \Pr\left(P_{j1} < a_j, P_{j2} > b_j, P_{j3} > c_j\right)$$

where

$$P_{j1} = G_j - \sqrt{\frac{N}{\left[\left(\widehat{u_j^X}\right)^2 * \widehat{\sigma_{rj}^2} + \left(\widehat{u_0^X}\right)^2 * \widehat{\sigma_{r0}^2} + 2\right]}} (u_j^Y - u_0^Y)$$

$$P_{j2} = \frac{\overline{X_{m_1}^{(j)}}}{t} - \frac{\overline{X_{m_1}^{(h)}}}{t} - \left(\frac{u_j^X * \sigma_X}{t} - \frac{u_h^X * \sigma_X}{t}\right)$$

$$P_{j3} = \frac{\overline{X_{m_1}^{(j)}}}{t} - \frac{\overline{X_{m_1}^{(l)}}}{t} - \left(\frac{u_j^X * \sigma_X}{t} - \frac{u_l^X * \sigma_X}{t}\right)$$

$$a_j = w - \sqrt{\frac{N}{\left[\left(\widehat{u_j^X}\right)^2 * \widehat{\sigma_{rj}^2} + \left(\widehat{u_0^X}\right)^2 * \widehat{\sigma_{r0}^2} + 2\right]}} \left(u_j^Y - u_0^Y\right)$$

$$b_j = -\left(\frac{u_j^X * \sigma_X}{t} - \frac{u_h^X * \sigma_X}{t}\right)$$

$$c_j = -\left(\frac{u_j^X * \sigma_X}{t} - \frac{u_l^X * \sigma_X}{t}\right)$$

$$j \neq h, j \neq l, h \neq l, j, h, l \in \{1, 2, 3\}$$

5.7.2 R Code for Calculation of Stopping Boundaries

##This program is used for finding the critical value for the final test statistic to control type I error rate#

##The distribution of the final test statistic under H0 is proposed as Equation 5.2 in section "Type I error rate control"##

##stopping boundary determined by: interim time(1/2 used for Table 5.2) and rho##

##have to guess the stopping boundaries, and try the program until the "integral" in output achieves 1-alpha.##

##the critical value associated is the one to control type I error rate at level alpha.##

```
library(cubature)
rho = **#rho takes value between 0 and 1##
mtime = **#interim information time, mtime takes value
between 0 and 1##
r1 = sqrt(0.5*mtime)*rho
w = c(**, ..., **) ##the numbers to try for the true stopping
boundary##
res = c()
for (j in 1:length(w)){
a = w[j]
f = function(p){
3*((2*pi)^(-1.5)*(3-2*r1^2)^(-0.5)*exp(-0.5*(1/(3-2*r1^2))*
(3*p[1]^2-2*r1*p[1]*p[2]-2*r1*p[1]*p[3] + (2 -r1^2)*p[2]^2 +
(2-r1^2)*p[2]^2 + (2*r1^2-2)*p[2]*p[3] + (2-r1^2)*p[3]^2)))
}
intenum=adaptIntegrate(f, lowerLimit=c(-18, 0, 0), upperLimit=
c(a, 18, 18))
intenum2=cbind(intenum, a)
res=rbind(res, intenum2) #the stopping boundary could be
found as the number that associated with 1-alpha in column
"integral"in "res"##
```

5.7.3 Derivation Details for $\widehat{\sigma^2_{rj}}$

$$
\begin{aligned}
\sigma^2_{rj} &= Var\left(\frac{\overline{Y^{(j)}}/\sigma_Y}{\overline{X^{(j)}}/\sigma_X}\right) \\[2mm]
&\approx \frac{\sigma^2_X}{\sigma^2_Y} * \left(\frac{E^2\overline{Y^{(j)}}}{E^2\overline{X^{(j)}}}\left[\frac{Var\left(\overline{Y^{(j)}}\right)}{E^2\overline{Y^{(j)}}} - 2\frac{Cov\left(\overline{X^{(j)}},\overline{Y^{(j)}}\right)}{E\overline{X^{(j)}} * E\overline{Y^{(j)}}} + \frac{Var\left(\overline{X^{(j)}}\right)}{E^2\overline{X^{(j)}}}\right]\right) \\[2mm]
&= \frac{\sigma^2_X}{\sigma^2_Y}\left[\frac{(\sigma^2_Y/n) + \left(u^Y_j\right)^2}{(\sigma^2_X/n) + \left(u^X_j\right)^2}\left(\frac{(\sigma^2_Y/n)}{(\sigma^2_Y/n) + \left(u^Y_j\right)^2} - 2\frac{(1/n)\rho\sigma_X\sigma_Y}{u^X_j * u^Y_j} + \frac{(\sigma^2_X/n)}{(\sigma^2_X/n) + \left(u^X_j\right)^2}\right)\right]
\end{aligned}
$$

(5.4)

Equation 5.4 holds, because an approximation for the variance of ratio proposed in Stuart and Ord [19],

$$
Var\left(\frac{Y}{X}\right) = \frac{E^2Y}{E^2X}\left[\frac{Var(Y)}{E^2Y} - 2\frac{Cov(X,Y)}{EX * EY} + \frac{Var(X)}{E^2X}\right]
$$

Naturally,

$$
\widehat{\sigma^2_{rj}} = \frac{\widehat{\sigma^2_X}}{\widehat{\sigma^2_Y}}\left[\frac{(\widehat{\sigma^2_Y}/n) + (\widehat{u^Y_j})^2}{(\widehat{\sigma^2_X}/n) + (\widehat{u^X_j})^2}\left(\frac{(\widehat{\sigma^2_Y}/n)}{(\widehat{\sigma^2_Y}/n) + (\widehat{u^Y_j})^2} - 2\frac{(1/n)\widehat{\rho}\widehat{\sigma_X}\widehat{\sigma_Y}}{\widehat{u^X_j} * \widehat{u^Y_j}} + \frac{(\widehat{\sigma^2_X}/n)}{(\widehat{\sigma^2_X}/n) + (\widehat{u^X_j})^2}\right)\right]
$$

Acknowledgments

The authors would like to thank Ruth Foley for her professional editing and Dr. Jared Christensen, Dr. Bo Huang, and Joseph Wu for providing technical review and useful comments.

References

1. Stallard N., Todd S. 2003. Sequential designs for phase III clinical trials incorporating treatment selection. *Statist. Med.*, 22(5):689–703.
2. Kelly P.J., Stallard N., Todd S. 2005. An adaptive group sequential design for phase II/III clinical trials that select a single treatment from several. *J Biopharm Statist.*, 15(4):641–58.

3. Stallard N., Friede T. 2008. A group-sequential design for clinical trials with treatment selection. *Statist. Med.*, 27(29):6209–27.
4. Bauer P., Kieser M. 1999. Combining different phases in the development of medical treatments within a single trial. *Statist. Med.*, 18(14):1833–48.
5. Sampson A.R., Sill M.W. 2005. Drop-the-loser design: Normal case (with discussions). *Biometr. J.*, 47:257–81.
6. Chang M., Chow S.C., Pong, A. 2006. Adaptive design in clinical research—Issues, opportunities, and recommendations. *J. Biopharm. Statist.*, 16:299–309.
7. Gallo P. 2006. Operational challenges in adaptive design implementation. *Pharm. Statist.*, 5:119–24.
8. Todd S., Stallard N. 2005. A new clinical trial design combining phases 2 and 3: Sequential designs with treatment selection and a change of endpoint. *Drug Inf. J.*, 39(2):109–18.
9. Stallard N. 2010. A confirmatory seamless phase II/III clinical trial design incorporating short-term endpoint information. *Statist. Med.*, 29(9):959–71.
10. Friede T., Parsons N., Stallard N., Todd S., Valdes M.E., Chataway J., Nicholas R. 2011. Designing a seamless phase II/III clinical trial using early outcomes for treatment selection: An application in multiple sclerosis. *Statist. Med.*, 30(13):1528–40.
11. Shun Z., Lan K.K., Soo Y. 2008. Interim treatment selection using the normal approximation approach in clinical trials. *Statist. Med.*, 27(4):597–18.
12. Liu Q., Pledger G.W. 2005. Phase 2 and 3 combination designs to accelerate drug development. *J. Am. Statist. Assoc.*, 100(470):493–502.
13. Li G., Wang Y., Ouyang S.P. 2009. Interim treatment selection in drug development. *Statist. Biosci.*, 1(2):268–88.
14. Li G., Zhu J., Ouyang S.P., Xie J., Deng L., Law G. 2009. Adaptive designs for interim dose selection. *Statist. Biopharm. Res.*, 1(4):366–76.
15. Di S.L., Glimm E. 2011. Time-to-event analysis with treatment arm selection at interim. *Statist. Med.*, 30(26):3067–81.
16. Jenkins M., Stone A., Jennison C. 2010. An adaptive seamless phase II/III design for oncology trials with subpopulation selection using correlated survival endpoints. *Pharm. Statist.*, 10(4):347–56.
17. Chang M. 2011. *Modern Issues and Methods in Biostatistics*. New York: Springer.
18. Wang J., Chang M., Menon S., Wang L. 2013. Biomarker informed adaptive seamless phase II/III design. Submitted to *Statist. Med.*
19. Stuart A., Ord K. 1998. *Kendall's Advanced Theory of Statistics*. 6th Edition. New York: Wiley.

6

Fitting the Dose: Adaptive Staggered Dose Design

Joseph Wu, Sandeep Menon, and Mark Chang

CONTENTS

6.1 Introduction

The extensive application of advanced molecular technology has generated a vast amount of data on human biology in a very short time. For example, the Human Genome Project, completed in 2003, has successfully sequenced approximately 3 billion base pairs and identified a majority of the genes in the human genome [1]. Shortly thereafter, the advancement of the next generation sequencing methods has also made genomic sequencing more efficient but at much lower cost [2]. The availability of genetic and genomic information has allowed teams of scientists to further pinpoint the genetic predispositions to common but complex diseases such as cancer, cardiovascular diseases, and diabetes. With the cost of sequencing a personal genome further dwindling in the near future, it is predicted that we may be able to formally incorporate our genomic, epigenetic, and even proteomic information in a real-time fashion into our personal health care. Specifically, this has signaled the coming of the field of personalized medicine [3].

To facilitate the widespread practices of personalized medicine, it is important for clinical drug development to further refine the characterization of the efficacy and risk profiles among different patient subgroups. As an example for safety, it is well-known that the relative abundance of drug-metabolizing enzymes such as cytochrome P450 (CYP450) varies from person to person, and therefore adverse reactions to the same drug dosage can also be very different. As for efficacy, about 30% of women who are diagnosed with breast cancer have an overexpression of the epidermal growth factor receptor 2 (HER2) and do not respond to the standard therapy. However, an antibody drug, *trastuzumab*, can reduce the recurrence of a tumor in these women by 52% when used in combination with chemotherapy [4,5]. These scenarios tell us that, when personal genomic profiles are available, physicians and allied medical professionals trained in personalized medicine can together help their patients make better decisions and tailor their treatment to further optimize its efficacy and reduce its risks.

The possibility of practicing personalized medicine requires dedicated collaboration of many scientific disciplines. One such discipline is the application of efficient clinical trial methods that can expedite the profiling of efficacy and risks of a drug among patients with different biological backgrounds. In particular, we want to find and match the right doses to the right patient subgroups.

6.2 Motivations and Concepts

Suppose we have several possible doses that may benefit a particular patient subgroup; the main question in this context is, how can we quickly identify the best dose when we only have a limited sample of patients? In other situations, we may want to compare several modes of drug administration or regimens instead of actual doses. Without loss of generality, we will refer to doses from now on. In this case, a single trial design that combines dose selection and confirmation is desirable. This idea has led to the development of a class of adaptive trial designs that seamlessly combines both the selection of a therapeutic dose out of multiple doses and the confirmation of the selected dose. There are two major approaches in these trial designs: (i) two-stage ranking and selection procedures and (ii) multistage group sequential procedures.

Sampson and Sill described an early proposal of the two-stage ranking and selection procedure which they called the "drop-the-losers" design [6]. The drop-the-losers design is a statistical design that has two stages of a trial separated by a data-based decision. In this design, *J* experimental treatments and a control are administered in the first stage. At interim, the empirically best treatment is selected for continuation into the second stage, along with the control. At the end of the second stage, inference comparing the selected treatment and the control is conducted using data from both stages. Recently, other modified two-stage designs were also proposed [7,8]. In these designs, ranking of the estimated effects is performed at the end of the first stage and, based on the result, they allow the selection of one or two doses to be continued to the second stage. They also allow for early termination of the study if at least one dose shows statistical significance at the end of the first stage.

Multistage group sequential procedures are statistical designs that discard inferior treatments based on result of hypothesis testing at interim. Follmann et al. [9] extended the two-arm group sequential design to multiple arms and provided critical values that could strongly control the type I error. Other similar designs that used the efficient score statistics developed by Whitehead [10] also appear in the literature. These designs allow for sequential monitoring for any type of outcome—binary, normal, and survival [11,12]. The calculation of stopping boundaries remains the major difficulty in implementing multistage group sequential methods. A recent design by Chen et al. [13] suggests two methods of calculating the efficacy boundaries. The first method is called joint monitoring in which all dose-control comparisons are monitored simultaneously by one single alpha spending function. The second method is called marginal monitoring, where a marginal alpha level and an alpha spending function are specified for each dose-control comparison. The evaluation of stopping boundaries is still computationally intensive in these two methods.

Besides the two main approaches described previously, other innovative approaches are also found in the literature. Bretz et al. [14] propose combining multiple comparisons and parametric modeling techniques in selecting both a model and a dose that gives target level of efficacy. Although the above adaptive approaches have made significant improvement in increasing the statistical power and reducing the expected sample size, the derivation of the distribution of test statistics and the computation of stopping boundaries remain involved, particularly when the procedures require data-dependent ranking. Wu et al. have proposed a staggered dose design that starts off with only one or a subset of the doses, and, depending on interim results, adds remaining doses to the trial if the previous doses do not show evidence of efficacy [15]. This design also actively incorporates information from previous dose–response studies and allows for explicit prioritization of doses. This chapter is to describe this design and to characterize its performance.

When planning a trial, sometimes the clinical team may not consider all candidate doses to be of equal importance, but would be interested in studying these doses one after the other starting with doses with assumed better responses and proceeding to doses with assumed inferior responses if the earlier doses do not show statistical evidence of efficacy. After incorporating prior evidence of dose–response relationship, investigators are willing to consider J doses, which can be arranged in decreasing order of priority. We can represent this order of priority with $j = 1, 2, 3, ..., J$ with 1 being of the highest priority and J the lowest priority. We can denote the actual prioritized dose levels as $d_1, d_2, ..., d_J$. It is important to emphasize that this order of priority does *not* necessarily suggest an increasing $(d_1 < d_2 < \cdots < d_J)$ or decreasing $(d_1 > d_2 > \cdots > d_J)$ dosage. This *a priori* ordering is based on previous knowledge and offers additional flexibility for the team to explore the doses one after the other, knowing that we only have a limited number of patients in a dose selection and confirmation trial. Traditional fixed dose parallel group design treats all doses as equally important and the experiment randomizes patients equally to all of the doses. This type of design can be particularly inefficient when an informative prior model on the dose–response relationship exists or if this experimental drug belongs to a class of drug whose dose–response model is clearly established. The designs in current literature described in earlier paragraphs, although making improvement in dose selection, do not consider the option of adaptively inserting new doses.

This new design allows the option of adding new doses adaptively. Instead of starting off with all doses, patients are allocated to fewer doses, and at each interim stage, inferior doses are dropped and new doses are added at the same time. This new design, *adaptive staggered dose procedure*, may further reduce the expected sample size while gaining information about the efficacious doses more quickly. One major condition is that the clinical team has to provide an assumed best case of dose ordering by ranking the J candidate doses in decreasing order of assumed responses based on their clinical judgment or previous evidence on dose–response. The gain in trial efficiency necessitates this assumed dose ordering because optimal doses will be studied earlier than suboptimal doses. If the ordering is right, this design may perform better than both the drop-the-losers design and the fixed dose parallel group design in terms of reduced expected sample size and perhaps experimental time. If the *a priori* ordering is weak, this proposed design can perform as good as the drop-the-losers design in most scenarios but generally still better than the fixed dose parallel group design under assumed conditions.

6.3 Adaptive Staggered Dose Design

6.3.1 General Design

In a late-phase pivotal trial, if the objective is to select one or two optimal doses from J possible doses, these J doses can be staggered by the investigators in the order of *decreasing* priority $j = 1,2,\ldots,J$ as $\{d_1,d_2,\ldots,d_J\}$. It is worth noting that $\{d_1,d_2,\ldots,d_J\}$ are not necessarily in increasing or decreasing order of dosage. Also, it is generally assumed that these doses are well within the range of acceptable safety. However, if the team decides that it is important to escalate the doses for simultaneous assessment of safety and efficacy, a dose escalation order can be adopted, and in this case, $d_1 < d_2 < \cdots < d_J$. Additionally, we want to compare these doses with a control dose d_0 $(j = 0)$ and adopt a fixed randomization ratio of 1:R for control to each of the experimental doses. We study a primary biomarker endpoint which is assumed to follow a normal distribution with a known variance $\sigma^2 = 1$ common across the doses. We let Y_{ji} represent this normal outcome in the ith subject receiving dose d_j such that

$$Y_{ji} \sim N(\theta_j, 1) \tag{6.1}$$

It is also common to assume that the mean θ is related to the dose d monotonically such that $\theta_j = f(d_j)$ exists.

To illustrate this design, we consider looking at a maximum of D experimental doses $(D < J)$ at each of the K *global* stages. Therefore, we do not start off with all J doses but a subset containing the first D doses, $\{d_1,d_2,\ldots,d_D\}$. Depending on the assessment of efficacy at interim stages, we drop doses from the D doses that show convincing futility or lack of efficacy and simultaneously add new doses according to the dose ordering such that D current doses are maintained to the next interim stage. If the interim results demonstrate that at least one dose shows evidence of efficacy, the trial can be stopped early and no more doses will need to be added. Therefore, a maximum of D doses may be selected before or at the final Kth stage or none of the J doses shows efficacy at the final stage. If no dose is selected at the end of the experiment, this clinical drug development can be halted. We restrict the number of patients allocated to each experimental dose by setting the same minimum and maximum numbers of subjects allocated. For example, if we let c be the cohort size per dose and per stage, then the minimum number of subjects will be c and the maximum number of subjects will be cM, where M is the maximum number of *per-dose* stages. However, the control dose will always have c/R subjects randomized at each stage. It is important to stress that only the control subjects that are randomized *simultaneously* with the corresponding experimental dose are compared to the experimental subjects. This ensures comparability between the control subjects and the experimental subjects in all known and unknown prognostic factors except the doses assigned.

6.3.2 Specific Design

We consider a specific case of the general design described earlier, where we study only one dose at a time $(D = 1)$, with a maximum of two per-dose stages $(M = 2)$, and the number of global stages of $K = 2J$. Setting $K = MJ$ allows

An adaptive staggered dose procedure for dose selection

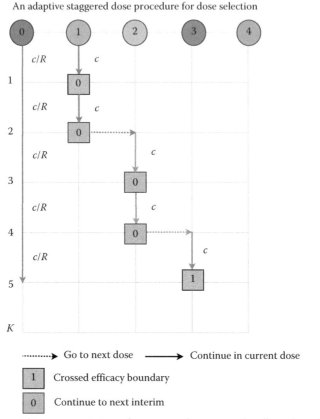

·········▶ Go to next dose   ⟶ Continue in current dose

| 1 | Crossed efficacy boundary |

| 0 | Continue to next interim |

This experiment stops when any one dose crosses the efficacy boundary.

FIGURE 6.1
(See color insert.) A graphical illustration of the proposed adaptive staggered dose procedure with $J = 4$, $D = 1$, $M = 2$, $R = 2$, and $K = 2J = 8$.

the experiment to fully explore each of the doses with an equal amount of information, if added to the trial. Figure 6.1 illustrates this specific adaptive staggered dose algorithm for $J = 4$ and a control to dose randomization ratio of 1:R at each stage. The number of global stages K is necessarily bounded, $J \leq K \leq MJ$. The lower-bound J ensures that each of the J doses will have at least one per-dose stage, while the upper bound ensures that each dose will have at most M per-dose stages. If the hypotheses are

$$H_{j0} : \theta_j \leq \theta_0, H_{ja} : \theta_j > \theta_0 \tag{6.2}$$

for $j = 1,2,\ldots,J$, then the standardized test statistic for dose d_j, conditioned on the outcomes of previous doses, will be

$$Z_{jm} = \frac{\bar{Y}_{jm} - \bar{Y}_{0m}}{\sqrt{(R+1)/cm}} \tag{6.3}$$

where $\bar{Y}_{jm} = \sum_{i=1}^{cm} Y_{ji}/(cm)$ and $\bar{Y}_{0m} = \sum_{i=1}^{(cm)/R} Y_{0i}/(cm/R)$ for $m = 1,2$. We should stress that Y_{0i}'s are the normal responses only for control subjects that are randomized simultaneously with the experimental subjects for dose d_j. The control subjects randomized simultaneously with subjects to the previous doses, $d_1,\ldots,d_{j-1}$, will not be included in the calculation of this test statistic since they may not be comparable in prognostic factors. The conditional distributions of these statistics are

$$Z_{j1} \sim N\left(\frac{\theta_j - \theta_0}{\sqrt{(R+1)/c}}, 1\right), \quad (Z_{j1}, Z_{j2})' \sim N_2\left(\left(\begin{array}{c} \dfrac{\theta_j - \theta_0}{\sqrt{(R+1)/c}} \\ \dfrac{\theta_j - \theta_0}{\sqrt{(R+1)/2c}} \end{array}\right), \Sigma = \left(\begin{array}{cc} 1 & \dfrac{1}{\sqrt{2}} \\ \dfrac{1}{\sqrt{2}} & 1 \end{array}\right)\right)$$

$$\tag{6.4}$$

Under this specific design, the decision rule for dose d_j at the kth interim is described as follows:

- If, whether $m = 1$ or 2, the test statistic for dose d_j is $Z_{jm} > b_k$ where b_k is the efficacy boundary for the kth interim analysis, then it is declared statistically significant and H_{j0} is rejected. This trial will stop and the remaining doses $\{d_{j+1},\ldots,d_J\}$ will not enter the trial.

- If, when $m = 1$, the test statistic for dose d_j at its first per-dose interim is $a_k < Z_{j1} \le b_k$, where a_k ($a_k < b_k$) is the futility boundary for the kth interim analysis, then it will continue to its second per-dose stage with an additional cohort of c subjects allocated. If, when $m = 2$, the test statistic is $Z_{j2} \le b_{k+1}$, where $a_{k+1} = b_{k+1}$, then this dose has reached its maximum allowable samples of $2c$ and it will be dropped due to lack of efficacy. At the same time, a new dose d_{j+1} in the next priority will be added to the experiment.

- If, when $m = 1$, the test statistic for dose d_j is $Z_{j1} \le a_k$, then it is dropped due to convincing futility and H_{j0} is accepted, and a new dose d_{j+1} in the next priority will be added to the experiment.

Therefore, at any global stage k, only one dose is being considered. This trial design allows early termination if: (1) any one dose is declared efficacious; (2) all of the J doses are declared futile; or (3) no dose is declared efficacious at the end of the Kth (final) stage.

Table 6.1 summarizes the definitions of the parameters of this adaptive staggered dose design. Under this design, we can achieve greater gain in

TABLE 6.1

Definitions of Adaptive Staggered Dose Selection Design Parameters

Parameter	Definition
J	Total number of experimental doses considered in the entire trial
D	Maximum number of experimental doses under study at each interim stage $(D < J)$
M	Maximum number of interim stages allowable to each experimental dose (i.e., *per-dose stage*)
c	Cohort sample size allocated to an experimental dose per interim stage
K	Total number of interim stages including final stage of the entire trial (i.e., *global* stage)
R	Randomization ratio of control dose to experimental dose is 1:R

design efficiency if we have strong prior knowledge of the dose–response relationship. In this adaptive staggered dose design, we do not allocate subjects to all of the doses at the beginning. At the end of the trial, if we cannot select a significantly efficacious dose, then this trial will stop and the candidate drug will not proceed to the next phase of development. Since the trial can stop at any global stage for futility or efficacy, the number of stages the trial requires before termination is therefore a random variable as is the sample size used. For a prespecified K, the total number of planned subjects for this entire trial is therefore equal to $cK(1/R + 1)$. We will examine the operating characteristics of this proposed design in the next section.

6.4 Other Design Specifications

6.4.1 Family-Wise Type I Error

For the specific design described in the previous section, we want to discard interim futility analysis for the moment and focus on efficacy for each dose. In this case, we let $a_k = -\infty$ and hence $Pr(Z_{jm} \leq a_k) = 0$ for all k. Therefore, each dose will always go through all M per-dose stages as no futility analysis is performed on the doses. Investigators can still drop a dose before its Mth per-dose interim stage, if safety or other unpredictable issues arise, without inflating the family-wise type I error, and this can provide additional flexibility. In this setting, dose d_j is considered at two global interim stages: $k = 2j - 1$, if k is odd, or $k = 2j$ if k is even (see Figure 6.1).

For this specific design without futility analysis, we denote the probability of rejecting the null hypothesis H_j0 for dose d_j at the kth interim as $\psi_{j,k}$. Under H_{j0}, the standardized test statistics for dose d_j will have the following distributions, using Equation 6.4 for all j

$$Z_{j1} \sim N(0,1), \qquad (Z_{j1}, Z_{j2})' \sim N_2 \left(\begin{pmatrix} 0 \\ 0 \end{pmatrix}, \ \Sigma = \begin{pmatrix} 1 & \dfrac{1}{\sqrt{2}} \\ \dfrac{1}{\sqrt{2}} & 1 \end{pmatrix} \right) \qquad (6.5)$$

Since these distributions, under the null hypothesis, are the same for all doses, we can simply replace Z_{j1} with Z and (Z_{j1}, Z_{j2}) with (Z_1, Z_2). As we have seen, when no futility analysis is performed, the probability of rejecting H_{j0} given that it is true can be shown to be

$$\psi_{j,k} = \begin{cases} Pr(Z > b_k) & \text{if } j = 1, k = 1 \\ Pr(Z_1 \leq b_{k-1}, Z_2 > b_k) & \text{if } j = 1, k = 2 \\ \left\{ \displaystyle\prod_{i=1}^{(k-1)/2} Pr(Z_1 \leq b_{2i-1}, Z_2 \leq b_{2i}) \right\} Pr(Z > b_k) & \text{if } j > 1, k = 2j - 1 \\ \left\{ \displaystyle\prod_{i=1}^{(k-2)/2} Pr(Z_1 \leq b_{2i-1}, Z_2 \leq b_{2i}) \right\} Pr(Z_1 \leq b_{k-1}, Z_2 > b_k) & \text{if } j > 1, k = 2j \end{cases}$$

$$(6.6)$$

The family-wise type I error for this trial is therefore

$$\psi = \sum_{j=1}^{J} (\psi_{j,2j-1} + \psi_{j,2j}) \qquad (6.7)$$

and we are interested in preserving it under a target alpha level, Sup $\psi \leq \alpha$. Under this design, we can assert that by controlling the probability of false-positive conclusion under the *global null hypotheses*—when all H_{j0}'s are true, we can control the family-wise type I error in the strong sense. This assertion is proved in the Appendix.

6.4.2 Calculation of Stopping Boundaries

As multiple interim looks during an experiment are well-known to cause inflation of type I error, and therefore among other methods, flexible *alpha spending functions* are commonly used to monitor the test statistic in the classical group sequential design [16,17]. However, it is important to distinguish the use of alpha spending function in the traditional group sequential setting versus in this adaptive, staggered dose design setting. In the traditional two-arm trial setting, the alpha spending function is applied to monitor one test statistic as information accrues through the stages in order to control type I error. However, in this adaptive staggered dose selection design, since earlier doses are investigated at earlier stages and later doses at later stages, the use of a single alpha spending function across all global stages jointly monitors the test statistics of all of the doses. For the kth interim, if $\alpha(t)$ represents the alpha spending function with t ($0 < t < 1$) being the information fraction, then the doses and their corresponding hypotheses can be monitored through the following:

$$\psi_{j,k} = \alpha(t_k) - \alpha(t_{k-1}) \tag{6.8}$$

where $t_k = k/(2J)$ and $k = 1, 2, \ldots, 2J$ since c, cohort size per stage and per dose, is a constant.

Some well-known alpha spending functions used in traditional group sequential designs are the Pocock, O'Brien and Fleming, and Lan and DeMets. More flexible schemes such as the Rho alpha spending function can also be used in this adaptive design. Rho alpha spending is a one-parameter function and offers more flexibility by simply adjusting the parameter ρ in

$$\alpha(t) = \alpha t^{\rho} \tag{6.9}$$

When $\rho < 1$, it allocates more alpha to the earlier stages, hence favoring earlier doses, while for $\rho > 1$, it favors the later doses by pushing the trials to later stages. In fact, Pocock's approach is similar to the former and O'Brien and Fleming's approach to the latter. The choice of a suitable value for ρ reflects how optimistic or conservative the investigators are toward the ordering of the doses, as well as how informative the dose–response relationship $\theta_j = f(d_j)$ they are willing to assume. This will be discussed in more detail in the next sections via extensive simulation. Another alternative to monitoring the doses is to assign different alpha spending functions $\alpha_j(t)$'s for different doses d_j's since we know exactly which dose is investigated at the kth stage. In this case, the alpha spending function for dose d_j, $\alpha_j(t)$ will depend on the alpha levels of the previous doses, $(\alpha_1, \alpha_2, \ldots, \alpha_j{-}1)$. Therefore, again, the choice of the nominal alpha level α_j for each dose can be prespecified with regard to the strength of the dose ordering. Given the general form of the type I error in Equation 6.6, and a chosen alpha spending function in Equation 6.8, we can numerically solve for the set of efficacy stopping boundaries, $b = (b_1, b_2, \ldots, b_k, \ldots, b_K)$ using the null distributions in Equation 6.5.

6.4.3 Statistical Power

Based on the stage-wise type I error defined in Equation 6.6, we can derive the stage-wise statistical power, denoted as $\xi_{j,k}$, for dose d_j at the kth global stage. Under the alternative hypothesis of a dose–response model, $\theta_j = f(d_j)$, the stage-wise statistical power can be shown as

$$
\xi_{j,k} =
\begin{cases}
1 - \Phi\left(\omega_{j,k}\right) & \text{if } j = 1, k = 1 \\[2mm]
\displaystyle\int_{\omega_{j,k}}^{\infty} \Phi\left(\sqrt{2}\omega_{j,k-1} - t\right)\phi(t)dt & \text{if } j = 1, k = 2 \\[4mm]
\left\{\displaystyle\prod_{i=1}^{(k-1)/2}\left(\int_{-\infty}^{\omega_{i,2i}} \Phi\left(\sqrt{2}\omega_{i,2i-1} - t\right)\phi(t)dt\right)\right\}(1 - \Phi(\omega_{j,k})) & \text{if } j > 1, k = 2j - 1 \\[4mm]
\left\{\displaystyle\prod_{i=1}^{(k-2)/2}\left(\int_{-\infty}^{\omega_{i,2i}} \Phi\left(\sqrt{2}\omega_{i,2i-1} - t\right)\phi(t)dt\right)\right\} \\[4mm]
\left(\displaystyle\int_{\omega_{j,k}}^{\infty} \Phi\left(\sqrt{2}\omega_{j,k-1} - t\right)\phi(t)dt\right) & \text{if } j > 1, k = 2j
\end{cases}
$$

$$(6.10)$$

where

$$
\omega_{j,k} = b_k - \frac{f(d_j) - \theta_0}{\sqrt{(R+1)/c}} \quad \text{when } k = 2j - 1
$$

$$
\omega_{j,k} = b_k - \frac{f(d_j) - \theta_0}{\sqrt{(R+1)/2c}} \quad \text{when } k = 2j
$$

and Φ and ϕ are the cumulative density and the probability density functions of the standard normal distribution.

It can be noted that the stage-wise statistical powers depend on $\omega_{j,k}$, which in turn depends on both b_k and $f(d_j)$. If $f(d_j)$ is large for an early dose d_j, $\omega_{j,k}$ will be small, and hence the stage-wise statistical power, $\xi_{j,k}$, for this early dose will increase. As a result, this design will stop early for efficacy for these early efficacious doses. If we complement this with a more optimistic error spending function such as Pocock's or Rho with $\rho < 1$ error spending, b_k will be smaller and so will $\omega_{j,k}$ and the same reasoning follows.

In order to find c, the cohort size per stage and per dose, for a given power $\xi = \sum_{k=1}^{K} \xi_{j,k}$ of 80% or 90%, a dose ordering $\{d_1, d_2, \ldots, d_J\}$, and a dose–response model $f(d_j)$, we can use numerical integration using Equation 6.10. One of the major advantages of this adaptive staggered dose procedure is stopping the trial early if a dose showing evidence of efficacy is selected. In addition, the doses following the selected dose under the given dose ordering do not have to enter the trial, and therefore, saving patients from further allocation to potentially inferior doses. Under the proposed design, the number of stages a trial goes through before stopping for efficacy, denoted by K, is a random variable. The expected number of stages is thus given by

$$
E(K) = 2J - \left\{\sum_{j=1}^{J-1}\left((2J - 2j + 1)\xi_{j,2j-1} + (2J - 2j)\xi_{j,2j}\right)\right\} - \xi_{J,2J-1} \quad (6.11)
$$

We can see from Equation 6.11 that $E(\mathcal{K}) \ll 2J$ if the stopping probabilities $\xi_{j,k}$'s are large. The sample size S for this specific design is also random and its expectation is given by

$$E(S) = c\left(\frac{1}{R} + 1\right)E(\mathcal{K}) \tag{6.12}$$

as the control arm will always require an allocation of c/R subjects per stage. And finally, the probability of selecting dose, d_j, is therefore given by

$$\frac{\xi_{j,2j-1} + \xi_{j,2j}}{\xi} \tag{6.13}$$

for $j = 1,2,\ldots,J$.

6.5 Operating Characteristics

6.5.1 Numerical Studies

In this section, we want to investigate the operating characteristics of this proposed adaptive staggered dose procedure for dose selection. We consider the specific trial design illustrated in Figure 6.1 using the same design parameters: $J = 4$, $D = 1$, $M = 2$, $R = 2$, and $K = 2J = 8$. That means, in this specific procedure, we have four experimental doses, eight global stages, and only one dose being compared to the control at each interim stage. Each experimental dose will have a maximum of two per-dose stages. A fixed randomization ratio of 1:2 is used for the control dose to each of the experimental doses throughout the trial. In other words, if c is the cohort size for each experimental dose per stage, then the control will have a cohort of $c/2$ per stage.

Specifically, we are interested in numerically evaluating, for a given dose–response model, the cohort size c required to attain statistical power of 0.8 under different combinations of dose orderings and error spending schemes. This cohort size c will guide the investigation team to decide and plan for the recruitment of the total trial sample size under given prespecified scenarios. As we have seen earlier, this design allows for early stopping when an experimental dose is selected due to statistically significant evidence of efficacy. Due to early stopping, the number of global stages each trial requires is random and so is the sample size used. Therefore, we want to know their expectations using the cohort size corresponding to each of the dose orderings and error spending schemes. Also, since the experimental doses will be selected with different probabilities, we also want to characterize the variation of these dose selection probabilities under different dose orderings and error

TABLE 6.2

Five Selected Dose–Response Models with $\theta_0 = f(d_0) = 0$

Dose–response	$\theta_j = f(d_j)$	$(d_0, d_1, d_2, d_3, d_4) = (0,2,4,6,8)$
Flat	$\theta_j = 0.35$	(0.000, 0.350, 0.350, 0.350, 0.350)
Linear	$\theta_j = 0.04375 d_j$	(0.000, 0.088, 0.175, 0.263, 0.350)
Emax	$\theta_j = 0.4375 \dfrac{d_j}{2 + d_j}$	(0.000, 0.219, 0.292, 0.328, 0.350)
Logistic	$\theta_j = -0.015 + \dfrac{0.38}{1 + \exp(0.798(4 - d_j))}$	(0.000, 0.049, 0.175, 0.301, 0.350)
Umbrella	$\theta_j = 0.117 d_j - 0.0097 d_j^2$	(0.000, 0.194, 0.311, 0.350, 0.311)

spending schemes. Finally, we would like to compare this adaptive staggered dose design with the classical parallel group design using Dunnett's adjustment (Dunnett, 1955) [18] and the drop-the-losers (pick-the-winner) design described by Sampson and Sill (2005). We will describe each of the simulation settings below.

We chose the following dose levels, $d = 0,2,4,6$, and 8 for illustration. The first dose level of zero refers to the control dose, d_0, with $\theta_0 = f(d_0 = 0) = 0$ and the second to fifth are the four increasing dose levels of the experimental drug. We consider five dose–response models—flat, linear, emax, logistic, and umbrella, for our alternative hypothesis. Table 6.2 describes these five dose–response curves, $E(Y_{ji}) = \theta_j = f(d_j)$. These five curves are chosen because they are the commonly assumed dose–response models in clinical trials. They are plotted in Figure 6.2.

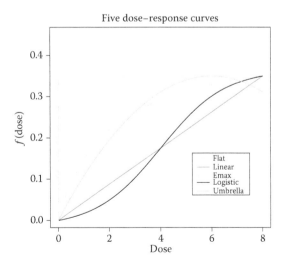

FIGURE 6.2

(**See color insert.**) Plot of five selected dose–response models with $\theta_0 = f(d_0) = 0$.

We consider looking into three ordering schemes for the four experimental doses—dose-escalation, informative, and uninformative orderings. In dose-escalation ordering, these four experimental doses are given the order of priority of $(1,2,3,4)$, such that $(d_1,d_2,d_3,d_4) = (2,4,6,8)$. In this case, the trial proceeds from the lowest dose to the highest dose. If a strong dose–response model based on preclinical or earlier clinical experience preexists, we can adopt an informative ordering. In informative ordering, we arrange the doses in the presumed order of decreasing efficacy. For example, for the umbrella dose–response model described above, we can give the four experimental doses the order of priority of $(4,2,1,3)$, then $(d_1,d_2,d_3,d_4) = (6,4,8,2)$. In this case, we prefer to explore $f(d_1 = 6) = 0.35$ first and $f(d_4 = 2) = 0.194$ last. In uninformative ordering, we will use all of the 24 ($J! = 4!$) permuted orderings and take the average of all the calculated cohort sizes. This is the expected cohort size required if we randomly pick an ordering out of the 24 permuted orderings with equal probabilities. This simulates the situation where there is no prior knowledge of the dose–response relationship.

Next, we select six different error spending plans. We include the Pocock, the O'Brien and Fleming, and Rho error spendings with parameter ρ pre-specified at 0.3, 1, and 3, and a final error spending that fixes a constant efficacy stopping boundary b_k across all $K = 8$ stages. For Rho error spending, we choose the above values of ρ to examine how a wider spectrum of error spending can affect the cohort size, the expected number of stages to stop the trial and the probabilities of dose selection. The family-wise type I error is set at one-sided $\alpha = 0.05$ for all of the selected error spending plans.

6.5.2 Simulation Studies

To assess the relative advantages of this proposed adaptive staggered dose procedure, we will compare the statistical power of this design with those of the parallel group design using Dunnett's adjustment and the drop-the-losers design given the same expected trial sample size. We use the expected total trial sample size under uninformative ordering as the trial sample size in this comparison. We denote this as E(S) as in Equation 6.12. This is performed for the target power of 0.8 under the proposed design. In the parallel group design, we use a balanced allocation ratio for the control dose and the four experimental dose groups. Therefore, each arm will receive E(S)/5 subjects. If at least one dose is found to show statistical evidence of efficacy under Dunnett's multiplicity adjustment with $\alpha = 0.05$, then the trial will be declared a success.

For the drop-the-losers design, we have two stages. In the first stage, a balanced allocation ratio is used for the control dose and the four experimental dose groups with each group receiving w subjects. At interim, the experimental dose, compared to the control dose, that demonstrates the largest sample mean difference, will continue to the second stage with the control dose, while the remaining three experimental doses will be dropped from the trial without further randomization. This second stage will use a balanced allocation ratio to randomize the remaining subjects to both the selected dose and the control dose, with each receiving another w subjects. Therefore, w is equal to $E(S)/7$. There is no testing of hypothesis at the first interim stage, but only dose selection. However, the test statistic at the final stage comparing the selected dose and the control dose will use all $2w$ subjects allocated in both stages. The efficacy stopping boundary for the final stage, evaluated by simulation, will keep the family-wise type I error at $\alpha = 0.05$. If this selected dose shows evidence of efficacy, then this drop-the-losers trial is a success. We simulate data from normal distribution with common known unit variance ($\sigma^2 = 1$) and the number of simulated trials is 10,000 unless otherwise stated. All of the numerical evaluations and simulations are conducted in the open-source $\mathcal{R}$ software.

6.5.3 Efficacy Stopping Boundaries

Table 6.3 shows the stage-wise efficacy boundaries and their corresponding alphas using the six selected error spending plans under the global null hypothesis. We have seen earlier that, without futility analysis at interim

TABLE 6.3

Six Selected Alpha Spending Schemes and Their Corresponding Stage-Wise Efficacy Stopping Boundaries (b_k) and Errors (α_k) for $J = 4$, $D = 1$, $M = 2$, $R = 2$, and $K = 2J = 8$

Error Spending Scheme	k	1	2	3	4	5	6	7	8
1. Constant efficacy boundary	b_k	2.442	2.442	2.442	2.442	2.442	2.442	2.442	2.442
	α_k	0.0073	0.0054	0.0072	0.0054	0.0071	0.0053	0.0070	0.0052
2. Pocock-type boundary	b_k	2.337	2.291	2.451	2.399	2.534	2.480	2.599	2.544
	α_k	0.0097	0.0081	0.0070	0.0061	0.0055	0.0049	0.0045	0.0041
3. O'Brien- and Fleming-type boundary	b_k	5.421	3.750	3.015	2.600	2.426	2.220	2.232	2.078
	α_k	2.96e − 08	8.84e − 05	0.0013	0.0042	0.0076	0.0104	0.0125	0.0139
4. Rho error spending $\rho = 0.3$	b_k	1.930	2.277	2.619	2.613	2.755	2.728	2.837	2.802
	α_k	0.0268	0.0062	0.0043	0.0034	0.0028	0.0024	0.0022	0.0020
5. Rho error spending $\rho = 1.0$ (i.e., constant error spending)	b_k	2.498	2.407	2.493	2.402	2.489	2.397	2.484	2.392
	α_k	0.0062	0.0063	0.0063	0.0063	0.0063	0.0063	0.0063	0.0063
6. Rho error spending $\rho = 3.0$	b_k	3.725	3.190	2.901	2.638	2.512	2.289	2.236	2.016
	α_k	9.77e − 05	0.0007	0.0019	0.0034	0.0060	0.0089	0.0124	0.0165

Note: Family-wise type I error is controlled at $\alpha = 0.05$. Nonbinding futility is adopted, $a_k = -\infty$ for all k.

stages, dose d_1 is studied at interim stages $k = 1,2$; dose d_2 at $k = 3,4$; and so on. The constant efficacy boundary scheme offers similar α_k spent for each of the four doses. Dose d_1 gets an alpha of 0.0127, d_2 of 0.0126, d_3 of 0.0124, and d_4 of 0.0122. In this case, we are not showing strong favoritism to any of the doses.

Under the Pocock-type boundary set, we are favoring the earlier doses by spending more alphas in the earlier stages, while under the O'Brien and Fleming-type boundary set, we are doing the opposite by spending more alphas in later stages. The boundary set under Rho error spending with $\rho = 0.3$ has similar properties to the Pocock-type boundary set, while that with $\rho = 3$ is similar to the O'Brien and Fleming-type boundary set. Similar to the constant boundary set, the boundary set under Rho error spending with $\rho = 1$ also has the same α_k spent for each of the four doses. Each dose gets an alpha spending of 0.0125. This is similar to the constant efficacy boundary scheme except the fact that constant efficacy boundary favors the first per-dose stage $m = 1$ slightly more than the second per-dose stage $m = 2$ for each of the doses, that is, $\alpha_1 > \alpha_2$, $\alpha_3 > \alpha_4$, and so on.

6.5.4 Cohort Sizes and Planned Trial Sample Size

Tables 6.4 and 6.5 display the cohort sizes under this proposed adaptive procedure to obtain statistical power of 0.8. For all dose–response models except the flat model, the required cohort size is smaller when a trial uses informative ordering and error spending schemes that favor earlier stages, namely, Pocock and Rho with $\rho = 0.3$. Considerable saving in patient resources in terms of sample size and time can be achieved under these optimistic scenarios. When prior knowledge of the dose–response relationship is strong, we can plan the trial by putting presumably efficacious doses first and applying an optimistic error spending function that favors earlier stages. On the other hand, if we couple an informative ordering with an error spending plan that favors later stages and doses, such as O'Brien and Fleming and Rho with $\rho = 3$, we will have to increase the cohort size to maintain the same statistical power. O'Brien and Fleming error spending performs the worst in this case due to its strong favoritism on the later stages. In this case, this type of error spending plan is not complementary to the informative dose ordering.

For these same dose–response models except the flat model, the constant efficacy boundary and Rho with $\rho = 1$ have similar results with the latter showing only a small advantage. It can be seen that for these two error spending plans, informative ordering does not offer additional advantage over dose-escalation ordering. It is apparent that the flat dose–response model is immune to dose ordering and all error spending plans perform similarly under this model. Tables 6.4 and 6.5 also show the total planned sample sizes using these cohort sizes for statistical power of 0.8. It is important to note that since this adaptive procedure allows for stopping the trial early for efficacy, the expected sample sizes can be substantially smaller than the planned total sample size.

TABLE 6.4

Cohort Size Per Stage c, Expected Global Stage to Stop for Efficacy E(K), Expected Trial Sample Size $(c(1 + R)/R)E(K)$, and Dose Selection Probabilities Given Power of 80% for Pocock, O'Brien, and Fleming, and Constant Boundary Error Spending Plans

Dose Response		Pocock's Error Spending			Constant Boundary Error Spending			O'Brien and Fleming Error Spending		
		Escalation	Informative	Uninformative	Escalation	Informative	Uninformative	Escalation	Informative	Uninformative
1. Flat	Cohort size	45	45	45	46	46	46	49	49	49
	Expected stage	4.3	4.3	4.3	4.4	4.4	4.4	5.8	5.8	5.8
	Expected sample size	289	289	289	307	307	307	430	430	430
	Selection probabilities	(0.48, 0.26, 0.15, 0.10)	(0.48, 0.26, 0.16, 0.10)	(0.25, 0.25, 0.25, 0.25)	(0.42, 0.28, 0.18, 0.12)	(0.42, 0.28, 0.18, 0.12)	(0.25, 0.25, 0.25, 0.25)	(0.05, 0.34, 0.37, 0.24)	(0.05, 0.34, 0.37, 0.24)	(0.25, 0.25, 0.25, 0.25)
2. Linear	Cohort size	92	81	87	87	87	87	72	140	98
	Expected stage	6.0	3.3	4.5	6.2	3.3	4.6	6.7	4.3	5.7
	Expected sample size	835	396	583	804	433	606	721	901	833
	Selection probabilities	(0.09, 0.20, 0.34, 0.37)	(0.01, 0.04, 0.16, 0.79)	(0.04, 0.12, 0.29, 0.55)	(0.06, 0.19, 0.36, 0.39)	(0.01, 0.05, 0.17, 0.76)	(0.04, 0.11, 0.28, 0.57)	(0.00, 0.11, 0.42, 0.47)	(0.04, 0.13, 0.39, 0.44)	(0.03, 0.10, 0.27, 0.60)
3. Emax	Cohort size	61	58	60	60	60	60	56	75	66
	Expected stage	5.0	3.8	4.3	5.2	3.9	4.5	6.2	5.3	5.8
	Expected sample size	466	330	386	467	355	406	518	593	571
	Selection probabilities	(0.27, 0.32, 0.25, 0.17)	(0.04, 0.11, 0.25, 0.60)	(0.12, 0.23, 0.30, 0.35)	(0.21, 0.32, 0.28, 0.19)	(0.05, 0.13, 0.27, 0.55)	(0.12, 0.23, 0.30, 0.35)	(0.01, 0.26, 0.42, 0.30)	(0.12, 0.31, 0.45, 0.13)	(0.11, 0.22, 0.30, 0.36)
4. Logistic	Cohort size	85	75	81	81	81	81	66	127	91
	Expected stage	6.1	3.3	4.5	6.2	3.4	4.6	6.6	4.3	5.7
	Expected sample size	779	373	540	751	408	562	652	817	774
	Selection probabilities	(0.05, 0.19, 0.44, 0.31)	(0.01, 0.04, 0.21, 0.75)	(0.02, 0.11, 0.36, 0.51)	(0.03, 0.18, 0.45, 0.33)	(0.01, 0.04, 0.23, 0.72)	(0.10, 0.10, 0.36, 0.52)	(0.00, 0.10, 0.50, 0.40)	(0.02, 0.10, 0.50, 0.37)	(0.01, 0.10, 0.35, 0.54)
5. Umbrella	Cohort size	63	59	61	61	61	61	58	77	67
	Expected stage	4.9	3.8	4.3	5.1	3.9	4.5	5.9	5.3	5.8
	Expected sample size	465	335	395	468	361	414	517	608	582
	Selection Probabilities	(0.22, 0.39, 0.28, 0.11)	(0.03, 0.23, 0.61, 0.13)	(0.10, 0.27, 0.36, 0.27)	(0.17, 0.38, 0.31, 0.14)	(0.04, 0.24, 0.56, 0.16)	(0.10, 0.27, 0.36, 0.27)	(0.00, 0.32, 0.46, 0.21)	(0.09, 0.40, 0.13, 0.37)	(0.10, 0.27, 0.37, 0.27)

Note: These are all numerically evaluated.

TABLE 6.5

Cohort Size Per Stage c, Expected Global Stage to Stop for Efficacy $E(K)$, Expected Trial Sample Size $(c(1 + R)/RE(K))$, and Dose Selection Probabilities Given Power of 80% for Rho Error Spending Plans Using $\rho = 0.3,1,3$

Dose Response		Rho Error Spending $\rho = 3.0$			Rho Error Spending $\rho = 1.0$			Rho Error Spending $\rho = 0.3$		
		Escalation	Informative	Uninformative	Escalation	Informative	Uninformative	Escalation	Informative	Uninformative
1. Flat	Cohort size	51	51	51	44	44	44	48	48	48
	Expected stage	3.8	3.8	3.8	4.5	4.5	4.5	5.6	5.6	5.6
	Expected sample size	295	295	295	300	300	300	405	405	405
	Selection probabilities	(0.60, 0.20, 0.12, 0.08)	(0.60, 0.20, 0.12, 0.08)	(0.25, 0.25, 0.25, 0.25)	(0.41, 0.28, 0.19, 0.13)	(0.41, 0.28, 0.19, 0.13)	(0.25, 0.25, 0.25, 0.25)	(0.14, 0.29, 0.32, 0.25)	(0.14, 0.29, 0.32, 0.25)	(0.25, 0.25, 0.25, 0.25)
2. Linear	Cohort size	111	84	98	85	85	85	72	122	93
	Expected stage	5.9	2.9	4.2	6.2	3.4	4.7	6.7	3.9	5.5
	Expected sample size	985	372	610	790	429	597	726	718	764
	Selection probabilities	(0.14, 0.17, 0.32, 0.37)	(0.01, 0.03, 0.11, 0.86)	(0.04, 0.12, 0.29, 0.54)	(0.06, 0.19, 0.36, 0.39)	(0.01, 0.05, 0.17, 0.76)	(0.04, 0.11, 0.28, 0.57)	(0.01, 0.10, 0.38, 0.51)	(0.04, 0.10, 0.26, 0.61)	(0.03, 0.10, 0.26, 0.61)
3. Emax	Cohort size	73	64	68	59	59	59	56	71	64
	Expected stage	4.6	3.4	3.9	5.2	4.0	4.5	6.1	4.9	5.6
	Expected sample size	505	325	396	461	351	402	514	527	531
	Selection probabilities	(0.37, 0.27, 0.21, 0.15)	(0.03, 0.08, 0.18, 0.71)	(0.13, 0.23, 0.30, 0.34)	(0.21, 0.32, 0.28, 0.19)	(0.05, 0.13, 0.27, 0.55)	(0.12, 0.23, 0.30, 0.35)	(0.04, 0.25, 0.39, 0.32)	(0.12, 0.25, 0.35, 0.27)	(0.11, 0.22, 0.30, 0.37)
4. Logistic	Cohort size	104	78	91	78	79	79	66	113	86
	Expected stage	6.0	3.0	4.2	6.2	3.4	4.7	6.6	3.9	5.5
	Expected sample size	942	355	567	729	404	553	658	667	709
	Selection probabilities	(0.08, 0.17, 0.43, 0.32)	(0.00, 0.02, 0.15, 0.82)	(0.03, 0.12, 0.36, 0.50)	(0.03, 0.18, 0.45, 0.34)	(0.01, 0.04, 0.23, 0.72)	(0.02, 0.11, 0.36, 0.52)	(0.02, 0.08, 0.46, 0.44)	(0.01, 0.08, 0.35, 0.55)	(0.01, 0.10, 0.35, 0.55)
5. Umbrella	Cohort size	74	65	69	60	60	60	58	73	65
	Expected stage	4.6	3.4	3.9	5.1	4.0	4.5	5.9	4.9	5.6
	Expected sample size	515	329	405	462	357	410	516	539	542
	Selection probabilities	(0.32, 0.34, 0.25, 0.10)	(0.02, 0.16, 0.72, 0.10)	(0.11, 0.27, 0.35, 0.27)	(0.17, 0.38, 0.31, 0.14)	(0.04, 0.25, 0.56, 0.16)	(0.10, 0.27, 0.36, 0.27)	(0.03, 0.31, 0.43, 0.23)	(0.09, 0.32, 0.29, 0.30)	(0.10, 0.27, 0.37, 0.27)

Note: These are all numerically evaluated.

6.5.5 Expected Stages and Expected Trial Sample Sizes

For all of the dose–response models except the flat model, informative dose ordering results in substantial reduction in the number of stages a trial requires for efficacy, regardless of which error spending function is used. This reduction in stages is particularly greater, $E(\mathcal{K}) < 4$, under Pocock, Rho with $\rho = 0.3$ and $\rho = 1$ error spendings. We can only achieve $E(\mathcal{K}) < 6$ if we use O'Brien and Fleming or Rho with $\rho = 3$ under informative ordering. Again, constant efficacy boundary and Rho with $\rho = 1$ perform similarly. As expected, the flat model does not depend on dose ordering, but Pocock or Rho with $\rho = 0.3$ error spending can offer an advantage to stop the trial early for efficacy better than the other error spending plans.

We can also see from these tables that dose-escalation ordering does not perform well in reducing the expected number of stages a trial requires before stopping for efficacy. This is because the better doses are placed at the later stages, so trials that use dose-escalation ordering and error spending plans which favor later stages will tend to proceed through the later stages. Tables 6.4 and 6.5 also combine the results of cohort sizes and expected number of stages to obtain the expected trial sample sizes.

6.5.6 Probabilities of Dose Selection

Under dose-escalation ordering, the best dose is usually located last except in flat and umbrella dose–response models. Error spending functions that favor later stages such as O'Brien and Fleming or Rho with $\rho = 3$ tend to push the trial to these later stages and therefore increase the probabilities that these better doses are selected. On the other hand, error spending functions that favor earlier stages are unlikely to move a trial to later stages, and thus they decrease the probabilities that these better doses are selected. For example, for power of 0.8 under the linear model and dose-escalation ordering, if Rho error spending with $\rho = 0.3$ is used, the probability that $d_4 = 8$ with $\theta_4 = 0.35$ is selected is 0.37, but this probability increases to 0.51 if Rho with $\rho = 3$ is used.

Under informative ordering, the best dose is located first and when it is coupled with a complementary error spending function like Pocock or Rho with $\rho = 0.3$, the probabilities that these best doses being selected are higher. The probability of selecting dose $d_4 = 8$ with mean response of $\theta_4 = 0.35$ is 0.86 which is higher when we use $\rho = 0.3$. However, under the flat model, the later doses, although having a similar mean effect, are likely not selected. If one insists on fully exploring all of the experimental doses, a Rho error spending plan with $\rho = 3$ or higher can help a trial go through all the stages, allowing doses under the flat dose–response model to have comparable probabilities of being selected.

It is important to note that the probabilities of dose selection not only depend on the mean responses of the doses but also on the ordering of the doses and the error spending plan chosen for the trial. Generally, error spending plans that favor the later stages tend to push the trial all the way through the stages, and therefore most of the doses will be studied. This will increase the probability of selection for later doses.

6.5.7 Comparison of Statistical Power

Table 6.6 displays the statistical powers of the parallel group fixed dose design and the drop-the-losers design. It also shows the probabilities of dose selection under the drop-the-losers design. The statistical powers for these two designs are simulated using the expected trial sample sizes from the adaptive staggered dose procedure with power of 0.8. Therefore, we can compare these simulated powers to the 0.8 level.

For parallel group design using traditional Dunnett's adjustment, its statistical power is lower than that of the adaptive staggered dose procedure except under the following two error spending plans—O'Brien and Fleming and Rho with $\rho = 3$. As we have seen earlier, these are the error spending plans that favor later stages and therefore they need larger expected number of global stages for the trial to stop for efficacy. As a result, they also tend to require larger expected sample sizes under the proposed adaptive design and hence we will lose efficiency if we use this type of error spending functions.

When compared to the drop-the-losers design, the proposed adaptive procedure can outperform in statistical power when certain conditions are met. Figures 6.3 through 6.7 compare the statistical powers of all three designs using the same expected trial sample size from uninformative ordering. Their powers are plotted against the cohort size that gives the same expected trial sample size under the adaptive staggered dose design.

Under the flat, emax, or umbrella dose–response models, the adaptive procedure performs better than both parallel group and drop-the-losers designs when using an error spending that favors earlier doses such as Pocock or Rho with $\rho \leq 1$. This can be confirmed from Table 6.6. Under linear or logistic dose–response models, this adaptive design performs worse than the other two designs, except under informative ordering coupled with Pocock or Rho with $\rho \leq 1$. Generally, the adaptive design performs better than the parallel group and drop-the-losers designs when using informative ordering and optimistic error spending functions such as Pocock or Rho with $\rho \leq 1$. If one has to use the dose-escalation ordering, then the cohort size must be increased substantially in order to achieve comparable statistical power.

As for dose selection, under the drop-the-loser design, the probability of selecting $d_4 = 8$ with $\theta_4 = 0.35$ is 0.707, compared to 0.860 when we use Rho with $\rho = 0.3$ and informative dose ordering. The probability of selecting the optimal dose can be higher only if we use an optimistic error spending function and when knowledge of dose–response model is strong. If dose safety is not of great concern, assuming a monotonically increasing dose–response curve, dose de-escalation ordering is considered the best informative ordering and can result in higher probability of selecting the best dose.

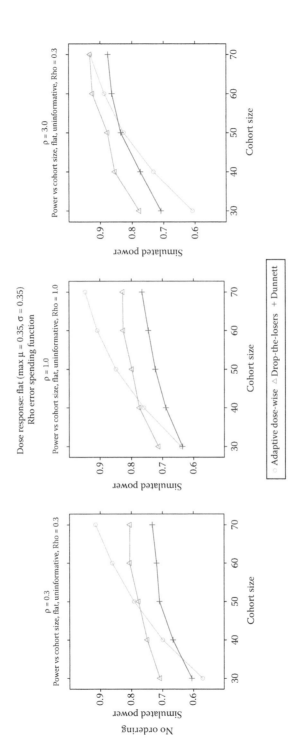

FIGURE 6.3
(See color insert.) Comparison of power under flat dose–response model (3000 simulated trials).

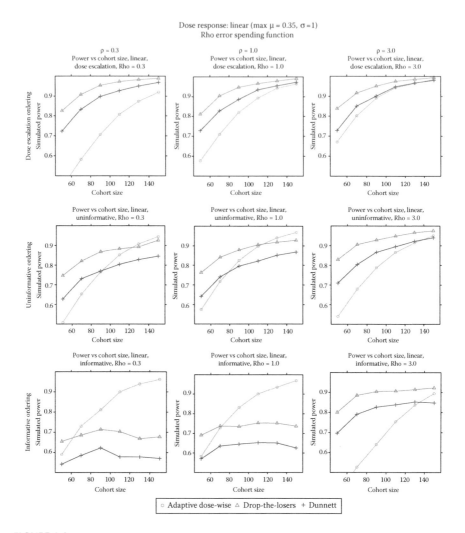

FIGURE 6.4
(See color insert.) Comparison of power under linear dose–response model (3000 simulated trials).

6.6 Discussion and Summary

Reflecting on the numerical and simulation results from the previous section, we can learn some important lessons about this adaptive staggered dose procedure. In order to achieve additional gain in trial efficiency, several conditions must be met. First, it is assumed that the doses chosen for the study are from a dose range of acceptable safety. Second, an informative ordering of the doses necessitates a strong and accurate prior knowledge of the dose–response

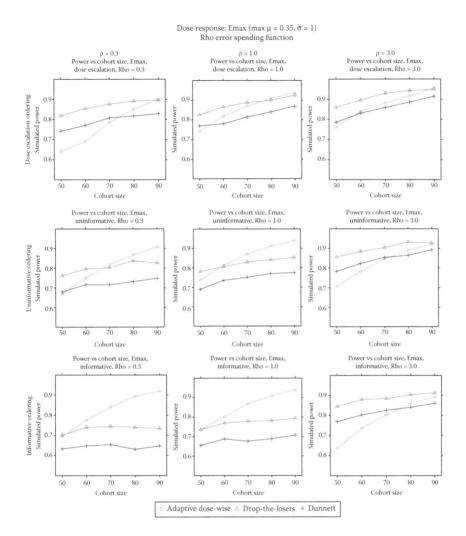

FIGURE 6.5
(See color insert.) Comparison of power under emax dose–response model (3000 simulated trials).

relationship from previous preclinical or clinical studies on a similar class of drugs, so that potentially efficacious doses are explored as early as possible. Third, an application of an optimistic error spending function such as Pocock or Rho with $\rho \leq 1$ allows early efficacious doses to be selected.

By randomizing patients in an adaptive staggered dose fashion instead of randomizing to all of the doses at the same time, we can learn about efficacy more quickly from one dose to another. If a dose shows evidence of futility, we can drop it and move onto the next dose; but if it shows evidence of efficacy, we do not need to expose patients to the remaining and potentially

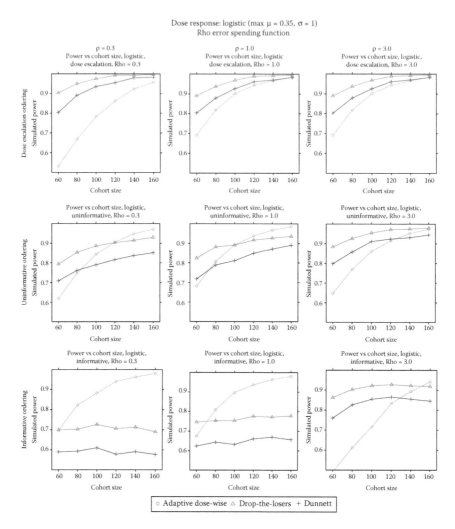

FIGURE 6.6
(**See color insert.**) Comparison of power under logistic dose–response model (3000 simulated trials).

inferior doses. As a result, we may be able to save patient resources earlier by stopping for efficacy earlier. For example, in some oncology trials, where the recruitment period is extended and patients enter a trial at a staggered rate, we can learn and make decisions quickly by focusing patient resources on fewer but potentially more efficacious doses first rather than allocating them to many doses, some of which may be inefficacious.

As we have seen from the earlier plots, the power curves for the adaptive procedure are steeper as cohort size increases. Even under unfavorable ordering such as dose-escalation ordering, we may be able to use an error spending

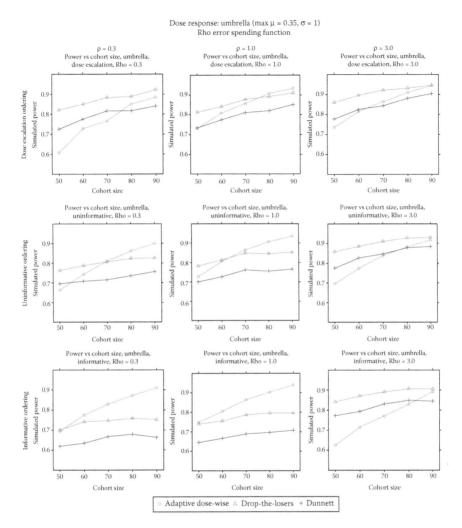

Dose response: umbrella (max μ = 0.35, σ = 1)
Rho error spending function

FIGURE 6.7
(See color insert.) Comparison of power under umbrella dose–response model (3000 simulated trials).

scheme that favors later stages such as O'Brien and Fleming or Rho with ρ > 1 *and* a larger cohort size to offset the loss of statistical power due to the use of dose-escalation ordering. However, this may risk selecting a suboptimal dose too early and failing to explore the other more efficacious doses.

This adaptive procedure has potential but preventable drawbacks. First, it can be likely to randomize more patients to the control arm than to the new test treatment. This is particularly undesirable if the trial continues to later stages due to unsuccessful earlier doses. One way to overcome this undesirable condition, while maintaining a blinded randomization to avoid potential

TABLE 6.6

Powers from Parallel Group Fixed Dose Design with Dunnett's Adjustment and Drop-the-Losers Design Using Expected Sample Sizes from Tables 6.4 and 6.5 under Uninformative Ordering

Dose Response		Pocock's Spending	Constant Boundary	O'Brien and Fleming	Rho Spending ρ = 0.3	Rho Spending ρ = 1	Rho Spending ρ = 3
1. Flat	Parallel group	0.695	0.711	0.841	0.700	0.708	0.806
	Drop-the-losers	0.782	0.798	0.908	0.780	0.791	0.885
	Selection probabilities	(0.26, 0.24, 0.25, 0.25)	(0.25, 0.25, 0.25, 0.25)	(0.25, 0.250.25, 0.25)	(0.24, 0.26, 0.25, 0.25)	(0.25, 0.26, 0.25, 0.25)	(0.25, 0.25, 0.25, 0.25)
2. Linear	Parallel group	0.759	0.777	0.897	0.783	0.770	0.866
	Drop-the-losers	0.867	0.868	0.949	0.867	0.863	0.925
	Selection probabilities	(0.01, 0.05, 0.24, 0.70)	(0.01, 0.06, 0.23, 0.71)	(0.00, 0.040.21, 0.74)	(0.01, 0.05, 0.23, 0.71)	(0.01, 0.05, 0.25, 0.69)	(0.00, 0.05, 0.22, 0.73)
3. Emax	Parallel group	0.700	0.725	0.855	0.718	0.720	0.826
	Drop-the-losers	0.793	0.815	0.916	0.805	0.810	0.900
	Selection probabilities	(0.07, 0.21, 0.31, 0.41)	(0.01, 0.20, 0.32, 0.40)	(0.06, 0.18, 0.32, 0.43)	(0.07, 0.20, 0.33, 0.41)	(0.07, 0.20, 0.33, 0.41)	(0.07, 0.19, 0.33, 0.42)
4. Logistic	Parallel group	0.761	0.789	0.895	0.785	0.779	0.871
	Drop-the-losers	0.862	0.870	0.949	0.879	0.870	0.932
	Selection probabilities	(0.00, 0.05, 0.35, 0.60)	(0.00, 0.05, 0.34, 0.61)	(0.00, 0.04, 0.34, 0.63)	(0.03, 0.05, 0.33, 0.62)	(0.00, 0.04, 0.35, 0.61)	(0.00, 0.04, 0.34, 0.62)
5. Umbrella	Parallel group	0.710	0.732	0.854	0.711	0.728	0.839
	Drop-the-losers	0.798	0.810	0.920	0.807	0.811	0.893
	Selection probabilities	(0.05, 0.27, 0.42, 0.26)	(0.05, 0.26, 0.43, 0.27)	(0.04, 0.26, 0.43, 0.26)	(0.05, 0.26, 0.41, 0.27)	(0.05, 0.27, 0.41, 0.27)	(0.04, 0.26, 0.43, 0.27)

Note: Dose selection probabilities from drop-the-losers design. The number of simulated trials is 10,000.

bias, is to change the randomization ratio using a higher R such as 1:3 or 1:4. These ratios may reduce the overall power. Therefore, a trade-off may exist in reducing the number of patients allocated to the control and maximizing statistical power. Second, as discussed earlier, if one insists on using the dose-escalation ordering because of safety issues, this adaptive staggered dose procedure may not be efficient compared to other designs. Third, this adaptive design may take longer to complete as doses are studied one after the other, especially if earlier doses do not show evidence of efficacy.

Therefore, if a drug trial is to use this adaptive staggered dose procedure for dose selection, it is strongly suggested to perform statistical simulations to understand its operating characteristics under all plausible dose–response models. Since the operating characteristics depend on the chosen design parameters, by trying different sets of these design parameters, we can better understand their comparative performance in dose selection. Investigators can choose the trial among those studied that can optimize the trial efficiency under the most probable scenario. Using simulations, the team can also determine the cohort sizes and plan the trial sample sizes to achieve their target statistical power accordingly.

As we have discussed, this adaptive procedure has demonstrated some desirable features in increasing trial efficiency. To further improve this design and to overcome some of the potential drawbacks identified earlier, several possible solutions can be proposed. For example, by increasing R, we can randomize fewer patients to the control arm and more to the experimental doses. This will further reduce the overall expected sample size but may affect the statistical power to some extent. Another solution is to use $D = 2$, that is, to use a design that looks at two concurrent experimental doses at the same time. In this case, if $J = 4$, we can conduct the experiment by randomizing patients to the control and the first two experimental doses given the dose ordering. When either one or both of these two doses do not show evidence of efficacy, the next dose or the remaining two doses can be added to the experiment for randomization in order to maintain two concurrent doses. In this case, we randomize fewer patients to the control dose. Another modification in the trial design is to use a different number of maximum per-dose stages M. However, higher M means additional interim analyses, which can be costly. Therefore, the investigators should carefully consider the availability of resources when choosing the design parameters.

Previously, we have mentioned the use of separate alpha spending functions for each of the doses instead of using one single alpha spending function. In that case, we can have better control over how the alpha is spent on each of the doses. Further work is needed in generalizing this adaptive staggered dose design to other types of endpoints such as binary or time-to-event endpoints. A dose-searching algorithm based on this adaptive procedure can also be developed for the selection of an optimal drug combination given two experimental drug compounds. As a result, the application of this adaptive staggered dose procedure can be easily modified depending on the objectives of a specific trial.

Appendix A: Proposition of Strong Control of Type I Error

Proposition

Given an adaptive staggered dose procedure with the following parameters: $D = 1$, $M = 2$, and without interim futility analysis, the α-level efficacy stopping boundaries under the global null hypotheses are sufficient to provide strong control of family-wise type I error under α.

Proof.

Suppose there is a subset of the experimental doses, $\mathcal{J} \subset \{d_1, d_2, \ldots, d_J\}$, indexed by J, such that $\mathcal{J} = \{d_{\mathcal{J}} : H_{\mathcal{J}a} : \theta_{\mathcal{J}} > \theta_0 \text{ is true}\}$, it is sufficient to show that the following inequality is true in order to prove the above proposition

$$Pr(Z_{\mathcal{J}1} < b_k, Z_{\mathcal{J}2} < b_{k+1}) < Pr(Z_1 < b_k, Z_2 < b_{k+1})$$

Since given a dose ordering, if at least one dose $d_{\mathcal{J}} \in \mathcal{J}$ ($\mathcal{J} < j$) precedes any null dose d_j whose H_{j0} is true, the probability of rejecting H_{j0} depends on the probability on the left-hand side above according to Equation 6.6. The probability of rejecting H_{j0} if it is true, however, is not affected by doses $d_{\mathcal{J}} \in \mathcal{J}$ ($\mathcal{J} > j$) that follow d_j given the dose ordering. Since $(Z_{\mathcal{J}1}, Z_{\mathcal{J}2})$ follows the distribution in Equation 6.4 and (Z_1, Z_2) in Equation 6.5, given the same stopping boundaries, (b_k, b_{k+1}), and $\theta_{\mathcal{J}} - \theta_0 > 0$, the probability on the left-hand side is smaller than the one on the right and the probability $\psi_{j,k}$ in Equation 6.6 is also smaller, thus controlling the family-wise type I error under α.

Acknowledgments

The authors would like to thank Ruth Foley for her professional editing and Dr. Mayetri Gupta, Jing Wang, and Revathi Ananthakrishnan for providing technical review and useful comments.

References

1. International Human Genome Sequencing Consortium. 2004. Finishing the euchromatic sequence of the human genome. *Nature*, 431(7011):391–45.
2. Schuster, S.C. 2008. Next-generation sequencing transforms today's biology. *Nature Methods*, 5(1):16–8.

3. Personalized Medicine Coalition. *The Case for Personalized Medicine*, 3rd Edition. Available online at http://www.personalizedmedicinecoalition.org/about/about-personalized-medicine/the-case-for-personalized-medicine

4. Piccart-Gebhart, M.J., Procter, M., Leyland-Jones, B., et al. 2005. Trastuzumab after adjuvant chemotherapy in HER2-positive breast cancer. *NEJM*, 353:1659–72.

5. Romond, E.H., Perez, E.A., Bryant, J., et al. 2005. Trastuzumab plus adjuvant chemotherapy for operable HER2-positive breast cancer. *NEJM*, 353:1673–84.

6. Sampson, A.R. and Sill, M.W. 2003. Drop-the-losers design: Normal case. *Biometrical Journal*, 47:257–68.

7. Li, G., Zhu, J., Ouyang, S.P., Xie, J., Deng, L. and Law, G. 2009. Adaptive designs for interim dose selection. *Statistics in Biopharmaceutical Research*, 1(4):366–376.

8. Wang, Y., Lan, K.K.G., Li, G. and Ouyang, S.P. 2011. A group sequential procedure for interim treatment selection. *Statistics in Biopharmaceutical Research*, 3(1):1–13.

9. Follmann, D.A., Proschan, M.A. and Geller, N.L. 1994. Monitoring pairwise comparisons in multi-armed clinical trials. *Biometrics*, 50(2):325–36.

10. Whitehead, J. 1977. *The Design and Analysis of Sequential Clinical Trials*, Revised 2nd Edition. Chichester: Wiley.

11. Stallard, N. and Todd, S. 2003. Sequential designs for phase III clinical trials incorporating treatment selection. *Statistics in Medicine*, 22:689–703.

12. Stallard, N. and Friede, T. 2008. A group-sequential design for clinical trials with treatment selection. *Statistics in Medicine*, 27:6209–27.

13. Chen, J., DeMets, D.L. and Lan, K.K.G. 2010. Some drop-the-loser designs for monitoring multiple doses. *Statistics in Medicine*, 29:1793–807.

14. Bretz, F., Pinheiro, J.C. and Branson, M. 2005. Combining multiple comparisons and modeling techniques in dose-response studies. *Biometrics*, 61:738–48.

15. Wu, J., Menon, S. and Chang, M. 2013. An adaptive staggered dose design for dose selection for a normal endpoint. Submitted to *Journal of Biopharmaceutical Statistics*.

16. Armitage, P., McPherson, C.K. and Rowe, B.C. 1969. Repeated significance tests on accumulating data. *Journal of Royal Statistical Society*, Series A 132:235–44.

17. Lan, K.K.G. and DeMets, D.L. 1983. Discrete sequential boundaries for clinical trials. *Biometrika*, 70:659–63.

18. Dunnett, C.W. 1955. A multiple comparison procedure for comparing several treatments with a control. *Journal of the American Statistical Association*, 50(272):1096–121.

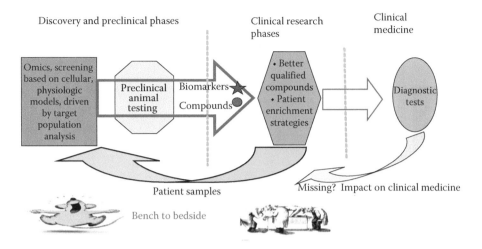

FIGURE 1.1
BMs connect discovery to clinical research and create a continuous feedback for innovation.

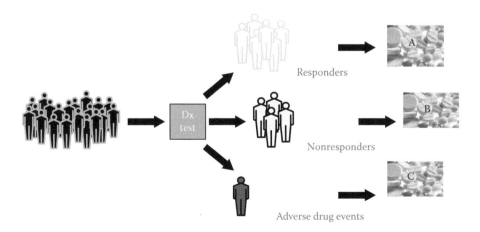

Choose the RIGHT DRUG at the RIGHT DOSE for the RIGHT PERSON

FIGURE 1.2
Personalized medicine concepts foresee greater use of diagnostics in therapeutic decision making. Classical treatments assume a homogenous patient before testing a new drug.

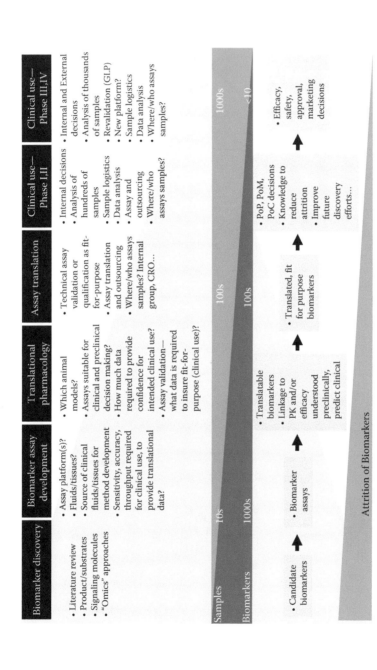

FIGURE 1.3

A schematic of a workflow for the discovery and development of a "fit-for-purpose disease-related biomarkers." This process requires a well-planned and executed research plan.

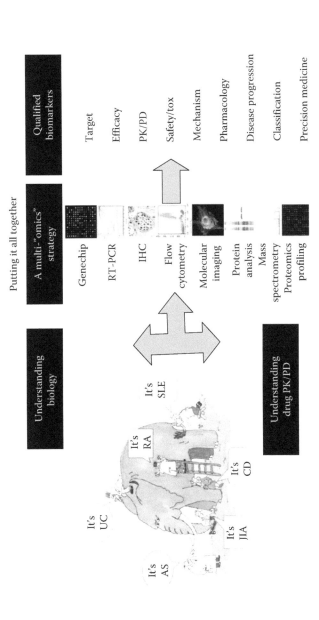

Putting it all together

Understanding biology

It's
UC

It's
AS

It's
RA

It's
SLE

It's
JIA

It's
CD

Understanding drug PK/PD

A multi-"omics" strategy

Genechip

RT-PCR

IHC

Flow cytometry

Molecular imaging

Protein analysis
Mass spectrometry
Proteomics profiling

Qualified biomarkers

Target

Efficacy

PK/PD

Safety/tox

Mechanism

Pharmacology

Disease progression

Classification

Precision medicine

FIGURE 1.4

Putting it all together, a multidimensional and a multi-omics strategy for the discovery of BMs attempting to identify specific signatures for complex diseases including inflammatory and autoimmune disease, which has many overlapping symptoms, begins with understanding the biology of disease as well as understanding the response to drug and finally putting all the pieces together in a unified picture as illustrated. It is also recommended that the correlations largely should derive from cross-sectional observations using a multi-omics strategy to develop robust and validated BMs in diseases that do not clearly define the pathogenesis of the individual disease process. (The source of the elephant is: Himmelfarb, J. et al. 2002. *Kidney Int* **62**(5): 1524–1538; doi:10.1046/j.1523-1755.2002.00600.x; Right panel adapted from Rabia Hidi, SGS Biomarkers webinar, 10.07.10)

Industry and academia need to increase collaborative efforts

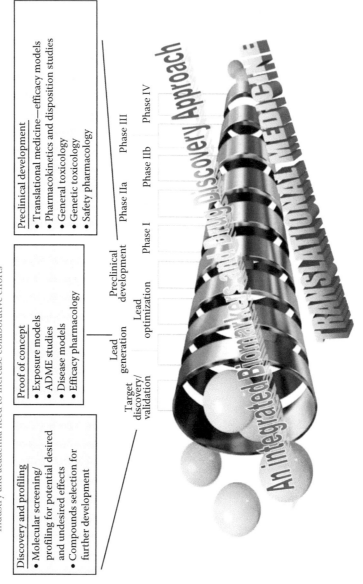

Discovery and profiling
• Molecular screening/ profiling for potential desired and undesired effects
• Compounds selection for further development

Proof of concept
• Exposure models
• ADME studies
• Disease models
• Efficacy pharmacology

Preclinical development
• Translational medicine—efficacy models
• Pharmacokinetics and disposition studies
• General toxicology
• Genetic toxicology
• Safety pharmacology

Target discovery/ validation | Lead generation | Lead optimization | Preclinical development | Phase I | Phase IIa | Phase IIb | Phase III | Phase IV

An integrated Biomarkers and Drug Discovery Approach

TRANSLATIONAL MEDICINE

FIGURE 1.5

To accelerate the successful drug discovery process and reduce attrition, industry and academia must work collaboratively.

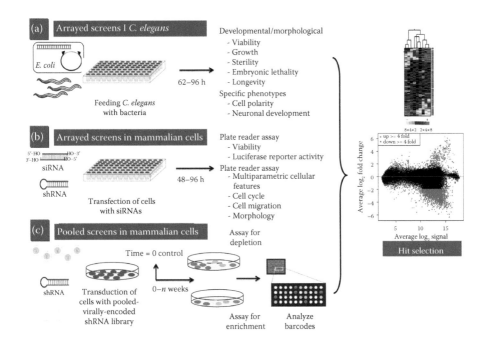

FIGURE 2.1

Arrayed or pooled-RNAi screening g workflows. (a) Screening in *C. elegans*. Feeding *C. elegans* with dsRNA-producing bacteria is accomplished by seeding bacteria into 96 well plates. Developmentally synchronized worms are then added into each well of the 96-well plate and depending on the assay, worms are scored for phenotypic aberrations within 2–4 days. (b) Arrayed RNAi screens. Each RNAi reagent targeting a unique gene is dispensed (or spotted) in each well of a multiwell dish (96-, 284-, or 1536-well plate or spotted on glass slides) and assayed 72–96 h posttransfection. RNAi reagent libraries can comprise synthetic siRNAs, plasmid- or virus-encoded shRNAs. Various assay readouts are used to determine the effect of RNAi on the phenotype of interest such as the measurement of cell viability, luminescent or fluorescent reporter assays as well as high-content image analysis using throughput microscopes may be used to measure cellular phenotypes in screens. (c) Vector-derived RNAi screens in pooled format: Pooled vector libraries can be used to transduce target cell population in a single tissue culture dish using pooled-viral vectors encoding libraries of shRNAs targeting multiple genes or entire genome. Transduced cells are selected and expanded and then assayed for a defined period of time. After selecting for the desired phenotype, genomic DNA is isolated from reference (time = 0) and assayed populations, and analyzed for the identification of genes whose inhibition by RNAi knockdown causes the specific phenotype such as changes in general cell morphology, cell proliferation, or cellular death. The relative abundance of each shRNA or a random 60-mer barcode specific to each shRNA can be identified and quantified by labeling the PCR product with fluorescent dyes (e.g., Cy5 or Cy3). The PCR products are then hybridized to custom designed cDNA microarrays containing barcode or shRNA complementary oligonucleotides. Alternatively, next-generation sequencing can be used to indentify barcode or shRNA sequences responsible for the desired phenotype. The relative abundance of barcodes obtained from the cells that were exposed to selective pressure is compared to that detected in control cells that have been exposed to the same shRNA library, but not to the selective pressure (e.g., drug treatment or genetic mutations). (Adapted from Simpson KJ, Davis GM, Boag PR, 2012. *Nat Biotechnol* **29**(4): 459–470.)

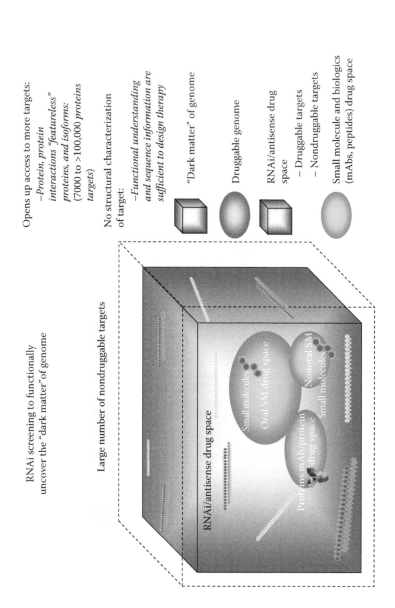

RNAi screening to functionally
uncover the "dark matter" of genome

Opens up access to more targets:
–Protein, protein
interactions "featureless"
proteins, and isoforms:
(7000 to >100,000 proteins
targets)

No structural characterization
of target:
–Functional understanding
and sequence information are
sufficient to design therapy

"Dark matter" of genome

Druggable genome

RNAi/antisense drug
space
– Druggable targets
– Nondruggable targets

Small molecule and biologics
(mAbs, peptides) drug space

Large number of nondruggable targets

RNAi/antisense drug space

Small molecules
Oral SM drug space

Nonoral SM
drug space
Small molecules

Proteins mAb/protein
drug space

FIGURE 2.2

RNAi screens can uncover previously unknown and unknowable large number of nondruggable targets and automatically reveal information on their functional activity. RNAi screening provides access to entire genome icluding the noncoding genome which constitutes the majority of genome. It provides opportunities to more previously unknown or knowable targets, molecular pathways and mechanisms, cellular functions, protein–protein interactions, "featureless" proteins, isoforms, and factors contributing to disease the biological and physical manifestations of disease.

Druggable genome gene classification

Gene families	No. of genes	% of druggable genome
Ligases	949	13.9
Cell surface and nuclear receptors	722	10.6
Kinases	719	10.6
Ion channel and transporters	639	9.4
Cell adhesion and Cytoskeleton	496	7.3
GPCR	479	7.0
Apoptosis	437	6.4
Proteases	379	5.6
Growth factors/receptors	375	5.5
Oxidoreductases	338	5.0
Nucleic acid binding	310	4.6
Phosphatases	293	4.3
Ion channels	285	4.2
Assorted functional genes	228	3.3
Cell regulation	227	3.3
Metabolism and cell traffic	217	3.2
Hydrolases	204	3.0
Transferases	184	2.7
Cytokines and chemokines	106	1.6
Transfer and carrier proteins	71	1.0
Nuclear hormone receptors	46	0.7
Drug-metabolizing enzymes (CYP450, etc.)	54	0.8
Drug transporters		
Total	6809	100

FIGURE 2.3

Human druggable genome that can be studied using RNAi. The table illustrates number of genes that can be targeted by RNAi reagent collections that permit the study of the function of entire pathway, specific gene families, pathways, mechanisms, and specific cellular functions. For example, drug-metabolizing enzymes (DMEs) and drug transporters (DTs) are molecular determinants of pharmacokinetic property of a drug and their expression is controlled by nuclear receptors (NRs). Due to the complex nature of studying the function of individual DMEs, DTs, and NRs, RNAi can be used in addition to chemical inhibitors and inhibitory antibodies to characterize their specific roles in drug metabolism and transport, gene regulation, and drug–drug interactions. Additionally, RNAi may be employed to modulate DT expression to overcome multidrug resistance. Top right panel illustrates human druggable genome and gene classification. Bottom right panel illustrates percentage of gene families within druggable genome that can be probed by RNAi reagent collections. (Adapted from Hopkins AL, Groom CR, 2002. *Nat Rev Drug Discov* **1**(9): 727–730; Wishart DS et al. 2008. DrugBank: A knowledgebase for drugs, drug actions and drug targets. *Nucleic Acids Res* **36** (Database issue): D901–906,), Selectbiosciences.com, SigmaAldrich.com, and Dharmacon.com.

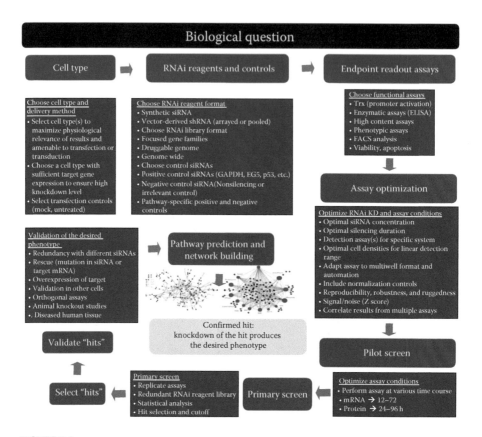

FIGURE 2.4

Guideline for a successful pilot study for RNAi screen. RNAi screening workflow begins with choice of diseases to target, choice of cell type, choice of delivery and screening method as well as RNAi reagent format and genome-coverage, followed by experimental design (scope, redundancy, throughput, controls), selection or development of a cell-based assays to monitor RNAi effect, such as phenotypic assays (growth advantage, cell viability, mobility, etc.), reporter-based assays (GFP, labeled antibodies, fluorescent dyes), transcriptional and enzymatic assays (luciferase), antibody and microscopy-based assays (e.g., protein modification (phospho-specific abs). This is followed by primary screen with appropriate controls and data analysis and statistical tools for hit selection. After the primary screen, candidate genes are mapped into pathways and gene networks to provide better understanding of the functions of these genes in biological system. Finally, the candidate hit-genes are validated using a variety of approaches. Assay optimization and a pilot screen is necessary to optimize the conditions and identify issues before embarking on the primary screen. Additionally, analytical and statistical tools must be identified or developed for proper analysis of large data sets, hit selection, gene annotation, pathway prediction, and gene network building.

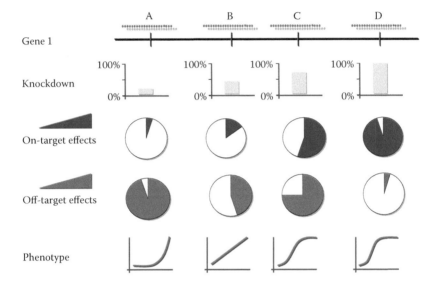

FIGURE 2.5
Examples of variables that impact RNAi screens. For a phenotypic RNAi screen involving X number of genes, the ranking of any one gene will be influenced by the knockdown efficiencies of the RNAi reagents (e.g., knockdown efficiency siRNAs D > C > B > A for that gene, their off-target effects (A > C > D > B), and on-target effects (D > C > B > A), and the dose-response curves linking the activity of that gene and the phenotype being measured (e.g., loss of viability). (Adapted from Kaelin WG, Jr, 2012. *Science* **337**(6093): 421–422.)

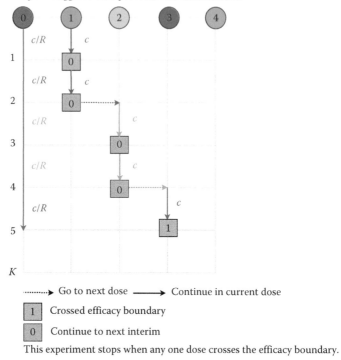

An adaptive staggered dose procedure for dose selection

........▶ Go to next dose ──────▶ Continue in current dose

| 1 | Crossed efficacy boundary

| 0 | Continue to next interim

This experiment stops when any one dose crosses the efficacy boundary.

FIGURE 6.1
A graphical illustration of the proposed adaptive staggered dose procedure with $J = 4$, $D = 1$, $M = 2$, $R = 2$, and $K = 2J = 8$.

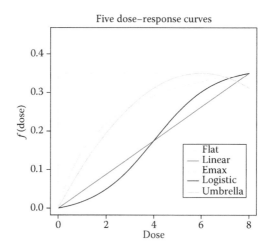

FIGURE 6.2
Plot of five selected dose–response models with $\theta_0 = f(d_0) = 0$.

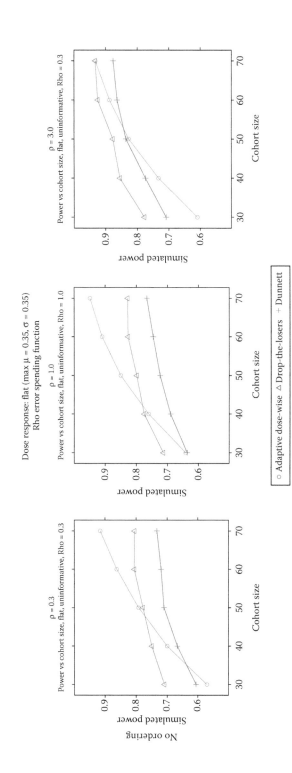

FIGURE 6.3
Comparison of power under flat dose–response model (3000 simulated trials).

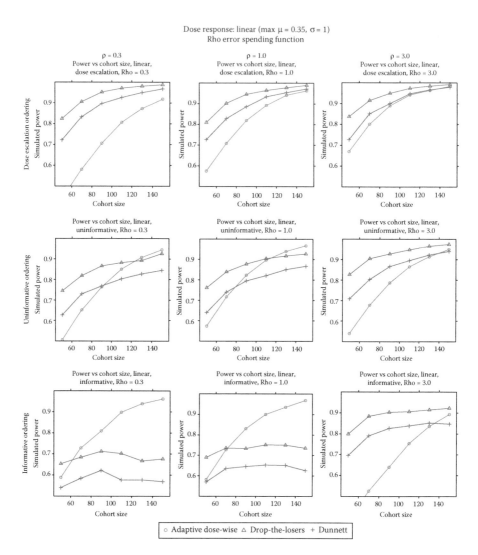

FIGURE 6.4
Comparison of power under linear dose–response model (3000 simulated trials).

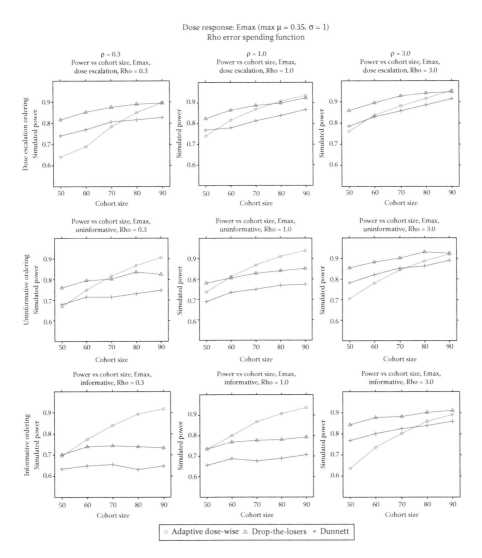

FIGURE 6.5

Comparison of power under emax dose–response model (3000 simulated trials).

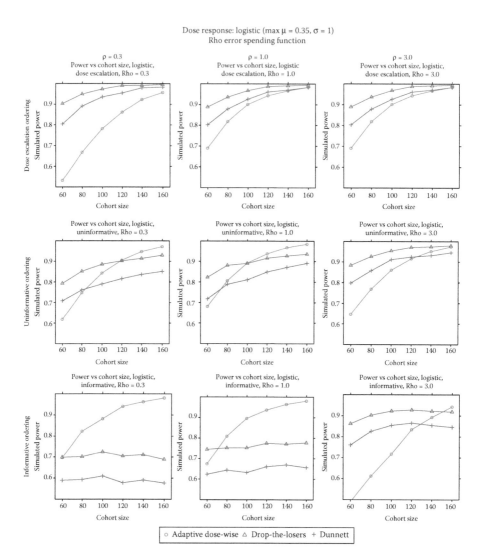

Dose response: logistic (max μ = 0.35, σ = 1)
Rho error spending function

○ Adaptive dose-wise △ Drop-the-losers + Dunnett

FIGURE 6.6
Comparison of power under logistic dose–response model (3000 simulated trials).

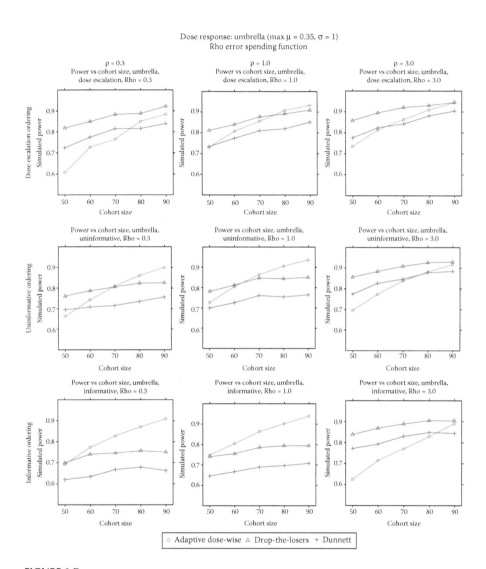

FIGURE 6.7

Comparison of power under umbrella dose–response model (3000 simulated trials).

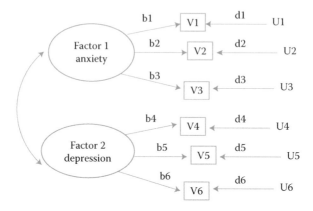

FIGURE 10.1
Path model for a six-variable, two-factor model with correlated factors.

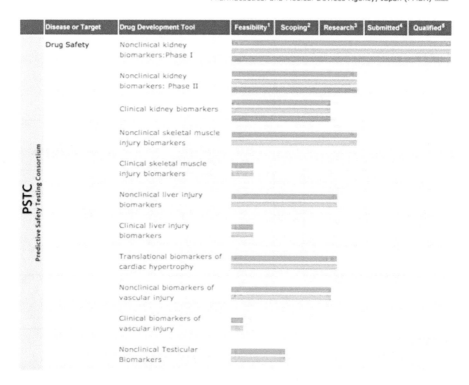

FIGURE 11.1
Drug Safety Biomarkers submitted by the Predictive Safety Testing Consortium (PSTC). (From http://www.fda.gov/NewsEvents/Newsroom/PressAnnouncements/2008/ucm116911.htm, reproduced with permission from PSTC.)

7

Evidence-Based Adaptive Statistical Decision and Design Strategies for Maximizing the Efficiency of Clinical Oncology Development Programs with Predictive Biomarkers

Cong Chen and Robert A. Beckman

CONTENTS

7.1 Introduction

The future of oncology drug development lies in identifying subsets of patients who will benefit from particular therapies, using predictive biomarkers. Increasingly, national health authorities and insurers are demanding value from medicines. For example, the United Kingdom's National Institute for Clinical Excellence (NICE) demands a cost of less than or equal to 30,000 British pounds per quality-adjusted life year (QALY). Most cancer medicines are far more expensive than this. The low value of cancer medicines is largely driven by two factors: (1) the low average benefit of cancer medicines because they benefit only a subset of the population, and (2) the high cost of oncology drug development due to its high failure rate, and to the need for large pivotal trials to detect small average benefits.

Predictive biomarkers, or "responder identification" biomarkers, are molecular or other characteristics of a patient or a patient's malignancy that predict increased benefit from a particular drug. Predictive classifiers, which may be constructed from one biomarker or a composite of biomarkers, identify patients more likely to benefit. With increasing knowledge of the molecular biology of cancer, the number and potential of these predictive biomarkers and classifiers is increasing.

Examples of predictive biomarkers of importance in oncology include her2neu expression for trastuzumab therapy, sensitizing mutations in the epidermal growth factor receptor (EGFR) gene for gefitinib and erlotinib therapy, ras wild-type status for therapy with cetuximab or panitumumab, BRAF V600E mutation for vemurafenib, and ALK mutation for crizotinib.[1–10] However, examples of failure of predictive biomarkers also exist. Since most of them occur in phases 1 and 2, they are often underreported after discontinuation of the development programs. In these cases, biomarker use added cost, complexity, and time, and narrowed the treated population unnecessarily. A notable setback that has caught a lot of attention was the failure of EGFR expression to predict efficacy by EGFR-directed antibodies. This anomaly may have been due to insufficient sensitivity, biased sampling, loss of antigen expression with storage, or tumor evolution between the time the biopsy was obtained and when the therapy was applied,[11,12] but these issues affect any real-world attempt to test a predictive biomarker hypothesis. Thus, predictive biomarker classifiers, and the assays used to test them, must be robust to these pitfalls.

The great promise of predictive biomarkers, together with inconsistent results, and the significant investment of time and money required, has led to variable attitudes ranging from uncritical enthusiasm to harsh skepticism.[13–16] The skepticism is well expressed by Ratain and Glassman: "Whereas 'wins' have occurred here,... most attempts to identify such biomarkers have been nothing more than expensive fishing expeditions. Drug response is multifactorial; patient populations are heterogeneous; potential markers are innumerable; and scientific underpinnings to marker development are imperfect." (p. 6546)[16]

These issues and legitimate concerns may hinder the development of a field that is increasing in promise with increasing molecular understanding of cancer. The lack of consensus on interdisciplinary drug development teams about if, when, and how to apply predictive classifiers is manifest in many clinical trials we still observe today that lack a meaningful use of these classifiers. Beckman et al.[14] advocate the application of predictive biomarker classifiers in exact proportion to the evidence supporting their clinical value. This chapter supplements with a greater level of statistical details for practitioners to follow. Biomarker development can be divided into an exploration phase and a confirmation phase.[17] This chapter focuses on the confirmation phases (i.e., phases 2 and 3), and it will be clear that a lot of the discussions are applicable to a general late-stage oncology drug development programs with or without a predictive biomarker.

7.2 From Exploration to Phase 2 Proof of Concept

When a new drug is transitioned from the exploration phase, which normally includes preclinical experiments and phase 1/2a dose finding and preliminary assessment of antitumor activity, to the phase 2 POC phase, it carries with a lot of excitement and often times a set of candidate predictive biomarkers. How to test these biomarker hypotheses with rigor is often an intriguing issue. These biomarkers are often identified based on tumor shrinkage ("response") in preclinical and early clinical experiments (so much so that the term "responder ID hypothesis" is commonly used). Moreover, these experiments often lack active controls and only compare response between biomarker positive (BM+) samples and biomarker negative samples, making the relevance to clinical settings less clear. This section provides guidance for increasing the quality of transition.

7.2.1 A Moratorium on Fishing, and the Importance of Prioritization and Iteration

To demonstrate the value of a predictive biomarker classifier, it must be validated against patient clinical benefit beginning with the phase 2 POC trial, and continuing, if indicated by the data, through to a phase 3 pivotal trial that definitively validates the biomarker classifier as a predictor of clinical benefit, resulting in simultaneous health authority approval for both the drug and the associated diagnostic test for patient selection ("codiagnostic" or "in vitro diagnostic [IVD]"). By incorporating formal statistics into the predictive classifier evaluation in a phase 2 study, we are able to optimally manage risk across a portfolio of drugs and putative biomarker classifiers.

Formal statistical analysis precludes the "fishing expeditions" as described by Ratain and Glassman, in which a large number of biomarkers are informally tested in an "exploratory" fashion. In this exploratory approach, many possible biomarker hypotheses are being simultaneously tested. The possibility that one of these hypotheses will appear to be true based on chance alone is extremely high. Moreover, if the hypotheses are not specified prospectively, but rather after the study data are available, the chance of crafting an artifactually successful predictive biomarker hypothesis is even higher. There are methods available to control the overall type I error rate or false discovery rate, but all at the expense of reduced power for individual hypotheses. Therefore, we require that one primary predictive biomarker hypothesis must be specified in advance. The POC study is formally powered around the subgroups defined by this biomarker classifier. Ideally, it will be specified prior to the start of the POC study, since it is helpful in the design of that study, but if necessary, its specification can be delayed until just before the samples are analyzed at the end of the study, the "prospective retrospective" approach.[18]

The time just prior to the end of phase 2 sample analyses is also the latest time by which assays to determine biomarker status must be available to stratify randomization by the predictive biomarker classifier in phase 3. Ideally, these assays will be analytically validated in terms of sensitivity, specificity, reproducibility, accuracy, and linearity[19] at this time. Such analytically validated assays require only validation against clinical data to be approved as IVDs, and are termed "IVD candidates." If absolutely necessary, the phase 2 samples can be analyzed with a nonanalytically validated "research use only" assay and the IVD candidate assay can be delivered at the time of analysis of phase 3 samples (interim or final analysis), but this entails the risk of misleading results from the phase 2 biomarker evaluation.

The primary predictive biomarker hypothesis is chosen based on data from preclinical studies, phase 1 clinical studies, phase 2a exploratory studies, and neoadjuvant studies where the tissue for exploratory biomarker work can be readily obtained, and where applicable, experimental medicine studies in patients or volunteers. It should be the hypothesis that is best supported by the scientific rationale and data to that point. Moreover, studies of tissue banks should have determined the expected prevalence of BM+ and negative subgroups in the proposed POC indications.

Given the intricacies of cancer biology, choosing one primary hypothesis will not be a foolproof exercise. As a backup, additional predictive biomarker hypotheses may be tested in an exploratory fashion in the POC study. If the primary hypothesis is false, perhaps, one of these exploratory hypotheses will generate promising data. Such new findings represent a lower level of evidence and should be validated in a second POC study, which could be the phase 2 part of a seamless phase 2/3 study, designed with the new hypothesis as primary. Such iteration should not be viewed as failure. It will require persistence to successfully unravel the complexities of biomarker-directed cancer therapy. Just as backup compounds are available in the event of failure of a lead compound in development, backup predictive biomarker-based hypotheses, which need to be validated with a subsequent iteration of phase 2, should be planned for and expected.

7.2.2 Endpoints for Phase 2 POC Studies

We strongly argue for the use of randomized-controlled studies for phase 2 POC trials, and recommend progression-free survival (PFS) to be the primary endpoint in most cases. PFS is an interval-censored time-to-event variable. When it is used as the primary endpoint, it should be analyzed with an appropriate interval-censored method to make inference the most efficient and least biased.[20,21] However, we recognize that response rate may also be considered especially in single-arm phase 2 studies of patients with advanced or metastatic diseases who have exhausted all treatment options, whereas PFS may be confounded with patients' performance status. In contrast to response, PFS is a continuous variable and is informative in all patients, which is particularly helpful with targeted therapies that may not influence response rate. It may also be expected to correlate more closely than response does with the primary variable of interest in phase 3 that is often overall survival (OS) so much so that it is sometimes accepted by the regulatory agencies as the primary endpoint of pivotal trials for drug approvals.[22–25] RECIST 1.1 is often used as a response criterion for defining disease progression (and response). The cutoff point for definition of disease progression therein is debatable and there is a loss of information due to dichotomization of an otherwise continuous variable in tumor size change. In the future, a more biologically meaningful definition of progression may be developed,[26] incorporating heterogeneity of lesion response within the same tumor,[27] continuous variations in tumor volume, and distinctions between solid masses and those with central necrosis. Currently, however, unless an improved version of the criterion is developed and well accepted in practice, disease progression as conventionally defined drives physicians' decision on whether to continue a treatment and, as such, has an intrinsic impact on clinical benefit of an investigational treatment.

When response rate (or its variant) is used as the primary endpoint in an uncontrolled study for evaluation of an investigational predictive biomarker, extra caution must be exerted in interpreting the study results as historical response rate is often unknown in the biomarker-classified population. For example, it was generally believed that BRCA mutation was a predictive biomarker in ovarian cancer patients for a new class of investigational therapies called PARP inhibitors.[28] The jury is still out whether this hypothesis holds, but, the fact that doxorubicin (a likely comparator in pivotal trials that has been in the market for many years) seems to also work better in this population[29] than in nonmutant patients complicates the issue. Without knowing the prognostic value of a predictive biomarker and how these patients respond to existing therapies, it is dangerous to jump from response data in an uncontrolled phase 2 study to a pivotal one. This uncertainty makes randomized controlled designs especially pertinent to development of therapies with predictive biomarkers.

A number of alternative early efficacy endpoints based on tumor size measurement or certain biomarker level (e.g., carcinoembryonic antigen and CA125) have generated a lot of interest in recent years, including percent change from baseline in tumor size or the level of a biomarker at a landmark (e.g., week 8). Compared to PFS, these endpoints can be assessed even earlier but have some fundamental issues. First, some patients may not have an assessment at the landmark due to early discontinuation or death. Handling of missing data is tricky, and different analyses may lead to different (and sometimes conflicting) conclusions. Second, unlike in a preclinical trial where study animals can be treated at the same time and have same follow-up, the follow-up time of patients in a clinical trial is different by the time of landmark analysis in that some may have died or have reached disease progression. A landmark analysis that ignores these data or does not fully account for them is deemed naive and less efficient. Third and most important, the underlying assumption of a landmark analysis is that the clinical benefit of an investigational treatment can be largely explained by the early endpoint.[30–34] Unfortunately, the data that support this assertion are much less robust than that for PFS. After all, had the assumption held, continued treatment beyond the landmark would have made little difference to patients, deviating from the conventional paradigm!

Despite their limitations, the early endpoints may still be considered from a cost-effectiveness standpoint,[35] especially in disease settings when patients' prognosis is favorable with a long time to disease progression (or disease relapse). While it may still be challenging to decide whether a treatment difference based on such an early endpoint predicts clinical benefit of the study therapy, it is less controversial as to whether an early kill decision can be made based on lack of treatment difference or whether a dose–response may be used to assist with a dose-selection decision.

Regardless of which endpoint is chosen, for the purpose of design, the most important measure is the relative effect size between a candidate phase 2 endpoint and the phase 3 clinical endpoint. The relative effect size should be estimated from a meta-analysis[36–38] of multiple large randomized and controlled trials in similar disease settings. Each trial is considered as a unit in the meta-analysis. If data from only one large trial are available, each center in the trial may be considered as a unit and the bootstrap technique may be applied as appropriate for estimation. There is a tendency to use single-arm trials to evaluate the "surrogacy" of an investigational endpoint by correlating the posttreatment change of an early endpoint with outcome in a clinical endpoint. This is a fundamentally flawed approach because, in the absence of a control, the correlation if any is confounded with prognostic factors.

7.3 Phase 2 POC Design and Decision Strategy

Given that there are typically nearly 1000 approved and experimental therapies for cancer actively tested in clinical trials at any one time, that they may have one or more candidate predictive biomarkers, that they can be combined in twos and threes, that different schedules may be used, and that many clinical indications and lines of therapy are available, the number of potential POC trials that could potentially be performed is enormous. The possibilities only increase when one looks at possible subsets defined by biomarker classifiers, where one must take into account approximately 30,000 genes in the human genome and the genetic instability and consequent heterogeneity of cancer.[39–41] Although preclinical information offers prioritization of these possibilities, there still remains a very large number of potentially useful POC studies, which far exceed the availability of patients, and funding from either public or private sources.

Statisticians traditionally design randomized POC studies with the concepts of type I and II error in mind. These refer, respectively, to the false-positive and false-negative rates due to chance findings as a result of the finite sample size in a POC trial. False-positive results lead to phase 3 trials that are undertaken in error and will likely lead to negative results at great expense. False-negative results lead to the wrong conclusion that an effective drug is ineffective for the indication, resulting in a loss of opportunity. Traditionally, phase 2 POC studies are designed to have a type I error of 10% and a type II error of 20% (the "power" is 100% minus the type II error; thus, 80% power in this case). So engrained is this tradition that POC studies with <80% power are often termed "underpowered," even though the traditional powering still allows significant room for error, and "perfect" POC trials would require infinite sample sizes. But, in fact, there is no absolute scientific basis for selecting particular type I and II error rates in POC trials. These are simply a function of risk tolerance, which is in turn a function of strategy. Indeed, we observe an alternative style of smaller "underpowered" trials being executed in many cases.

Chen and Beckman[42–44] investigated whether optimal type I and II error rates could be objectively defined by requiring that the efficiency of phases 2 and 3 development be maximized. Given the fact that the possible expenditure on POC trials of interest in oncology usually exceeds available patient and financial resources, efficiency was defined as the risk-adjusted number of truly effective drug/indication combinations identified by POC trials and developed to approval (benefit) divided by the risk-adjusted number of patients utilized in phase 2 and phase 3 trials (cost). In addition to type I and II error rates, Beckman et al.[14] defined type III error based on the opportunity cost if a valid hypothesis is not tested due to resource limitations. The benefit–cost ratio analysis helps address the following essential questions pertinent to all POC trials with or without a predictive biomarker: Is it better to perform larger POC trials, to minimize the adverse consequences of type I and II error, or to perform smaller POC trials, so that more valuable hypotheses can be tested under a fixed POC trial budget? How to set the cost-effective go-no-go bars to phase 3?

7.3.1 Basic Statistics on Phase 2 to Phase 3 Transition

Consider a typical phase 2 POC trial with two arms (the experimental arm and the control arm). Denote by Δ the target effect size (treatment effect divided by standard deviation) for the primary endpoint of the study. The target effect size is often obtained from a back-calculation so that the corresponding effect size to the phase 3 primary endpoint $\gamma\Delta$ is clinically meaningful whereas γ is the relative effect size between the two. For example, when the relative effective size is estimated to be 0.5 between PFS and OS in log hazard-ratio (HR) scale from a meta-analysis, a 25% hazard reduction in OS would correspond to a 44% hazard reduction in PFS. Therefore, $\Delta = -\log(1–0.44) = -\log(0.56)$ in this case. If the variance of γ estimate is large, Δ may be increased to account for the uncertainty. When γ does not have a reliable estimate, a working Δ may be obtained under the conventional assumption that the median OS improvement is the same as the median PFS improvement. For example, when a 2-month OS improvement is of clinical interest in phase 3 and the median PFS for the control arm is 3 months, Δ may be chosen to be $-\log(0.6)$ by noticing that the target HR for PFS is $3/(3 + 2)$ under the usual assumption of exponential distribution. In this case, if the median OS is 6 months in the control arm, the relative effect size would be 0.56 (i.e., $\log(6/(6 + 2))/\log(3/(3 + 2))$). We call an estimate of relative effect size so obtained a *canonical* estimate. Target effect size for endpoints other than PFS can be similarly derived.

Denote by (α, β) the doublet of one-sided type I error rate and type II error rate of the trial. The total sample size for the trial is approximately

$$N = 4(Z_{1-\alpha} + Z_{1-\beta})^2/\Delta^2 \tag{7.1}$$

where $Z_{(\cdot)}$ denotes the respective quantile of the standard normal distribution. When a time-to-event variable is the primary endpoint of interest, Δ refers to logarithm of HR (control arm vs. experimental arm) and N refers to number of events. A go decision to continue the program for later development in a phase 3 confirmatory trial is made if the one-sided *p*-value from the POC trial is less than α favoring the experimental arm. Notice that the standard error for estimate of the treatment difference is $2/\sqrt{N}$ that is equal to $\Delta/(Z_{1-\alpha} + Z_{1-\beta})$ from the sample size formula and the cutoff point for the empirical bar relative to Δ in a go decision is $Z_{1-\alpha}/(Z_{1-\alpha} + Z_{1-\beta})$. Clearly, the empirical bar increases when type I error rate decreases or when type II error rate increases. It is > 0.5 when $\alpha < \beta$ and > 1 when $\beta > 0.5$.

In the oncology therapeutic area, a single confirmatory trial accompanied with a supportive POC trial usually meets the minimum requirements for regulatory registration purposes. Denote by C_2 the cost for a POC trial and by C_3 the cost for the future phase 3 confirmation trial in the same population. In the first-line lung cancer setting, a typical POC trial with $(\alpha, \beta) = (0.1, 0.2)$ for the detection of a 40% hazard reduction in terms of PFS may need 100–150 patients with a minimum follow-up of 4–6 months. A confirmatory trial in the same setting with $(\alpha, \beta) = (0.025, 0.1)$ for the detection of a 25% hazard reduction in terms of OS may need 600–800 patients with a minimum follow-up of 8–10 months. When cost is proportional to sample size, the relative cost of a POC trial to a confirmatory trial (i.e., C_2/C_3) is around 20% in this setting. Phases 2–3 cost ratio may be different in different settings. For simplicity, we consider C_3 to be fixed, that is, the design of the phase 3 trial is independent of strength of the signal from the POC trial. Various extensions can be found in Refs. [42–44].

7.3.2 Benefit–Cost Ratio Analysis of a Single POC Trial

Let us start with a simple question. Given a fixed budget for conducting a typical POC trial with $(\alpha, \beta) = (0.1, 0.2)$ as described above, what is the optimal (α, β) to be most cost-effective? There are infinitely many ways to choose (α, β) as long as the choice satisfies the sample size constraint $Z_{1-\alpha} + Z_{1-\beta} = Z_{1-0.1} + Z_{1-0.2}$. Each choice corresponds to a different go-no-go criterion to the confirmatory trial. A self-evident choice is $(0.2, 0.1)$ by the equivalence of (β, α) to (α, β) in Equation 7.1. However, a type I error rate of 0.2 or indeed, any number for this matter could be easily challenged. Many clinical researchers[45–48] have provided qualitative guidance for how to properly size POC trials and make go-no-go decisions. Here, we provide quantitative guidance. To answer the above question, consider the following benefit–cost ratio function that involves phase 2 design parameters ($p, \alpha, \beta, B, C_2, C_3$) whereas p is the probability of the study drug being truly active (often called probability of success [POS] in practice; at this stage, in the absence of phase 2 data, an estimate of this parameter from the development team is required) with an effect size equal to the target effect (the probability of no treatment effect is assumed to be $1-p$) and B is the benefit of a successful proof of concept (POC) for a truly active drug:

$$R_1 = \frac{Bp(1 - \beta)}{C_2 + C_3[p(1 - \beta) + (1 - p)\alpha]} \qquad (7.2)$$

The numerator represents the benefit adjusted with POS and type II error (the benefit of a truly inactive drug is assumed to be zero). It represents the expected number of active drugs correctly identified by the POC study, multiplied by the benefit per drug, and thus, is a simple surrogate for overall benefit. The denominator represents the summation of the cost for the POC trial and the expected cost for the phase 3 trial multiplied by the probability of a positive outcome, true or false, from the POC trial. Thus, the denominator represents the total expected cost of the overall late development program, where the phase 3 trial happens if and only if the POC trial gives a true positive or a false-positive outcome. Hence, the ratio function defined in Equation 7.2 directly measures the cost-effectiveness of the design. Maximization of R_1 is equivalent to maximizing of the return in benefit in the face of limited resources, rendering the design strategy the most cost-effective one from a portfolio management standpoint. Whenever the decision maker is confronted with a fixed total research budget across a number of opportunities that may lead to benefit, optimization of the benefit–cost ratio will produce the maximum benefit for that fixed budget.

Notice that the benefit term B does not have an impact on optimization, making our proposed approach more robust to uncertainties in benefit assessment, in contrast to the conventional decision-theoretic approach that often uses benefit minus cost as the utility function. In addition, the optimal choice of (α, β) depends on (C_2, C_3) only via C_2/C_3. Therefore, it can be easily obtained by maximizing Equation 7.2 subject to the sample size constraint for fixed $(p, C_2/C_3)$. However, actual values of (B, C_2, C_3) are relevant if the R_1 value is used for choosing which trials to conduct among many opportunities.[41-43] Apparently, a minimum requirement for a trial to be included in a portfolio of trials is $R_1 > 1$ when B, C_2, and C_3 are determined reasonably accurately and expressed in comparable units.

Table 7.1 provides optimal design parameters for a typical POC trial with fixed sample size under $(\alpha, \beta) = (0.1, 0.2)$ for different POS levels and

TABLE 7.1

Optimal Designs of a POC Trial with Fixed Sample Size under $(\alpha, \beta) = (0.1, 0.2)$

POS (p)	C_2/C_3	Optimal α (%)	Optimal β (%)	Empirical Bar Relative to Δ
0.1	0.2	6.7	26.7	0.71
0.1	0.3	8.8	22.0	0.64
0.1	0.4	10.7	18.9	0.59
0.2	0.2	7.2	25.3	0.69
0.2	0.3	9.6	20.7	0.62
0.2	0.4	11.5	17.8	0.56
0.3	0.2	8.0	23.7	0.66
0.3	0.3	10.4	19.3	0.59
0.3	0.4	12.6	16.4	0.54

C_2/C_3 values. As expected, the empirical bar associated with optimal (α, β) decreases with increasing POS and C_2/C_3. In the first-line lung cancer setting where C_2/C_3 is around 0.2, the optimal empirical bars are in the range of 0.66–0.71Δ, the optimal α levels are in the range of 6.7–8.0%, and the optimal β levels are in the range of 23.7–26.7%. As a comparison, the starting point of $(\alpha, \beta) = (0.1, 0.2)$ would be approximately optimal at $C_2/C_3 = 0.3$ when POS is 0.3, and the associated optimal empirical bar for a go decision would be lower at 0.60Δ.

7.3.3 Benefit–Cost Ratio Analysis of Multiple POC Trials

Let us consider a more complicated problem. Suppose that there is a fixed budget (C_2) for conducting k POC trials with $(\alpha, \beta) = (0.1, 0.2)$. But, there are more trials with different POS and benefit that are of similar interest. What is the optimal resource allocation strategy and optimal design parameters? These POC trials may be for the same drug in different indications, for the same indication in different subgroups classified by a predictive biomarker or other baseline characteristics, or for different drugs. Let $(p_i, \alpha_i, \beta_i, B_i, C_{2i}, C_{3i})$ be the design parameters associated with the ith trial $(i = 1,\dots,k)$ similarly defined as in R_1. Consider the following general version of the benefit–cost ratio function to Equation 7.2:

$$R_2 = \frac{\sum_{i=1}^{k} B_i p_i (1 - \beta_i)}{\sum_{i=1}^{k} \{C_{2i} + C_{3i}[p_i(1 - \beta_i) + (1 - p_i)\alpha_i]\}} \tag{7.3}$$

From the expression of R_2, it is clear that only relative benefit is needed for optimization. To illustrate, we assume that cost structure and treatment effect for detection are the same for the k POC trials so that trials with same type I and II error rates have the same cost. We further assume that the costs for the corresponding phase 3 trials are also the same and fixed, that is, $C_{3i} = C_3$ $(i = 1,\dots,k)$. In practice, these assumptions can clearly be relaxed. After the simplification, the optimal type I/II error rates (α_i, β_i) and resource allocation ratio (C_{2i}/C_2) only depend on relative benefit B_i, POS p_i, and the ratio of total POC trial resources to cost of a single phase 3 trial, C_2/C_3. They are solved by maximizing Equation 7.3 subject to the following constraints $(i = 1,\dots,k)$:

$$Z_{1-\alpha_i} + Z_{1-\beta_i} = \sqrt{C_{2i}/C_2}(Z_{1-0.1} + Z_{1-0.2}) \tag{7.4}$$

$$\sum_{i=1}^{k} C_{2i} = C_2 \tag{7.5}$$

Once optimal type I/II error rates are obtained by maximizing R_2, optimal empirical bars follow immediately.

Let us illustrate with an example. We assume that there is a budget for one typical POC trial under $(\alpha, \beta) = (0.1, 0.2)$ but there are two POC trials with different POS ($p_1 = 0.3$ and $p_2 = 0.2$) and same benefit ($B_1 = B_2$) of interest. Figure 7.1 presents the optimal resource allocation ratio and empirical bar for the two POC trials as a function of C_2/C_3. Just as in the single-trial case, the empirical bar associated with optimal (α, β) decreases with increasing POS and C_2/C_3. The figure shows that if the budget for the POC trials is around 20% that of a phase 3 confirmatory trial as in the first-line lung cancer setting, both POC trials should be conducted with approximately 60% of the resource allocated to the one with 30% POS and the remaining 40% of the resource to the one with 20% POS. The corresponding (α, β) is (10%, 32%) for the trial with 30% POS and is (5%, 68%) for the one with 20% POS. This analysis also suggests more and smaller trials with higher empirical bars to be more cost-effective in this setting. (However, when the number of POC studies approaches a threshold, the benefit–cost ratio flattens out and gradually decreases once the number exceeds it.[44]) The cutoff point in terms of C_2/C_3 value for deciding whether to conduct one or two trials is at about 17% (the cutoff point would be considerably lower if the two trials had the same POS level—results are not shown here). If the relative phase 2 budget is lower than that, it is more cost effective to just conduct the trial with higher POS.

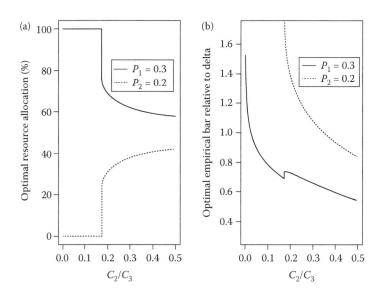

FIGURE 7.1

Optimal resource allocation (a) and empirical bars for a go decision (b) for two POC trial candidates of different POS when there is budget for a typical POC trial under $(\alpha, \beta) = (0.1, 0.2)$. C_2 represents the budget for POC trials and C_3 represents the cost for a phase 3 trial.

7.3.4 Discussion

When a predictive biomarker classifier is validated in a POC study, we are really testing two POC hypotheses: POC for the drug, and POC for the biomarker classifier. This would in principle double the size of the POC study since one needs to perform statistical tests on both BM+ and biomarker negative patient subgroups, and often leads to a debate as whether to only study the BM+ population in POC to save the cost. Two statistical designs are often referenced in this context when the assay is ready: the biomarker-enriched design and the biomarker-stratified design.

A biomarker-enriched design is the most efficient if there is very high confidence in the hypothesis. The argument to include biomarker negative patients assumes a certain degree of "equipoise"; that is, uncertainty about the truth or falsity of the predictive biomarker hypothesis. Equipoise is often underestimated in real situations, where the predictive biomarker hypothesis was invented by people in the development team, who may have difficulty objectively recognizing the inconsistent translation of preclinical results to the clinic. Moreover, publication bias leads to more frequent and prominent publication of biomarker success stories than cautionary tales. The surprising failure of EGFR expression to clearly segregate those who would benefit from anti-EGFR antibody therapy from those who would not argues that even the most "obvious" predictive biomarker hypotheses require validation. It must be remembered that even the best-supported hypothesis will be limited by preanalytic variability and by assay performance under real-world clinical conditions. Therefore, we would recommend the biomarker-enriched design only rarely.

In the biomarker-stratified design, enrollment is stratified by the biomarker status and the results are evaluated in each independent stratum. This is the most efficient design when there is equipoise concerning the predictive biomarker hypothesis. Clinical validation of a predictive biomarker classifier should generally involve the use of at least some patients who are biomarker negative to verify that the diagnostic test can distinguish between those who will benefit and those who will not, since the test will in the future be used to deny therapy to biomarker negative patients. From the benefit–cost ratio standpoint, the optimal strategy depends on phase 2 budget, phase 3 cost, and perceived POS. The sample sizes for each subpopulation would be smaller than in a typical POC trial after optimization for cost-effectiveness. Optimal cost-effectiveness with less power also corresponds to a higher bar for go-no-go decisions that determine whether a drug will advance to phase 3 development.

Throughout this section, the relative effect size between the phase 2 endpoint and the phase 3 endpoint (OS) is treated as known for simplicity. When the variance is taken into account, it can be shown that the POC trials associated with greater uncertainty on relative effect size should have smaller sample size and higher bars for a go decision.[35] This and other findings in this section based on the benefit–cost analysis are all sensible and consistent with intuition. However, intuition alone would not be able to pinpoint the optimal decision points. It is our general opinion that, for clinical drug development to become a real science, it is imperative to make the decision process more objective and quantitative. It may be an overkill to apply the analysis to the design of every POC trial, but the conclusion from our analysis provides a valuable general guidance for portfolio management of oncology drug candidates.

In the next section, we show how to further incorporate prior assumptions on relative effect size into inference.

7.4 Information Basis for Transition from Phase 2 to Phase 3

While the type I error rate of a POC study is predetermined from a benefit–cost ratio analysis or a conventional approach, the actual go-no-go decision and the decision on which population to study in phase 3 (e.g., BM+ population or overall population) are subject to revision after all phase 2 data are collected. Continuous adaptation in response to data is a cornerstone of our proposed strategy for development of drugs with or without a predictive biomarker. Nonetheless, frequent adaptation in oncology is hampered by the fact that the primary endpoint of greatest interest, OS, takes significant time to collect. More rapid endpoints are of interest only to the degree that they have some predictive ability for survival.

Transition from phase 2 to phase 3 can occur as early as after accrual for phase 2 has completed (i.e., seamless phase 2/3 design[49]), or more typically after phase 2 has reached its primary milestone (e.g., target number of PFS events has occurred). Oftentimes, the follow-up of the study effectively stops as patients may be allowed to crossover and minimal data are collected after the milestone. While the information (and value) of a trial is ultimately measured, sadly, by the number of deaths, it quickly becomes an afterthought to keep following-up patients for survival. There are some reasons behind this practice. The team is in a celebratory mood after a positive phase 2 and is busy preparing for phase 3. Continued follow-up becomes a lower priority especially when it is less clear what to do next if the OS result does not look favorable. (e.g., Should preparation of phase 3 be put on hold?) When patients are allowed to crossover, there is also a concern that it will dilute the "true" treatment effect to be expected in phase 3 although confounding effect of subsequent therapy is always unavoidable.

Regardless of the follow-up strategy, we typically have more data on the phase 2 endpoint than on OS. To accelerate transition from phase 2 to phase 3, it is critical to use all the information in a prespecified analysis to make the decision more objective and efficient. In this section, we provide a general method to synthesize all key information into a single statistic and illustrate its application in a real example. For ease of presentation, PFS is used as the phase 2 primary endpoint.

7.4.1 A Simple Synthesis Method for Joint Estimation of OS Effect

Define $\hat{\gamma}$ as the mean estimate of the ratio of OS effect to PFS effect in the log HR scale, and $\hat{\sigma}_\gamma$ (>0) as the corresponding estimate of the standard error. The historical relationship in effect size is adequately captured in the doublet ($\hat{\gamma}, \hat{\sigma}_\gamma$) under the asymptotic normality assumption. Further, let $\hat{\Delta}_{OS}$ and $\hat{\Delta}_{PFS}$ be the respective log HR estimates of OS and PFS effect from the phase 2 POC trial. Their respective variance estimates are $\hat{\sigma}^2_{OS}$ and $\hat{\sigma}^2_{PFS}$, and an estimate of the correlation between $\hat{\Delta}_{OS}$ and $\hat{\Delta}_{PFS}$ is ρ that is readily available from an appropriate resampling analysis or from the SAS procedure PROC PHREG for multiple failure data analysis by invoking, for example, the Wei-Lin-Weissfeld method.[50]

The estimation of ($\hat{\gamma}, \hat{\sigma}_\gamma$) is not our focus, but it plays a critical role in study design. We provide two examples of ($\hat{\gamma}, \hat{\sigma}_\gamma$) from the literature for illustration purpose. In the first-line metastatic colorectal cancer disease setting treated with chemotherapy, the relative effect size is estimated as the regression slope of OS effect on PFS effect for several randomized clinical trials with moderate-to-large size.[22] It was estimated to be 0.54 with standard error of 0.10 on the hazard reduction scale. The estimate of intercept was negligible, and inclusion of it or not in the linear model did not change the point estimate of the regression slope. Since hazard reduction approximates $-\log(HR)$, (0.54, 0.10) represents a reasonable estimate of ($\hat{\gamma}, \hat{\sigma}_\gamma$) in the first-line metastatic colorectal cancer disease setting under chemotherapy treatment. In an adjuvant colon cancer setting,[51] the regression slope is estimated to be 0.89 with standard error of 0.061 on HR scale for trials of fluorouracil-based regimes. The intercept was estimated to be 0.12, which implies that HR of OS = 0.12 + 0.89*HR of PFS or one-HR of OS = -0.01 + 0.89*(one-HR of PFS), that is, the intercept term would be negligible at -0.01 on hazard reduction scale under the same regression slope. This is consistent with findings from Ref. [51] in that the regression slope was estimated to be 0.90 on the log(HR) scale for trials of different regimens whereas the intercept term is negligible at 0.03. On the basis of these data, (0.89, 0.061) represents a reasonable estimate of ($\hat{\gamma}, \hat{\sigma}_\gamma$) in the adjuvant colon cancer setting when treated with chemotherapy. We note that the relationship between PFS and OS may change when the broad mechanisms and biological effects change. Thus, the relative effect sizes for chemotherapy may be different than those for cytostatic-targeted therapy, antiangiogenic therapy, or immunotherapy.

By the definition of $\hat{\gamma}$, a natural estimate of the OS effect based on the relative effect size estimate and $\hat{\Delta}_{PFS}$ is $\hat{\Delta}_P = \hat{\gamma} \hat{\Delta}_{PFS}$. The overall variance of $\hat{\Delta}_P$ is $Var(\hat{\Delta}_P) = \hat{\gamma}^2 \hat{\sigma}^2_{PFS} + \hat{\Delta}^2_{PFS} \hat{\sigma}^2_\gamma + \hat{\sigma}^2_\gamma \hat{\sigma}^2_{PFS}$. The distribution of $\hat{\Delta}_P$, as a product of two random variables, is not normal in general but behaves like a normal distribution especially when $\hat{\gamma}$ has a nonzero mean and a very small variance. Observe that $Var(\hat{\Delta}_P) > \hat{\gamma}^2 \hat{\sigma}^2_{PFS}$, which implies that $\hat{\Delta}^2_{PFS}/Var(\hat{\Delta}_P) = (\hat{\gamma}\,\hat{\Delta}_{PFS})^2/Var(\hat{\Delta}_P) < (\hat{\gamma}\,\hat{\Delta}_{PFS})^2/(\hat{\gamma}^2\,\hat{\sigma}^2_{PFS}) = \hat{\Delta}^2_{PFS}/\hat{\sigma}^2_{PFS}$. This shows that the estimated OS effect from PFS will always be less statistically significant than the PFS effect. Similarly, $\hat{\Delta}^2_P/Var(\hat{\Delta}_P) < \hat{\gamma}^2/\hat{\sigma}^2_{\gamma}$ and $\hat{\Delta}_P$ will be less statistically significant than $\hat{\gamma}$. Both are intuitive because additional uncertainty is introduced with the incorporation of relative effect size into the estimation.

With $\hat{\Delta}_{OS}$ available, a weighted estimator of the OS effect that naturally incorporates $\hat{\Delta}_{OS}$ is

$$\hat{\Delta}_J = w\hat{\Delta}_{OS} + (1 - w)\hat{\Delta}_P \tag{7.6}$$

When the correlation between $\hat{\Delta}_{OS}$ and $\hat{\Delta}_{PFS}$ is estimated to be ρ, the covariance of $\hat{\Delta}_{OS}$ and $\hat{\Delta}_P$ is $\hat{\gamma}\rho\hat{\sigma}_{OS}\hat{\sigma}_{PFS}$. The variance of $\hat{\Delta}_J$ is estimated to be

$$\begin{aligned} Var(\hat{\Delta}_J) &= w^2\, Var(\hat{\Delta}_{OS}) + (1 - w)^2\, Var(\hat{\Delta}_P) + 2w(1 - w)Cov(\hat{\Delta}_{OS},\hat{\Delta}_P) \\ &= w^2\,\hat{\sigma}^2_{OS} + (1 - w)^2 Var(\hat{\Delta}_P) + 2w(1 - w)\,\hat{\gamma}\,\rho\,\hat{\sigma}_{OS}\,\hat{\sigma}_{PFS} \end{aligned} \tag{7.7}$$

We will adopt a conventional inverse-variance-weighted estimate of w to our synthesized approach, which is defined as

$$w = Var(\hat{\Delta}_P)/(Var(\hat{\Delta}_P) + \hat{\sigma}^2_{OS}) \tag{7.8}$$

Equations 7.6 through 7.8 together provide the statistical properties of the proposed joint estimate of OS effect $\hat{\Delta}_J$. A more complicated joint estimate of the OS effect may be obtained by maximum likelihood estimation (MLE).[23] It is not our focus to find an optimal estimate of the OS effect and its statistical properties in this chapter. The joint estimate provides a reasonable starting point in practice. Notice that, purely from a statistical standpoint, a negative trend on the treatment effect in either PFS or OS does not automatically rule out a positive finding based on the synthesized approach. However, such a contradictory outcome, should it ever occur, will inevitably call into question the consistency of $(\hat{\gamma}, \hat{\sigma}_{\gamma})$ with the trial outcome. Whenever possible, the assumption on relative effect size needs to be checked from trial data before a conclusion can be made. To empirically validate the assumption on relative effect size, one may compare $\hat{\Delta}_{OS}$ to the 95% confidence interval (CI) of $\hat{\Delta}_P$, $(\hat{\Delta}_P - 1.96\sqrt{Var(\hat{\Delta}_P)}\,, \hat{\Delta}_P + 1.96\sqrt{Var(\hat{\Delta}_P)})$ whereas $\exp(\hat{\Delta}_P + 1.96\sqrt{Var(\hat{\Delta}_P)})$ is the lower bound of the 95% CI for estimated OS effect from PFS by noticing the greater the value, the lower the treatment effect. If it falls into the CI, a positive conclusion may be made with strong confidence. If it does not but

$\hat{\Delta}_{OS}$ is less than $\hat{\Delta}_P - 1.96 \sqrt{Var(\hat{\Delta}_P)}$ (i.e., observed OS effect is stronger than estimated from PFS data), and if the two estimates are in qualitative agreement with both suggesting a benefit, it represents a pleasant surprise and an even stronger conclusion may be made assuming that the OS effect is robust. Certainly, one may use other empirical approaches as appropriate to validate the assumption.

7.4.2 Application to a Phase 2/3 Seamless Design

We use a real example to illustrate the application of the synthesized approach to the design of an operationally seamless phase 2/3 design[49] of a drug candidate in platinum-resistant ovarian cancer patients.

In the phase 2 portion of the study, patients will be randomized to three treatment groups with equal allocation: test drug high dose, test drug low dose, and control. The primary endpoint for phase 2 is PFS. The phase 2 study will enroll about 210 patients and accumulate 135 PFS events to have sufficient power for each dose of the test drug to demonstrate superiority to the control in terms of PFS. After phase 2 is completed, one dose will be selected to move into phase 3. In the phase 3 portion, patients will be randomized to two treatment groups: test drug and control drug. The primary endpoint of phase 3 is OS. The phase 3 study will enroll about 720 patients and accumulate 508 deaths to have sufficient power to demonstrate that the test drug is at least noninferior to the control drug. This sample size also provides sufficient power to demonstrate that the test drug is superior to the control drug in terms of event rate for a particular adverse experience. Phase 2 data are unblinded for ease of dose-selection decision and are not included in the phase 3 analysis.

To make the phases 2–3 transition operationally seamless, an interim analysis will be conducted in phase 2. The enrollment of phase 2 will close when it is predicted that, approximately 4 months after this time point, there will be 135 PFS events. The interim analysis will take place approximately 1 month before the accrual completes to have enough time for data cleaning and analysis. The purpose of this interim analysis is to determine whether phase 3 enrollment can be initiated before final data of phase 2 are available. If a go decision is made, one arm of the test drug along with the control arm will immediately be carried to phase 3. If a go decision cannot be made at the interim analysis, phase 3 will be put on hold and a final decision will be made at the end of phase 2. Regardless of when the go decision is made, phase 2 follow-up continues until OS data are mature. The OS data will be used to help set the futility bar at an interim analysis of the phase 3 study.[43]

The go-no-go bar for the end of phase 2 data is calculated from a benefit–cost ratio analysis, and the go-no go for the interim analysis in phase 2 to trigger a seamless transition is backcalculated so that it gives 80% conditional probability that the go bar will be passed at the end of phase 2.

In our example, we assumed that the relative effect size has a normal distribution with mean of 0.6 and standard deviation of 0.2 based on a literature search. With this assumption on relative effect size, a 31% hazard reduction in PFS translates into a 20% hazard reduction in OS with a 95% CI of (7%, 31%), which was deemed reasonable by the team. A weight of 0.15 (i.e., $w = 0.15$) is given to the observed OS effect, which approximates the inverse-variance weight when the true treatment effect is in the parameter space of interest while the actual numbers of PFS and OS events are as expected from historical trials in the same disease setting.

Figure 7.2 shows the boundaries for the observed OS effect and PFS effect at interim analysis to trigger a seamless go decision to phase 3. If the empirical effects fall below both solid and dotted lines, phase 3 enrollment will be triggered while waiting for the phase 2 data to become mature. Figure 7.3 shows the corresponding boundaries at the final analysis that roughly correspond to a 9% hazard reduction based on the joint estimate of OS effect. Clearly, by appropriately taking all the key information into account, the synthesized approach does not leave any ambiguity to the decision rules, providing solid guidance for making a timely decision. When the derivation of go-no-go bars is further assisted with a benefit–cost ratio analysis to appropriately balance the risk and benefit, it is more objective than any conventional approach.

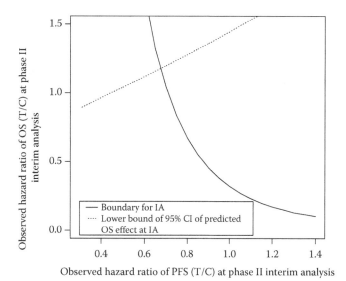

Observed hazard ratio of PFS (T/C) at phase II interim analysis

FIGURE 7.2

Criteria at interim analysis of phase 2 to trigger phase 3 enrollment. The higher the HR is, the smaller the treatment effect. An OS effect below the dotted line (i.e., $\exp(\hat{\Delta}_P + 1.96 \sqrt{Var(\hat{\Delta}_P)})$) indicates that it is either consistent with estimation from PFS effect or represents a pleasant surprise.

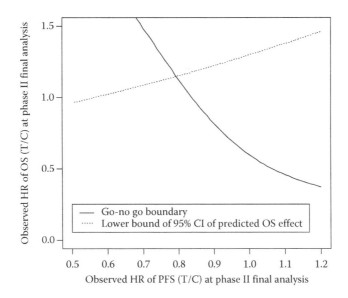

FIGURE 7.3
Optimal Go-No Go criteria at the end of phase 2. The higher the HR is, the smaller the treatment effect. An OS effect below the dotted line (i.e., $\exp(\hat{\Delta}_P + 1.96\sqrt{Var(\hat{\Delta}_P)})$) indicates that it is either consistent with estimation from PFS effect or represents a pleasant surprise.

7.4.3 Discussion

Our proposed approach assumes that a reasonably reliable estimate of the relative effect size is available. Clearly, after a simple modification, the synthesis method can be applied to POC studies with one population or more subpopulations. When there is reason to believe that the estimate in a BM+ population of a POC trial is different from that based on historical studies in unselected populations, one may conduct a sensitivity analysis by artificially inflating the variance estimate.[23] With or without a reliable estimate, one may use a plug-in method[52] or the inverse probability of censoring-weighted (IPCW) method[52,53] for an enhanced survival analysis to further improve the efficiency of inference. An enhanced analysis basically attempts to estimate the relationship between the phase 2 endpoint and OS using patients who have died, apply the estimated relationship to the prediction of OS for those who are alive, and then combine the observed OS effect and predicted OS effect into a single estimate. The information gain with an enhanced analysis is capped,[35] but could be substantial if the prior information on relative effect size is further incorporated into the analysis. This remains an open research topic yet to be fully investigated.

At the end of phase 2, just as before the initiation of phase 2, the same question arises as which population to study in phase 3. There are four options depending on assay availability and confidence in the predictive biomarker hypothesis: (1) enrichment design, (2) an all-comer study without any pre-specified retrospective analysis of a BM+ population, (3) an all-comer study with a prespecified retrospective analysis of the BM+ population, and (4) biomarker-stratified design. The first is appropriate when the biomarker is a clear predictor of treatment effect, and the second is appropriate otherwise. The last two options are the most appropriate when there is still great uncertainty about the predictive value of the biomarker, which represents a typical scenario in most cases and will be the focus of the next section. A decision analysis[14,55] may be used to assist with the decision on which option to choose.

7.5 Optimal Design of Phase 3 Trials with a Predictive Biomarker Hypothesis

Under either the third or the fourth option, two hypotheses are being tested simultaneously: (1) the drug is effective in the overall population, or (2) the drug is effective only in the BM+ population. The study enrolls the unselected population to be able to test both hypotheses. The total type I error rate for both hypotheses combined is set at 2.5% (one sided), as required by health authorities. This raises the question of how to divide up this false-positive rate between the two hypotheses. The hypothesis to which more of this type I error is assigned is effectively prioritized or emphasized in the final statistical analysis. Fredlin and Simon[56,57] proposed to assign 2% to the overall population and 0.5% to the biomarker population. Such a fixed α-split alpha approach is not efficient when the number of events in the biomarker population is uncertain. In the approach described below,[58] the split of the type I error is not fixed, but is adaptive to the actual number of events in the BM+ population and yet controlling the overall type I error rate at 2.5%.

7.5.1 Optimal α-Split with Respect to Target Treatment Effects

Suppose a two-arm phase 3 pivotal trial with 1:1 randomization is designed for detecting a treatment effect of Δ in log HR scale for OS at type I error rate α (one-sided) and type II error rate β. The trial is event driven and completes after the target number of events in the overall population is reached. Denote by I_3 the total information units, which are the total number of events as provided in Equation 7.1 divided by four. The Z-statistics from Cox-regression analysis will be used for hypothesis testing. Denote by r the proportion of events in the subpopulation classified by the predictive biomarker (i.e., the subpopulation has rI_3 units of information). Let (X_1, X_2) be the two Z-statistics for testing of the treatment effect in the two populations at the end of the trial. By definition, the two Z-statistics for the hypotheses have a correlation $\sqrt{r}$. The trial will be declared positive if the one-sided p-value is less than α_1

based on the overall population or less than α_2 based on the subpopulation. The overall type I error rate is controlled at $\alpha = 2.5\%$ under this α-split.

Under the above setup, when Δ_1 and Δ_1 are the target treatment effects in the overall population and the BM+ population, respectively, the overall power of the trial is $1 - \Phi_{\sqrt{r}}(Z_{1-\alpha_1} + \sqrt{I_3}\Delta_1, Z_{1-\alpha_2} + \sqrt{rI_3}\Delta_2)$ where $\Phi_s(,)$ denotes the cumulative distribution function of a standard bivariate normal vector with correlation s. We consider two adaptive approaches: (1) an exact method that incorporates the correlation coefficient $\sqrt{r}$ into α-control and (2) a conservative Bonferroni method that does not account for the correlation. Under the first approach, the two alphas are obtained by maximizing the power function under the constraint $1 - \Phi_{\sqrt{r}}(Z_{1-\alpha_1}, Z_{1-\alpha2}) = \alpha$; under the second approach, the two alphas are obtained by maximizing the power function under the constraint $\alpha_1 + \alpha_2 = \alpha$. Since the overall type I error rate conditional on r is controlled under either approach, the unconditional type I error rate is also controlled. The R code for the calculations is provided in the Appendix.

Figure 7.4 provides α_2 in terms of r under the two adaptive approaches and the corresponding overall study power for the overall study when the true hazard reduction is assumed to be 40% in the BM+ population and 30% in the overall population. Under this setup, the hazard reduction in the biomarker negative population ranges from 25% to 12% when r ranges from 30% to 60%. The power under Freidlin and Simon's fixed α-split approach ($\alpha_1 = 2.0\%$ and

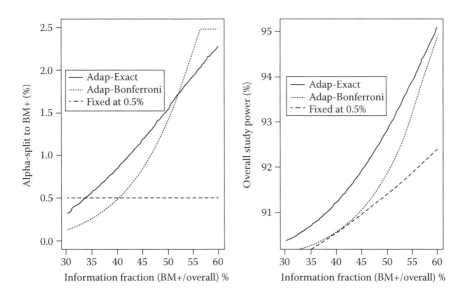

FIGURE 7.4
Comparison between fixed α-split approach and adaptive α-split approaches. The left panel provides α-split to the BM+ population and the right panel provides the corresponding overall study power. The target hazard reduction is 40% in the BM+ population and 30% in the overall population. The trial completes after 330 events are observed in the overall population.

$\alpha_2 = 0.5\%$) is also provided in Figure 7.4 for comparison. Clearly, the optimized exact approach always has the highest power, the fixed approach always has the lowest, and the optimized Bonferroni approach falls in between. By the construction of these approaches, one can prove that their relative performance stays the same under any assumption on treatment effects. As expected, as r increases, more alpha is allocated to the BM+ population under both adaptive approaches. The study power is always >90% under the adaptive approaches and it increases with r. However, the fixed α-split approach may have <90% power when r is small. The Bonferroni approach is more sensitive to r than the exact approach. When r approximately reaches 55%, the Bonferroni approach allocates all alpha to the BM+ population effectively suggesting to analyze the BM+ population first, but the exact approach does not go to that extreme. Notice that the improvement in power seems moderate under the adaptive approach, but this is only because the target power is already high. When the target power is lower, the improvement is more pronounced. Moreover, even when the power gain is small, the gain in efficiency of the study as measured by sample size is meaningful. For example, a 2–3% change in power from 90% corresponds to an 8–12% change in sample size, which is significant in the oncology drug development environment where cost and patient resources are an increasing concern, and all this is accomplished by a simple adjustment of α-split.

The adaptive α-splitting strategy, be it under the exact approach or under the Bonferroni approach, leads to a prespecified α-splitting function to the BM+ population as seen in Figure 7.4. The α-splitting function serves a similar role to the α-spending function in a group sequential design where r is often called the *information fraction*. The analogy is not surprising as a subgroup analysis is mathematically equivalent to an interim analysis. In this regard, the proposed adaptive α-splitting strategy can be easily embedded into a group sequential design that allows early stopping for efficacy at interim analyses. While controlling the overall type I error rate just as α-spending functions do in group sequential designs, the prespecified α-splitting function gives us tremendous flexibility to adaptively distribute alpha across the two populations with respect to r. Ability to adapt is an extremely desirable feature as typically r is unknown upfront. For trials that stratify randomization by the predictive biomarker classifier, while the number of BM+ patients is known, the number of events in the population is not because the prognostic significance of an investigational predictive biomarker is unclear. For trials that rely on retrospective analysis for testing the predictive biomarker hypothesis, missing data on biomarker measurements and lack of control on sample size of the BM+ population further add to the uncertainty. The use of exact calculation for α-splitting can also be found in Ref. [59]. The idea of using maximum power to optimize study design is not new. Previous researchers[60–62] have used it for designing psychological experiments. It is adopted here for addressing a totally different issue.

7.5.2 Optimal α-Split with Respect to External Information on Treatment Effects

When external information on treatment effects is available, it can be incorporated into optimization of the α-splitting strategy. Ideally, this external information is derived from extended follow-up of randomized phase 2 trials under the same disease setting in the same patient population. This is particularly useful in that OS data from a preceding phase 2 trial can be allowed to mature before the final phase 3 α-split is specified[14]; it allows a timely go-no go decision based on PFS and still allows a phase 3 adaptation based on mature phase 2 OS. The external information must be available prior to the phase 3 *analysis,* but need not be available prior to the phase 3 *start.* External information from less credible data sources should be used with caution.

Let $f(\Delta_1, \Delta_2)$ be the joint prior density function of $f(\Delta_1, \Delta_2)$ estimated from external data. Under the same setup as in the previous section, the predictive power of phase 3 with respect to the prior distribution of (Δ_1, Δ_2) is

$$1 - \int \Phi_{\sqrt{r}}(Z_{1-\alpha_1} + \sqrt{I_3}\Delta_1, Z_{1-\alpha_2} + \sqrt{rI_3}\Delta_2)f(\Delta_1, \Delta_2)d\Delta_1\Delta_2 \qquad (7.9)$$

whereas, again, r is the information fraction in the BM+ population that is the only information needed from phase 3. When $f(\Delta_1, \Delta_2) = 1$ at the target treatment effects, Equation 7.9 degenerates to the conventional study power as discussed in the previous section. We only consider exact control in this section so that the two alphas are obtained by maximizing Equation 7.9 under the constraint of $1 - \Phi_{\sqrt{r}}(Z_{1-\alpha_1}, Z_{1-\alpha_2}) = \alpha$. Just as in the previous section, because the overall type I error rate conditional on r is controlled under either approach, the unconditional type I error rate is also controlled.

Consider a phase 3 trial that targets a 25% HR in OS that completes after approximately 510 events are observed and in the end, half of the events are from the BM+ population ($r = 0.5$). Table 7.2 presents the optimal α-split when the number of events the prior is based on is 80 also with half from the BM+ population. Four assumptions are considered for the predictive biomarker effect: (1) no effect, (2) mild effect, (3) moderate effect, and (4) extreme effect

TABLE 7.2

Optimal α-Split That Maximizes Predictive Power with Respect to Prior Distribution of True Treatment Effect

Prior Point Estimates of Hazard Reduction		BM Effect	Number of Events Prior Is Based on		Optimal α-Split	
Overall (%)	BM+ (%)		Overall	BM+	Overall (α_1) (%)	BM + (α_2) (%)
25	25	No	80	40	1.9	0.9
25	30	Mild	80	40	1.7	1.2
15	25	Moderate	80	40	1.2	1.7
15	30	Extreme	80	40	0.9	2.0

TABLE 7.3

Comparison of Actual Study Power for Phase 3 under Various α-Splitting Strategies

True Hazard Reduction				Study Power			
Overall (%)	BM+ (%)	BM Effect	Optimal α-Split (%)	Modified Fredlin Simon ($\alpha_1 = 2.22\%$, $\alpha_2 = 0.56\%$) (%)	Original Fredlin Simon ($\alpha_1 = 2.0\%$, $\alpha_2 = 0.5\%$) (%)	Equal– Naive ($\alpha_1 = \alpha_2 =$ 1.25%) (%)	All comers ($\alpha_1 = 2.5\%$, $\alpha_2 = 0$) (%)
25	25	No	89	89	89	86	90
25	30	Mild	90	90	90	88	90
15	25	Moderate	61	54	52	57	45
15	30	Extreme	79	67	66	74	45

(treatment effect is entirely driven by the BM+ population). As expected, under the optimal α-splitting strategy, more α is allocated to the BM+ population for the improvement of predictive power when the biomarker effect becomes stronger. When the effect is not observed from the external data (i.e., estimated hazard reductions are 25% in both populations), more α is allocated to the overall population ($\alpha_1 = 1.9\%$) than to the BM+ population ($\alpha_2 = 0.9\%$). Apparently, it would be a preferred strategy to allocate all α to the overall population if the biomarker effect truly does not exist. However, given that uncertainty is unavoidable in practice, the method yields a sensible α-split based on limited prior information.

Table 7.3 provides a comparison of actual study power under various α-splitting strategies when the true treatment effects are the same as empirical estimates from the external data. We considered four non-data-driven strategies with fixed α-split: (1) Freidlin and Simon's original method without taking correlation into account ($\alpha_1 = 2.0\%$, $\alpha_2 = 0.5\%$); (2) modified Freidlin and Simon's method after taking correlation into account while keeping the same 4:1 ratio as in the original method ($\alpha_1 = 2.22\%$, $\alpha_2 = 0.56\%$); (3) equal distribution without taking correlation into account ($\alpha_1 = 1.25\%$, $\alpha_2 = 1.25\%$); and (4) allocate all alpha to the overall population ($\alpha_1 = 2.5\%$, $\alpha_2 = 0$). As expected, with the help of prior information, the optimal strategy is the most robust among all strategies considered. The modified Freidlin and Simon's method improves slightly over the original one. We conducted the same comparison under different assumptions on r. The findings are generally consistent (not shown here). Notice that, just like in the previous section, a similar α-splitting function can be generated under the proposed approach, which again is prespecified and guarantees control of the overall type I error rate at 2.5%, no matter what the actual r is.

7.5.3 Discussion

In this section, we have shown how to adaptively split alpha for improving the efficiency of the statistical design of a phase 3 study with two coprimary hypotheses, one of which is on the BM+ population. Only external data are considered. When interim data from phase 3 are used, a similar idea can be applied after proper multiplicity adjustment.[58] In this case, the allocation is determined by an independent review board according to rules that are prespecified, and that need to be agreed with health authorities in advance. The adaptation is only to the analysis strategy and does not affect patient selection or management. Type I error can still be strictly controlled even if all patients are included in the final analysis.

We have focused on type I error rate in this section. When treatment effect is statistically significant in both populations, the treatment-by-biomarker interaction effect may also need to be investigated.[63] Just as in a group sequential design crossing, the efficacy bar at an interim analysis does not guarantee drug approval because data maturity may be a review issue; the treatment-by-biomarker interaction effect could be a regulatory review issue at least as far as labeling is concerned even when the prespecified cut points for alpha are met for both populations.

Ideally, randomization is stratified by the predictive biomarker upfront (the *fourth* option). However, the turnaround time for tumor acquisition and biomarker testing often creates practical difficulties when there is an urgency to begin treatment, and in such cases, the *third* option is preferred. In addition, we may not have the assay or cut point ready at study initiation, and will have to rely on a retrospective analysis (the *third* option). In either case, the baseline imbalance has to be checked before testing the treatment effect in the BM+ population, and a sensitivity analysis has to be conducted to assess the impact of missing biomarker data on conclusions. As a base assumption, the data may be considered to be missing-at-random. However, this requires proper blinding of both the biomarker data and the clinical data. The procedures for data handling have to be prespecified and agreed upon by regulatory agencies to ensure the integrity of the study is not tampered or compromised.

The adaptive α-splitting strategy is different from conventional approaches for multiplicity adjustment. This opens the door to more research work along this line. Apparently, the utility function for maximization can be any function preferred by the user. For example, one could weigh the power for each of the two hypotheses by the respective population sizes. The general strategy can accommodate more than one biomarker subpopulation. Indeed, when the subpopulations are defined by different cutoff points of the same assay, the populations are nested within each other, just like interim analyses of a group sequential design.

7.6 Summary

We have devised decision and design strategies to adaptively integrate predictive biomarkers into oncology clinical development programs, in a data-driven manner in which these biomarkers are emphasized in exact proportion to the evidence supporting their clinical predictive value. Central to this paradigm is the prioritization of one predictive biomarker hypothesis that will be subjected to statistical validation as a predictor of clinical benefit in a randomized phase 2 POC study. The primary hypothesis and related assays to determine biomarker status should ideally be available at the beginning of this phase 2 study, but it is possible to wait until the sample analysis at the end. PFS or OS (for indications where life span is short) is the preferred endpoint for phase 2 POC studies, which may be optimally sized to include both BM+ and biomarker negative patients based on a benefit–cost ratio analysis. Continued survival follow-up of the phase 2 study is critical, given the uncertainty in relative effect size between a phase 2 endpoint and OS, especially in a biomarker selected population that has never studied before. The data not only help decide whether to go to phase 3, but also help determine several aspects of the phase 3 design. A synthesized method that incorporates prior information and within-trial data may be considered to help accelerate drug development from phase 2 to phase 3 after appropriately balancing the cost and benefit. Finally, an adaptive α-splitting approach can be used to incorporate external information from the phase 2 study and to account for uncertainty about the information fraction in the BM+ population in phase 3 studies that intend to declare success in either the overall population or the BM+ population.

Other equally critical issues such as dose selection in phase 2 and futility analysis in phase 3[64] are not discussed in this chapter. Some technical details and further extensions are omitted but can be found in the references. Research work is ongoing to investigate some of the new areas suggested in this chapter. Finally, this is not meant to be a review paper and some valuable references have not been included.

Appendix: R Code for Generating α-Splits under Proposed Approach

```
library(mvtnorm)
#r = information fraction in BM+ pop
#overall type I error rate-0.025 after accounting for
correlation
exact < -function(alpha2, alpha1, r){
alpha < -1-pmvnorm(lower = c(-Inf, -Inf), upper = c(qnorm(1-
  alpha1), qnorm(1-alpha2)), mean = c(0, 0),
            corr = rbind(c(1, sqrt(r)), c(sqrt(r), 1)))[1]
return(alpha-0.025)
}
```

```
#Adaptive - Bonferroni
obj1<-function(alpha1, r, hr1, hr2){
Info2<-(qnorm(0.025)+qnorm(0.1))^2/log(hr2)2
Info1<-Info2*r
beta1<-pnorm(sqrt(Info1)*log(hr1)-qnorm(alpha1))
alpha2<-0.025-alpha1
beta2<-pnorm(sqrt(Info2)*log(hr2)-qnorm(alpha2))
power<-1-pmvnorm(lower=c(-Inf, -Inf), upper=c(qnorm(beta1),
  qnorm(beta2)), mean=c(0,0),
            corr=rbind(c(1, sqrt(r)), c(sqrt(r), 1)))[1]
return(power)
}

#Adaptive - Exact
obj2<-function(alpha1, r, hr1, hr2){
Info2<-(qnorm(0.025)+qnorm(0.1))^2/log(hr2)^2
Info1<-Info2*r
beta1<-pnorm(sqrt(Info1)*log(hr1)-qnorm(alpha1))
alpha2<-uniroot(exact,c(0,0.025),alpha1=alpha1, r=r)$root
beta2<-pnorm(sqrt(Info2)*log(hr2)-qnorm(alpha2))
power<-1-pmvnorm(lower=c(-Inf, -Inf), upper=c(qnorm(beta1),
  qnorm(beta2)), mean=c(0,0),
            corr=rbind(c(1, sqrt(r)), c(sqrt(r), 1)))[1]
return(power)
}

optimal<-function(r, hr1, hr2){
test1<-optimize(obj1, c(0.00001,0.02499), r=r, hr1=hr1,
  hr2=hr2, maximum=TRUE)
test2<-optimize(obj2, c(0.00001,0.02499), r=r, hr1=hr1,
  hr2=hr2, maximum=TRUE)
return(c(test1$maximum, test2$maximum))
}

# Sample call when hazard reduction is 30% in overall
  population and 40% in biomarker positive
# population. The function generates optimal alpha-splits to
  the biomarker positive population
# and overall study power when 50% events are from biomarker
  positive population.
Optimal(0.5, 0.6, 0.7)
```

References

1. Cobleigh MA, Vogel CL, Tripathy D et al. Multinational study of the efficacy and safety of humanized anti-HER2 monoclonal antibody in women who have

HER2-overexpressing metastatic breast cancer that has progressed after chemotherapy for metastatic disease. *J. Clin. Oncol.* 1999; 17: 2639–2648.

2. Slamon DJ, Leyland-Jones B, Shak S et al. Use of chemotherapy plus a monoclonal antibody against HER2 for metastatic breast cancer that overexpresses HER2. *N. Engl. J. Med.* 2001; 344: 783–792.

3. Paez JG, Janne PA, Lee JC et al. EGFR mutations in lung cancer: Correlation with clinical response to gefitinib therapy. *Science* 2004; 30: 1497–1500.

4. Pao W, Miller V, Zakowski M et al. EGF receptor gene mutations are common in lung cancers from "never smokers" and are associated with sensitivity of tumors to gefitinib and erlotinib. *Proc. Natl. Acad. Sci. USA.* 2004; 101: 13306–13311.

5. Amado RG, Wolf M, Peeters M et al. Wild-type KRAS is required for panitumumab efficacy in patients with metastatic colorectal cancer. *J. Clin. Oncol.* 2008; 26: 1626–1634.

6. Lievre A, Bachet JB, Le Corre D et al. KRAS mutation status is predictive of response to cetuximab therapy in colorectal cancer. *Cancer Res.* 2006; 66: 3992–3995.

7. Bokemeyer C, Bondarenko I, Hartmann JT et al. KRAS status and efficacy of first-line treatment of patients with metastatic colorectal cancer (mCRC) with FOLFOX with or without cetuximab: The OPUS experience. *J. Clin. Oncol.* 2008; 26: Suppl. 15S, abstract 4000.

8. Van Cutsem E, Lang I, D'haens G et al. KRAS status and efficacy in the first-line treatment of patients with metastatic colorectal cancer (mCRC) treated with FOLFIRI with or without cetuximab: The CRYSTAL experience. *J. Clin. Oncol.* 2008; 26: Suppl. 15S, abstract 2.

9. Chapman PB, Hauschild A et al. Improved survival with vemurafenib in melanoma with BRAF V600E mutation. *N. Engl. J. Med.* 2011; 364: 2507–2516.

10. Kwak EL, Bang YJ, et al. Anaplastic lymphoma kinase inhibition in non-small-cell lung cancer. *N. Engl. J. Med.* 2010; 363(18): 1693–1703.

11. Yan L, Beckman RA. Pharmacogenetics and pharmacogenomics in oncology therapeutic antibody development. *Biotechniques* 2005; 39: 565–568.

12. Ransohoff DF, Gourlay ML. Sources of bias in specimens for research about molecular markers for cancer. *J. Clin. Oncol.* 2010; 28: 698–704.

13. Dalton WS, Friend SH. Cancer biomarkers—An invitation to the table. *Science* 2006; 312: 1165–1168.

14. Beckman RA, Clark J, Chen C. Integrating predictive biomarkers and classifiers into oncology clinical development programmes. *Nat. Rev. Drug Discov.* 2011; 10: 735–749.

15. Beckman RA, Dodion P. Analyze the current biomarker-guided development model. *Lecture/Debate, Center for Business Intelligence 2nd Annual Forum on Oncology Commercialization Strategies*, Philadelphia, Pennsylvania. January 12–13, 2009.

16. Ratain MJ, Glassman RH. Biomarkers in phase I oncology trials: Signal, noise, or expensive distraction? *Clin. Cancer Res.* 2007; 13: 6545–6548.

17. Orloff J, Douglas F, Pineiro J et al. The future of drug development: Advancing clinical trial design. *Nat. Rev. Drug Discov.* 2009; 8: 949–957.

18. Simon RM, Paik S, Hayes DF. Use of archived specimens in evaluation of prognostic and predictive biomarkers. *J. Natl. Cancer Inst.* 2009; 101: 1446–1452.

19. Dahle-Smith A, Petty RD. Developing predictive biomarkers in oncology: How can we achieve consistent success? In *Treatment Strategies–Oncology*, The Cambridge Research Centre, London, UK, 2010; pp. 47–54.

20. Sun X, Chen C, Li X, Song Y. A review of statistical issues with progression-free survival as an interval-censored time-to-event endpoint. *J. Biopharm. Stat.* 2013; 23(5): 986–1003.
21. Sun X, Chen C. Comparison of Finkelstein's method with the conventional approach for interval-censored data analysis. *Stat. Biopharm. Res.* 2010; 2(1): 97–108.
22. Tang PA, Bentsen SM, Chen EX, Siu LL. Surrogate endpoints for median overall survival in metastatic colorectal cancer: Literature-based analysis from 39 randomized controlled trials of first-line chemotherapy. *J. Clin. Onc.* 2007; 25: 4562–4568.
23. Chen C, Sun L. On quantification of PFS effect for accelerated approval of oncology drugs. *Stat. Biopharm. Res.* 2011; 3: 434–444.
24. EMEA CHMP. Methodological considerations for using progression-free-survival (PFS) as primary endpoint in confirmatory trials for registration, 2008, http://www.emea.eu.int.
25. Stone AM, Bushness W, Denne J et al. Research outcomes and recommendations for the assessment of progression in cancer clinical trials from a PhRMA working group. *Eur. J. Cancer* 2011; 47(12): 1763–1771.
26. Oxnard GR et al. When progressive disease does not mean treatment failure: Reconsidering the criteria for progression. *J. Natl. Cancer Inst.* 2012; 104: 1534–1542.
27. Beckman RA, Schemmann GS, Yeang CH. Impact of genetic dynamics and single-cell heterogeneity on development of nonstandard personalized medicine strategies for cancer. *Proc. Natl. Acad. Sci. USA* 2012; 109: 14586–14591.
28. Chan SL, Mok T. PARP inhibition in BRCA-mutated breast and ovarian cancers. *Lancet* 2010; 376 9737: 211–213.
29. Adams SF, Marsh EB et al. A high response rate to liposomal doxorubicin is seen among women with BRCA mutations treated for recurrent epithelial ovarian cancer. *Eur. J. Cancer* 2011; 47(12): 1763–1771.
30. Prentice RL. Surrogate endpoints in clinical trials: Definitions and operational criteria. *Stat. Med.* 1989; 8: 431–440.
31. Chen C, Wang HW. Proportion of treatment effect. *Encycl. Biopharm. Stat.* 2005; 1(1): 1–5.
32. Buyse M, Piedbois P. On the relationship between response to treatment and survival time. *Stat. Med.* 1996; 15: 2797–2812.
33. Molenberghs G et al. Statistical challenges in the evaluation of surrogate endpoints in randomized trials. *Control. Clin. Trials* 2002; 23: 607–625.
34. Buyse M, Molenberghs G. The validation of surrogate endpoints in randomized experiments. *Biometrics* 1998; 54: 1014–1029.
35. Chen C, Sun L, Chih C. Evaluation of early efficacy endpoints for proof-of-concept trials. *J. Biopharm. Stat* 2013; 23: 413.
36. Burzykowski T, Molenberghs G, Buyse M. *The Evaluation of Surrogate Endpoints.* Springer, 2005.
37. Whitehead A. *Meta-Analysis of Controlled Clinical Trials,* Chapter 4. Wiley, 2002.
38. Burzykowski T, Buyse M, Yothers G, Sakamoto J, Sargent D. Exploring and validating surrogate endpoints in colorectal cancer. *Lifetime Data Anal.* 2008; 14: 54–64.
39. Beckman RA. Efficiency of carcinogenesis: In the mutator phenotype inevitable? *Semin. Cancer Biol.* 2010; 20: 340–352.

40. Loeb LA, Bielas JH, Beckman RA. Cancers exhibit a mutator phenotype: Clinical implications. *Cancer Res.* 2008; 68: 3551–3557.
41. Beckman RA, Loeb LA. Genetic instability in cancer: Theory and experiment. *Semin. Cancer Biol.* 2005; 15: 423–435.
42. Chen C, Beckman RA. Optimal cost effective designs of proof of concept trials and associated go-no go decisions. *Proceedings of the American Statistical Association*, Salt Lake City, Utah, Biometrics Section, 2007.
43. Chen C, Beckman RA. Optimal cost-effective go-no go decisions in late stage oncology drug development. *Stat. Biopharm. Res.* 2009; 1: 159–169.
44. Chen C, Beckman RA. Optimal cost-effective Phase II proof of concept and associated go-no go decisions. *J. Biopharm. Stat.* 2009; 1: 424–436.
45. Rubinstein LV, Korn EL, Freidlin B et al. Design issues of randomized Phase II trials and a proposal for Phase II screening trials. *J. Clin. Oncol.* 2005; 23: 7199–7206.
46. Simon RM, Steinberg SM, Hamilton M et al. Clinical trial designs for the early clinical development of therapeutic cancer vaccines. *J. Clin. Oncol.* 2001; 19: 1848–1854.
47. Estey EH, Thall PF. New designs for Phase 2 clinical trials. *Blood* 2003; 102: 442–448.
48. Korn EL, Arbuck SG, Pluda JM et al. Clinical trial designs for cytostatic agents: Are new approaches needed? *J. Clin. Oncol.* 2001; 19: 265–272, 3154–3160 (correspondence).
49. Sun, L, Chen C. Advanced application of using progression-free-survival to make optimal go-no go decision in oncology drug development. *JSM Proceedings, Biopharmaceutical Section* 2012, Alexandria, VA: American Statistical Association.
50. SAS/STAT® Software: *Changes and Enhancements through Release 6.12*, Cary, NC: SAS Institute Inc., 1997.
51. Sargent D, Wieand S, Haller DG et al. Disease-free survival (DFS) vs. overall survival (OS) as a primary endpoint for adjuvant colon cancer studies: Individual patient data from 20, 898 patients on 18 randomized trials. *J. Clin. Oncol.* 2005; 23: 8664–8670.
52. Mackenzie T, Abrahamowicz M . Using categorical markers as auxiliary variables in log-rank test and hazard ratio estimation. *Can. J. Stat.* 2005; 33: 201–219.
53. Robins JM, Finkelstein DM. Correcting for noncompliance and dependent censoring in an AIDS clinical trial with inverse probability of censoring weighted (IPCW) log-rank tests. *Biometrics* 2000; 56: 779–788.
54. Robins JM. Information recovery and bias adjustment in proportional hazards regression analysis of randomized trials using surrogate markers. *Proceedings of Biopharmaceutical Section, American Statistical Association* 1993, San Francisco, CA; pp. 24–33.
55. Song Y, Chen C. Optimal strategies for developing a late-stage clinical program with a possible subset effect. *Stat. Biopharm. Res.* 2012; 4(3): 240–251.
56. Freidlin B, Simon RM. Adaptive signature design: An adaptive clinical trial design for generating and prospectively testing a gene expression signature for sensitive patients. *Clin. Cancer Res.* 2005; 11: 7872–7878.
57. Simon RM. The use of genomics in clinical trial design. *Clin. Cancer Res.* 2008; 14: 5984–5993.
58. Chen C, Beckman RA. Hypothesis testing in a confirmatory Phase III trial with a possible subset effect. *Stat. Biopharm. Res.* 2009; 1: 431–440.

59. Wang SJ, O'Neill RT, Hung HMJ. Approaches to evaluation of treatment effect in randomized clinical trials with genomic subset. *Pharm. Stat.* 2007; 6: 227–244.

60. Korn E. Projecting power from a previous study: Maximum likelihood estimation. *Am. Stat.* 1990; 44: 290–292.

61. Gillett R. An average power criterion for sample size estimation. *Statistician* 1994; 43: 389–394.

62. Gillett R. The expected power of *F* and *t* tests conditional on information from an earlier experiment. *Brit. J. Math. Stat. Psychol.* 1995; 48: 371–384.

63. Rothmann MD, Zhang JJ, Lu L, Fleming T. Testing in a prespecified subgroup and the intent-to-treat population. *Drug Inf. J.* 2012 March 1; 46(2): 175–179.

64. Li X, Chen C. Two-stage futility analysis in Phase II/III adaptive trials using time-to-event endpoints. *JSM Proceedings, Biopharmaceutical Section 2012,* Alexandria, VA: American Statistical Association.

8

Biomarker Identification in Clinical Trials

Ilya Lipkovich and Alex Dmitrienko

CONTENTS

8.1 Introduction

As emphasized in the draft FDA guidance on enrichment strategies for clinical trials (Food and Drug Administration, 2012), characterization of heterogeneity of subject responses to treatment is a critical component of drug development and regulatory decision making. The assessment of heterogeneous effects is performed based on a wide variety of covariates, including phenotypical, clinical, gene and protein expression markers, and so on (to simplify the terminology, they will be referred to as *biomarkers* in this chapter). It is important to distinguish between two types of biomarkers, namely, *prognostic* and *predictive* biomarkers. Prognostic biomarkers help select subgroups of subjects with different outcomes irrespective of the treatment they receive. In contrast, predictive biomarkers define groups of subjects who are likely to experience significant treatment benefit (*biomarker-positive* subjects) compared to subjects in the complementary groups (*biomarker-negative* subjects).

Predictive biomarkers guide the development of personalized medicine (tailored therapies), that is, treatments that target subgroups of subjects with particular characteristics, for example, subjects who are expected to derive substantial benefit from the experimental treatment compared to the control. There have been multiple examples of clinical development programs that utilize predictive biomarkers to evaluate targeted agents. Most commonly, biomarker-driven designs are used in oncology programs, but predictive biomarkers are beginning to play an increasingly important role in other therapeutic areas.

A variety of methods have been proposed in the clinical trial and biostatistical literature to facilitate the process of biomarker discovery. Biomarker search may be applied in a prospective or retrospective manner. A *prospective* search is commonly applied to the data collected using a Phase II trial database to select promising biomarkers. If one or more predictive biomarkers are identified, a multipopulation tailoring design may be considered in the Phase III program. A biomarker search may also be used in a *retrospective* setting mostly commonly at the end of a Phase III development program. If the overall outcome of the program is positive, the program's sponsor may be interested in identifying biomarkers that define subgroups of subjects with undesirable outcomes. These subjects can then be excluded from the final population. On the other hand, if there is no evidence of a positive treatment effect in the general population, a biomarker search may target biomarkers that define subgroups of subjects with a positive treatment effect.

This chapter provides a review of statistical methods used in the discovery of single biomarkers and combinations of biomarkers (known as *biomarker signatures*) in clinical trials that can be utilized in prospective and retrospective settings. The chapter begins with a high-level summary of general subgroup analysis methodology that is commonly used in biomarker discovery, including methods developed within the machine learning and data-mining communities. A novel subgroup search method, known as SIDES (subgroup identification based on differential effect search), is introduced to provide examples of flexible biomarker search tools. These include the regular SIDES procedure and its extended version, which employs a screening stage to facilitate the selection of strong predictive biomarkers (SIDEScreen procedure). A case study based on a real clinical trial is used to present key features of the SIDES and related procedures. Results of several simulation studies are presented to provide more information on the performance of the regular and extended SIDES procedures in different settings.

The regular SIDES and SIDEScreen procedures are implemented as an Excel add-in package (SIDESxl package). This package can be downloaded from the Multiplicity Expert web site at http://multxpert.com/wiki/Software.

8.2 Subgroup Search Methods

It is still fairly common to develop general guidelines and define good practices for performing subgroup analysis in clinical trials. This approach emphasizes the inherent risks of post hoc subgroup analysis, and the guidelines always state that unplanned subgroup analyses need to be interpreted "with caution." To give some examples, Brookes et al. (2001) developed a "checklist" of 25 rules, Rothwell (2005) proposed 21 rules, and Sun et al. (2010) listed seven existing and developed four additional criteria for assessing the credibility of subgroup analysis.

In this section, we provide a review of subgroup analysis methods used in biomarker discovery that rely on a data-driven (rather than guideline-driven) approach. The data-driven approach treats subgroup search as a special case of *model selection* and relies on key principles from machine learning and data mining. Specifically, instead of prespecifying a single data model, the data-driven approach is based on a relevant analytic strategy. The operating characteristics of this model selection strategy often can be optimized by using appropriate tuning (complexity) parameters and calibration may be performed based on the resampling methods.

Multiple methods that extend methodologies developed within different research areas, including machine learning, data mining, and causal inference, were recently proposed in the context of subgroup identification and biomarker discovery. To facilitate exposition of the methods, we will first introduce some notation.

Consider a clinical trial that was conducted to evaluate the efficacy and safety of an experimental therapy versus a control. Let y_i denote the outcome variable for the ith subject ($i = 1, \ldots, n$), which can be continuous, binary, or based on a time to event. Here, n is the total sample size in the trial. Further, T_i denotes the treatment arm indicator for the ith subject, that is, the subject was assigned to the control arm if $T_i = 0$ and to the experimental treatment arm if $T_i = 1$.

Suppose that k biomarkers, denoted by $X_1, \ldots, X_k$, were studied in the trial. Let $\mathbf{x}_i = \{x_{i1}, \ldots, x_{ik}\}$ denote a set of candidate biomarkers for the ith subject evaluated prior to the initiation of treatment. A subgroup $S(\mathbf{x})$ is defined by a rule that assigns a subject to the subgroup based on the vector of biomarker values $\mathbf{x}_i$, $i = 1, \ldots, n$. For example,

$$S(\mathbf{x}) = I\{c \leq x_{i1}, i = 1, \ldots, n\}$$

is composed of all subjects with elevated levels of the biomarker X_1.

Let $f(\mathbf{x}, t)$ denote the expected response of a subject as a function of the vector of observed biomarker values $\mathbf{x}$ and actual treatment assignment t. The expected *potential outcomes* are defined for each subject as $f(\mathbf{x}, 1)$ and $f(\mathbf{x}, 0)$. Further, let $z(\mathbf{x})$ denote a function that summarizes a treatment contrast at the subject's level, that is,

$$z(\mathbf{x}) = g(f(\mathbf{x}, 1), f(\mathbf{x}, 0)).$$

For example, $z(\mathbf{x})$ may be defined as the treatment difference, that is,

$$z(\mathbf{x}) = f(\mathbf{x}, 1) - f(\mathbf{x}, 0).$$

Subgroup analysis procedures developed for personalized medicine applications are commonly conceptualized within two frameworks:

- The first framework aims at identifying the right subject for a given treatment. To give an example, consider a trial's sponsor who is interested in developing a "salvaging strategy." This includes identification of subgroups of subjects who may still benefit from an experimental therapy versus a control, given that the therapy provides minimal or no benefit in the overall population.

- The second framework deals with identifying the right treatment for a subject. Consider, for example, the problem of finding the optimal treatment regimen or policy for a given subpopulation.

Although these two frameworks are closely related to each other, there are important differences, both philosophical and statistical. One of the differences in the statistical formulation of the two approaches is that the first approach entails searching for predictive biomarkers exhibiting *quantitative interactions* and modifying the overall treatment effect. The second approach requires the identification of predictive biomarkers that exhibit *qualitative interactions* leading to different optimal treatment strategies for different types of subjects. With a qualitative interaction, subjects with certain values of the biomarker (biomarker-positive subjects) experience a pronounced treatment effect, whereas subjects in the complementary subgroup (biomarker-negative subjects) benefit from the control.

To make this distinction more formal, let us assume that the true subject's response is formed as

$$f(\mathbf{x}, t) = h(\mathbf{x}) + tg(\mathbf{x}),$$

where $h(\mathbf{x})$ is the prognostic component and $g(\mathbf{x})$ is the predictive component. Then the first framework can be conceptualized as a situation where the average value of $g(\mathbf{x})$ over the entire covariate space is close to 0, rendering the overall treatment effect small, whereas a subgroup S may exist such that

$$E(g(\mathbf{x})|\mathbf{x} \in S) \geq c_1,$$

where c_1 is a positive constant that defines a clinically meaningful threshold.

The second framework of personalized medicine can be illustrated by the situation where qualitative interaction exists such that

$$E(g(\mathbf{x})|\mathbf{x} \in S_1) \geq c_1 \quad \text{and} \quad E(g(\mathbf{x})|\mathbf{x} \notin S_1) \leq c_2,$$

or

$$E(g(\mathbf{x})|\mathbf{x} \in S_1) \geq c_1 \quad \text{and} \quad E(g(\mathbf{x})|\mathbf{x} \in S_2) \leq c_2,$$

for two nonoverlapping subgroups S_1 and S_2 (c_2 is a negative constant). The subjects from S_1 benefit from the experimental treatment, whereas subjects from S_2 benefit from the control.

We first describe some methods that naturally fall within the first framework. Several classes of methods that can be used in subgroup search problems have been developed in the literature. The following is a high-level classification scheme to facilitate the discussion of commonly used approaches:

- *Global outcome modeling*: Modeling of the underlying outcome function $f(\mathbf{x}, t)$.
- *Global treatment effect modeling*: Modeling of the underlying treatment effect $z(\mathbf{x})$.
- *Local modeling*: Direct search for subgroups with a beneficial treatment effect, that is, identifying subgroups {$\mathbf{x} \in S$} with higher values of $z(\mathbf{x})$.

Examples of subgroup search methods based on the three approaches are provided below.

8.2.1 Global Outcome Modeling

Subgroup search methods in this class aim at fitting statistical models incorporating a large number of candidate covariates and treatment-by-covariate interactions using methods of penalized and ensemble regression. This often results in a complex "black box model," which is then used to evaluate the heterogeneity of the treatment effect and identify subgroups in which the treatment is highly effective. Subgroup search methods built around the concept of *potential outcomes* can be used to illustrate the global modeling approach.

Cai et al. (2011) proposed to model hypothetical outcomes using the proportional hazards, Cox regression, which incorporates subject-level variables, and developed a spline-based procedure to assess the treatment effect heterogeneity at the subject's level.

Penalized regression methods are often used when modeling the outcome as a function that includes the prognostic (main) effects of baseline covariates and their predictive effects (modeled as interactions with the treatment variable). Since the number of such potential interaction effects is substantial, fitting them within a standard likelihood-based framework may not be feasible. To address this problem, various penalized (a.k.a. regularization) methods placing constraints on the sizes of regression coefficients can be applied, which causes the interaction effects to shrink toward zero. With the LASSO penalty (least absolute shrinkage and selection operator, Tibshirani, 1996), some of the effects shrink exactly to 0, which leads to biomarker and subgroup selection methods. For example, Imai and Ratcovic (2013) proposed using a support vector machine (SVM) classifier (Vapnik, 1995) with separate LASSO-type constraints over the predictive and prognostic effects included in the model. This approach accounts for the fact that the predictive effects are inherently weaker and need to be treated differently from the prognostic effects.

Foster et al. (2011) developed a method called virtual twins that models potential outcomes using flexible machine learning methods. The underlying regression function $f(\mathbf{x}, t)$ is estimated in the first stage using random forests (Breiman, 2001) (other methods of ensemble regression can also be applied). Once a random forest has been fitted to the data, two predicted outcomes are obtained for the ith subject, assuming that the subject was in the treatment or control arms, respectively, that is,

$$\hat{f}(\mathbf{x}_i, 0) \quad \text{and} \quad \hat{f}(\mathbf{x}_i, 1), i = 1, \ldots, n.$$

A hypothetical treatment difference z_i is estimated for each subject as follows:

$$\hat{z}(\mathbf{x}_i) = \hat{f}(\mathbf{x}_i, 1) - \hat{f}(\mathbf{x}_i, 0).$$

The obtained treatment differences are used in the second stage of the virtual twins method as the outcome variables for a simple regression tree with the goal of identifying a subgroup, where $z(\mathbf{x}_i)$ is expected to be larger than some clinically meaningful threshold, say, c. The final subgroup is formed as the union of all terminal nodes of the tree where the predicted treatment differences are greater than c.

Bayesian methods for subgroup identification within the global modeling framework typically evolve around fitting complex models with terms involving biomarker-by-treatment interactions that are shrunk to zero via empirical Bayes or fully Bayesian methods. Such models can potentially handle a large number of candidate subgroups. Notable examples of Bayesian approaches in this context are Dixon and Simon (1991) and Hodges et al. (2007).

8.2.2 Global Treatment Effect Modeling

Methods in this category are attractive in that they bypass estimation of "main effects" (or identification of biomarkers with purely prognostic value) that "cancel out" and instead focus on directly estimating the treatment contrast. As a result, they may be more robust and less prone to model misspecification inevitable in global outcome modeling.

Negassa et al. (2005) and Su et al. (2009) proposed *interaction trees* for identification of subgroups and predictive biomarkers. This method essentially extends CART (classification and regression trees) methods introduced in Breiman et al. (1984) by incorporating a *treatment-by-split interaction* in the splitting criterion. Similar to other nonparametric methods based on recursive partitioning, this method supports subgroup identification within a very broad "model space." The model space in recursive partitioning consists of all possible configurations of selected variables and associated cutoffs, for example, a subgroup generated by an interaction tree may be defined as

$$S(\mathbf{x}) = I\{25 < x_{i1} \leq 40, x_{i2} = \text{'Male'}, i = 1,\ldots,n\},$$

where X_1 is the subject's age and X_2 is the subject's gender.

Interaction trees essentially classify all subjects into a collection of the nonoverlapping subgroups (terminal nodes). Subjects within the same terminal node have a similar treatment effect, which is typically estimated within the subgroup as a single treatment contrast. Therefore, interaction trees provide a piecewise constant fit for the underlying treatment effect $z(\mathbf{x})$.

Tian et al. (2012) proposed a simple yet ingenious general approach to the identification of predictive effects termed the *modified covariate* method. They observed that, for a continuous outcome variable, the treatment-by-covariate interaction effects can be fitted directly (without the need for modeling the main effects) by simply modifying the outcome variable by multiplying it by the treatment indicator $T = \{-1, 1\}$. However, as they show, this is equivalent to fitting a model to the original outcome variable while multiplying the (mean-centered) covariate vector by the treatment indicator. The authors argued that the modified covariate framework easily generalizes to different types of outcomes, for example, binary and survival outcome variables, and allows the incorporation of efficient estimation methods as well as dealing with high-dimensional data by regularization. This approach produces an estimated subject-specific predictive score that can be used to stratify populations by the expected treatment effect and identify subgroups of subjects who may experience enhanced treatment benefit or harm.

Bayesian subgroup analysis can also be performed by modeling the data at the treatment contrast level rather than at the treatment outcome level in a very straightforward manner. For example, Jones et al. (2011) presented a general framework for Bayesian subgroup analysis that subsumes the models proposed in Dixon and Simon (1991) and Hodges et al. (2007) as special cases. Within this framework, a hierarchical Bayesian model is posed for the treatment contrast in a candidate subgroup. The treatment effect is shared by all subjects within the subgroup (cell) and, to simplify the notation, the subgroup and subject indices will be dropped. The treatment effect is denoted by θ, which may be the mean difference, log-odds ratio, log-hazard ratio, and so on. The subgroup effects defined by single covariates are modeled simply by including their main effects, and the subgroup effects defined by m covariates would require $(m - 1)$-order interaction effects. As with any cell-means modeling, this approach works best with a relatively small number of covariates.

As an example, consider the process of modeling the treatment effect as a function of binary predictive biomarkers based on the subject's age (X_1), gender (X_2), and race (X_3). The resulting model for the treatment effect in this subgroup is defined as the sum of the overall effect, subgroup effects of the three biomarkers, and associated second- and third-order interactions as follows:

$$\theta = \mu + \gamma_1 I(x_1 < 50) + \gamma_2 I(x_2 = \text{'Male'}) + \gamma_3 I(x_3 = \text{'White'})$$
$$+ \delta_1 I(x_1 < 50) I(x_2 = \text{'Male'}) + \delta_2 I(x_1 < 50) I(x_3 = \text{'White'})$$
$$+ \delta_3 I(x_2 = \text{'Male'}) I(x_3 = \text{'White'}) + \alpha I(x_1 < 50) I(x_2 = \text{'Male'}) I(x_3 = \text{'White'}).$$

The subgroup effect, second- and third-order interaction effects, that is, $\gamma = (\gamma_1, \gamma_2, \gamma_3)$, $\delta = (\delta_1, \delta_2, \delta_3)$, and α are modeled using independent normal priors with zero means and separate variances, also modeled as random variables within the Bayesian hierarchical model, allowing for a differential amount of shrinkage for the associated subgroup effects. Note that modeling at the outcome level would require the inclusion of covariate-by-treatment interactions up to the fourth order, as well as all prognostic effects. The connection between the observed data and unobservable subgroup treatment effects θ on the left-hand side of the above equation occurs via the first level of the hierarchy. For example, when modeling a binary outcome using the same three biomarkers, we can assume that the observed log-odds ratio in each candidate subgroup is generated by independent normal distributions centered around θ, that is, $\hat{\theta} \sim N(\theta, \sigma_\theta^2)$.

8.2.3 Local Modeling

The last class of subgroup search methods focuses on direct search for treatment-by-covariate interactions and selecting subgroups with desirable characteristics, for example, subgroups with improved treatment effect $z(\mathbf{x})$. This approach obviates the need to estimate the response function over the entire covariate space and focuses on identifying specific regions of interest with a large treatment effect.

Examples include the responder identification procedure proposed by Kehl and Ulm (2006). This method extends the machine learning procedure of bump hunting (also known as the patient rule induction method or PRIM) developed by Friedman and Fisher (1999) to the problem of identifying subsets of subjects who experience a strong beneficial effect. This approach is based on an argument that, instead of estimating the response function $f(\mathbf{x},t)$ over the entire space of biomarker values and then selecting regions that may be "uninteresting" for the research goal, it may be more efficient to directly search for such regions:

> The problem of accurately approximating a general function of many arguments everywhere within some domain of input values, based on sampled data (with or without noise) remains a difficult one. Often function approximation is applied in situations for which the actual data analytic goal is far more modest; the interest is in some property of the target function. A common procedure in such situations is to attempt to estimate the target $f(\mathbf{x})$ everywhere in the input space and ascertain the property of interest from the resulting estimate of $f(\mathbf{x})$. Frequently however, this strategy can be counter-productive in that an alternative once focuses directly on estimating the property of interest may give rise to higher accuracy. (Friedman and Fisher, 1999)

One reason why this may be the case is that estimating the response function in potentially high-dimensional space would require careful tuning of various complexity parameters. It is clear that trying to estimate $f(\mathbf{x},t)$ well everywhere requires balancing of errors across the entire region and therefore may compromise the approximation quality in those special regions where the interest lies. For example, smoothing out a "bump" in the interest of achieving better approximation elsewhere would be counterproductive if, in fact, the bump was the most interesting part of the response function.

Another example of the direct search approach to subgroup identification is the SIDES method (Lipkovich et al., 2011), which will be the main topic of this chapter. The general SIDES method is presented in Sections 8.3 and 8.5.

It is worth noting that Bayesian approaches to subgroup identification within the local modeling framework were also developed. The methods proceed by identifying a set of candidate subgroups that are treated as "individual models" and assigning priors to each subgroup and applying

Bayesian model selection/averaging procedures (Sivaganesan et al., 2011; Berger et al., 2014). For example, in Berger et al. (2014), each submodel in the model space is constructed as a combination of possible predictive and prognostic (or baseline) effects using 10 different basic subgroup structures. Within each such structure, the predictive and prognostic components are modeled locally by subsetting on a small number of dichotomous biomarkers (up to one variable in the prognostic or/and predictive components). A continuous outcome variable in a "local" submodel M may be driven by a prognostic effect defined by the variable X_l and a predictive effect defined by the variable X_m, $l, m = 1, \ldots, k$, that is,

$$y_i | M = \mu + \alpha I(x_{il} = 0) + t_i \beta I(x_{im} = 0) + \varepsilon_i, \varepsilon_i \sim N(0, \sigma^2).$$

The authors then show how to elicit priors for each submodel in the model space for all possible combinations of prognostic and predictive effects. The final outcome prediction is based on averaging predictions from each model weighted by its posterior probability. The quantities of interest include the posterior distribution of treatment effect in each subgroup defined by the variables $X_1, \ldots, X_k$ as well as the distribution of the treatment effect for a subject with a specific biomarker profile.

8.2.4 Identification of the Right Treatment for a Subject

This section provides a brief overview of the second framework within the data-driven approach to subgroup search that lays emphasis on identifying optimal treatment for a given subject. Broadly, this includes any approach that specifically targets predictive biomarkers associated with qualitative (as opposed to quantitative) treatment-by-covariate interactions, which are closely related to the task of determining *optimal treatment regimes*. Gunter et al. (2011) proposed a method for identifying such qualitative biomarkers based on penalized regression.

Zhao et al. (2012) showed that estimating optimal individualized treatment policies can be framed as a classification problem where the optimal classifier corresponds to the optimal treatment regime. Within this framework, the treatment assignment variable plays a role of the outcome variable and a certain "outcome-based weight" is applied to each subject. Specifically, $w_i = y_i / \pi_i$ for treated subjects and $w_i = y_i / (1 - \pi_i)$ for untreated subjects, where

$$\pi_i = \hat{P}(T_i = 1 | \mathbf{x}_i)$$

is the estimated probability of assigning the ith subject to the experimental treatment arm (note that in a randomized treatment clinical trial, it can be simply estimated as the proportion of subjects with $T_i = 1$).

The idea is that the assigned weights take into account the subjects' observed outcomes in such a way that the misclassification costs will be minimized if subjects with desirable outcomes are assigned to the treatment arm that they were actually assigned to, and subjects who did not experience much benefit under their current treatment are assigned to the other treatment arm. Therefore, minimizing weighted misclassification costs will entail assigning a subject to the treatment that provides maximum benefits, given the subject's biomarker values. Any machine learning method can then be used for predicting binary or multinomial outcomes. For example, the machine learning method of SVMs was used in Zhao et al. (2012).

Zhang et al. (2012a) also considered estimating the optimal treatment regime as a classification problem under a somewhat more general framework. They proposed to fit a weighted classifier, for example, a CART or SVM model, to the class labels that are not the actual treatment labels but are rather formed by evaluating the sign of the treatment contrast estimated at the individual subject's level, that is, $I(z(\mathbf{x}_i) > 0)$. As in the virtual twins method (Foster et al., 2011), the treatment contrast is estimated using the framework of potential outcomes; however, combining the outcome model with the probability of the treatment model in a doubly robust augmented inverse probability-weighted estimator (AIPWE) is defined as follows (see also Zhang et al., 2012b):

$$\hat{z}_{\text{AIPWE}}(\mathbf{x}_i) = \frac{T_i}{\pi_i} y_i - \frac{1 - T_i}{1 - \pi_i} y_i - \frac{T_i - \pi_i}{\pi_i} \hat{f}(\mathbf{x}_i, 1) - \frac{T_i - \pi_i}{1 - \pi_i} \hat{f}(\mathbf{x}_i, 0).$$

The weighted classifier therefore will produce decision rules for discriminating subjects who benefit from the experimental treatment from those who benefit from the control treatment. The subject-specific weights are taken as the absolute values of the estimated treatment contrasts, that is, $|\hat{z}_{\text{AIPWE}}(\mathbf{x}_i)|$. Thus, the subjects for whom the choice of treatment does not make much difference exert less influence on the decision rule.

As shown in Zhang et al. (2012a), the outcome-weighted learning method developed in Zhao et al. (2012) can be considered a special case of their approach, when the treatment contrast $z(\mathbf{x})$ is estimated using the inverse probability-weighted estimator (IPWE) rather than AIPWE. The approach of Zhang et al. (2012a) can also be viewed as a generalization of the virtual twins method in that the AIPWE estimator of the hypothetical treatment difference, that is, $z(\mathbf{x}_i)$, subsumes the estimator of $z(\mathbf{x}_i)$ in that method. The advantage of AIPWE is that it is more efficient and is consistent even when the outcome model may be misspecified, but the treatment model is not. Note that this condition trivially holds for a randomized clinical trial where the probability of treatment assignment is known. When the data come from an observational study with nonrandom treatment assignment, the doubly robust AIPWE estimator protects against model misspecification as long as at least one of the two models (for outcome and treatment assignment) is correctly specified.

Recently, there has been a surge of literature on estimating optimal treatment regimes defined not only in terms of baseline biomarkers but also by utilizing evolving subject outcomes during the treatment period. This can be accomplished within the *reinforcement learning* framework (e.g., Q-learning), which originated in machine learning and is now applied to clinical research as well; see, for example, Zhao et al. (2009) and Schulte et al. (2013). Reinforcement learning utilizes data available from clinical trials where subjects could be rerandomized to a different treatment during the course of the study. In addition, this approach can be applied to observational studies where treatment switching occurs naturally, as physicians are trying to provide the best choice of treatment for each subject. Q-learning is based on estimating regression models for the outcome of interest, given each subject's information at each decision point, and is implemented through a backward recursive fitting procedure that is related to the dynamic programming algorithms (see Schulte et al., 2013, and references therein).

Sophisticated and computationally intensive resampling techniques are extensively used in many of the machine learning methods developed for biomarker discovery. Resampling-based methods are used to control the false-positive rates, reduce selection bias, or adjust for the bias in estimated treatment effects within subgroups. For example, Gunter et al. (2011) constructed a statistic that captures the amount of qualitative interaction in a particular subset of covariates. Further, the statistic is averaged over multiple bootstrap samples to remove the selection bias due to data overfitting. The resulting statistics are then thresholded with cutoffs that are calibrated using the null distributions of the above statistics to achieve a desired type I error rate. Similarly, in the virtual twins method presented above, an "honest" estimate of the treatment effect expected to be found in future data within the identified subgroup (in excess to that in the overall population) is constructed using k-fold cross-validation, as well as parametric and nonparametric bootstrap procedures.

8.3 Three SIDES Subgroup Search Procedure

This section introduces the SIDES method (Lipkovich et al., 2011) aimed at the identification of predictive biomarkers and biomarker signatures in clinical trial databases. This method can be used in prospective and retrospective settings and applied to the analysis of continuous, categorical, and time-to-event outcome variables. The general SIDES method features three novel aspects:

- Flexible direct search algorithm. The underlying algorithm focuses on direct search for treatment-by-biomarker interactions to identify subgroups of subjects who derive substantial benefit from the experimental therapy (and potentially desirable safety).

- Complexity control. A complexity criterion is used to control the size of the search space and produce results with straightforward clinical interpretation.
- Multiplicity control. A resampling-based multiplicity adjustment is employed to protect the probability of incorrect subgroup identification.

More information on the key features of this method is provided later in this section as well as in Sections 8.4 and 8.5.

We begin with the regular SIDES procedure and extensions of this procedure will be discussed in Section 8.5. The SIDES procedure has been successfully used in multiple development programs where the sponsor was interested in assessing the predictive ability of phenotypical or clinical variables. For example, Hardin et al. (2013) discussed an application of the SIDES procedure to a retrospective analysis of a large open-label study in subjects with type II diabetes mellitus who were randomized to receive two active treatments (twice-daily insulin lispro mix and once-daily insulin glargine). The predictive ability of 12 variables was examined in this study. The set of candidate markers included standard demographic variables such as subject's age, gender and baseline body-mass index, as well as clinical variables (use of metformin at baseline, baseline-fasting glucose level, baseline-fasting insulin level, baseline adiponectin level, etc.). The research concluded that there was substantial heterogeneity in treatment response based on the candidate biomarkers. In particular, younger subjects with higher levels of fasting insulin at baseline may benefit from a regimen that includes short-acting insulin-targeting postprandial glycemia.

Biomarker sets in a traditional subgroup search setting are relatively small. The regular SIDES procedure tends to demonstrate poor performance in "massive" biomarker identification problems with a large number of covariates, especially when most of the covariates are noninformative. This setting is quite common in modern clinical trials where hundreds of biomarkers may be collected in pharmacogenomics data sets. Extensions of the regular SIDES procedure are recommended to achieve a more robust performance in problems of this kind. The extended procedures, known as SIDEScreen procedures (Lipkovich and Dmitrienko, 2014), are introduced in Section 8.5.

8.3.1 Subgroup Search Algorithm

In the following, we will provide a high-level summary of the SIDES subgroup search algorithm. The algorithm will be illustrated in Section 8.4 using a case study based on a Phase III trial in subjects with colorectal cancer.

Using the same setting as in Section 8.2, consider a clinical trial database that includes one or more trials that were conducted to evaluate the efficacy and safety of an experimental therapy versus a control. The trial's sponsor is interested in performing a subgroup search based on a set of k candidate biomarkers, denoted by $X_1,...,X_k$, and identifying a set of subgroups with a greater response to the treatment compared to the overall population of subjects.

The SIDES subgroup search algorithm is defined in Table 8.1. The algorithm is applied recursively beginning with the overall population. Starting with the overall population, which is treated as the *parent group*, the algorithm optimally splits the overall group into two complementary *child subgroups* for each candidate biomarker. For example, if the biomarker X_j is continuous or ordinal, the child groups are defined as the biomarker-low and biomarker-high subgroups:

$$L_j(c_j) = \{x_{ij} \le c_j, i = 1,...,n\}, \quad H_j(c_j) = \{x_{ij} > c_j, i = 1,...,n\}, \quad j = 1,...,k,$$

where x_{ij} denotes the value of X_j for the ith subject (the biomarker-low and biomarker-high subgroups should not be confused with the biomarker-negative and biomarker-positive subgroups). It is important to note that continuous biomarkers do not need to be converted into categorical variables.

The cutoff c_j is selected by examining all possible values of the biomarker in the database that would result in nontrivial biomarker-low and biomarker-high subgroups. For a nominal biomarker with m different categories, the

TABLE 8.1

SIDES Subgroup Search Algorithm

Step 1. Initialize

A single zero-stage parent group is formed of all observations in the data set. Initialize the set of promising subgroups as an empty set, $\mathcal{P} = \emptyset$.

Step 2. Iterate (splitting the current l-stage parent group, $0 \le l \le L$)

If $l = L$, the current parent group becomes terminal and is not considered for further splitting; otherwise

1. Arrange the biomarkers from the "best" to "worst" in terms of the adjusted optimal value of the splitting criterion.

2. For each of the top M covariates, form two child subgroups based on the covariate's "best split" among all allowable splits. Select the subgroup with the larger positive treatment effect S_j and include it in the set of promising subgroups $\mathcal{P}$ provided the complexity criterion is met (if defined).

3. For each promising subgroup S_j, set S_j as the current parent group, let $l = l + 1$, and repeat step 2.

4. If no biomarker has allowable splits resulting in a promising subgroup, the current parent group becomes terminal and is not considered for further splitting.

Step 3. Finalize

Include a promising subgroup from $\mathcal{P}$ in the final set if the unadjusted treatment effect p-value is significant at a prespecified level and/or if the multiplicity-adjusted p-value computed using a resampling-based method is significant at a prespecified level.

optimal split of the parent group into child subgroups is found by optimizing the splitting criterion over all possible partitions of the m categories into two sets, which results in $2^{m-1} - 1$ nontrivial splits. To simplify the notation, we will assume in the following that all candidate biomarkers are continuous variables.

Let C_j define the *allowable set* of cutoffs for the biomarker X_j. A cutoff is included in this set if the size of the best of the child subgroups resulting from the split based on this cutoff is greater than a prespecified minimal sample size, denoted by $n_{\min}$ (the best subgroup is the one with the larger positive treatment effect, or the "promising subgroup," as will be defined later). The biomarker-specific cutoff is chosen from the allowable set by maximizing the differential treatment effect between the child subgroups based on an appropriate splitting criterion. We will assume that smaller values of the criterion are desirable, and thus, the optimal value of the cutoff for the biomarker X_j is defined as follows:

$$c_j^* = \arg\min{}_{c_j \in C_j} D(X_j, c_j),$$

where $D(X_j, c_j)$ is the splitting criterion. The commonly used splitting criteria are defined in Appendix A.

We would like to emphasize that optimality is understood in terms of the selected search criterion and therefore reflects local characteristics of the treatment effects within each parent group. This does not guarantee optimal identification of subgroups in terms of a global criterion that defines treatment benefit in the final subgroups.

Next, the optimal cutoffs are found for the candidate biomarkers based on a prespecified splitting criterion. Let L_j and H_j denote the resulting child subgroups and S_j denote the child subgroup with the larger positive treatment effect, known as the *promising subgroup*, for the biomarker X_j. Further, let d_j denote the optimal value of the splitting criterion for X_j. It is well known (see, e.g., Loh and Shih, 1997) that the optimal value of any splitting criterion found by an exhaustive search over the set of possible cutoffs is biased in favor of biomarkers with a larger number of levels. Since the number of levels varies across the candidate biomarkers, a multiplicity adjustment needs to be applied to perform a "fair" comparison of the biomarkers (see Appendix B for more information on computing adjusted values of splitting criteria). The adjusted values of the splitting criterion are denoted by

$$\tilde{d}_1, \tilde{d}_2, \ldots, \tilde{d}_k$$

and the candidate biomarkers are then ordered by the adjusted criterion. Specifically, the ordered criterion values are denoted by

$$\tilde{d}_{(1)} \leq \tilde{d}_{(2)} \leq \cdots \leq \tilde{d}_{(k)}$$

and the corresponding ordered promising subgroups are denoted by

$$S_{(1)}, S_{(2)}, \ldots, S_{(k)}.$$

To streamline the subgroup search, the algorithm retains only the best M subgroups, that is,

$$S_{(1)}, S_{(2)}, \ldots, S_{(M)},$$

the other promising subgroups are abandoned, where M is a prespecified constant. There are several reasons why it is important to pursue multiple child subgroups rather than selecting the top subgroup for each parent group. First, virtually identical subgroups of subjects are often described using different (but correlated) biomarkers; however, these biomarkers may have a different clinical interpretation. Therefore, retaining multiple subgroups helps ensure that most clinically meaningful biomarkers will not be missed. Second, from the machine learning perspective, a greedy "winner gets everything" principle often leads to unstable model selection. Alternative approaches based on different ensemble methods that capitalize on multiple sets of competing models are often used. For example, within the random forests method, predictions are averaged over multiple sets of trees grown from bootstrap samples. Similarly, the SIDES procedure pursues multiple branches by retaining several promising subgroups for a given parent group. In Section 8.5, we will take advantage of this feature of the SIDES procedure by computing variable importance scores over the collection of subgroups that are used for identifying important biomarkers.

The resulting M promising subgroups are examined to ensure that the restrictions on the magnitude of the treatment effect are met. The subgroup search algorithm focuses on subgroups with a strong treatment effect and a child subgroup is discarded if the treatment effect p-value exceeds a prespecified threshold.

8.3.2 Complexity Control

The selected child subgroups for a given parent are examined to determine if they meet the *complexity* criterion (this criterion was referred to as the continuation criterion in Lipkovich et al., 2011). This criterion helps control the size of the search space, that is, the total number of subgroups examined by the search algorithm. According to the complexity criterion, a child subgroup is considered promising and explored further only if the treatment effect in this subgroup is sufficiently large compared to the effect in the parent group. This approach is consistent with the objective of identifying a small set of subgroups with a strong treatment effect.

Formally, let $p_1, \ldots, p_M$ denote the one-sided treatment effect p-values in the promising subgroups retained by the algorithm, that is, $S_{(1)}, \ldots, S_{(M)}$.

Similarly, let p_0 denote the one-sided treatment effect p-value in the parent group. The complexity criterion is met if

$$p_j \leq \gamma p_0,$$

where γ is a prespecified complexity parameter with $0 < \gamma \leq 1$. This parameter determines the size of the overall search space. Indeed, if γ is infinitely large, there is no complexity control and subgroups are generated without any restrictions and $\gamma = 0$ corresponds to the most restrictive complexity control because no subgroups can be found in this case. The complexity parameter is typically set to a value between 0.1 and 1 and, as shown in Lipkovich et al. (2011), an optimal value of this parameter can be determined by cross-validation.

If a promising subgroup meets the complexity criterion, it is added to the list of parent groups and the algorithm is then applied to this subgroup. Note that subgroups at the second level are defined using two biomarkers, subgroups at the third level are defined using three biomarkers, and so on. Recursive partitioning continues until the SIDES subgroup search algorithm reaches the bottom level. This parameter is denoted by L and can be thought of as the subgroup depth, that is, it defines the number of times the algorithm can be recursively applied to parent groups starting with the overall population at $L = 0$. As a result, the algorithm can generate up to

$$M + M^2 + \cdots + M^L = \frac{M(1 - M^L)}{1 - M}$$

subgroups.

Figure 8.1 illustrates the SIDES subgroup search algorithm in a setting with $M = 2$ (up to two promising subgroups are chosen per parent) and $L = 2$ (subgroups are defined using up to two biomarkers). For the sake of simplicity, we assume that all biomarkers are continuous. Beginning with Level 1, the algorithm optimally splits the parent group based on the overall population by each biomarker. Since $M = 2$, two biomarkers that maximize the differential treatment effect (or, equivalently, minimize the splitting criterion) are selected. Suppose that the biomarkers X_1 and X_2 are selected. The biomarker-low and biomarker-high subgroups based on the biomarker-specific optimal cutoff are defined for each biomarker, that is, L_j and H_j, $j = 1, 2$. The optimal cutoffs are denoted by c_1 and c_2, respectively. A promising subgroup is chosen from each pair of child subgroups as the subgroup that exhibits the larger positive treatment effect. Figure 8.1 indicates that the following promising subgroups are identified at this level:

$$L_1, H_2.$$

If a promising subgroup satisfies the prespecified complexity criterion, it is retained and serves as a parent group at the next level. The other child subgroups identified in Figure 8.1, for example, H_1 and L_2, are abandoned.

Level 1

Parent = {All subjects}

Split by X_1		Split by X_2	
$L_1 = \{X_1 \le c_1\}$	$H_1 = \{X_1 > c_1\}$	$L_2 = \{X_2 \le c_2\}$	$H_2 = \{X_2 > c_2\}$
Retained	Abandoned	Abandoned	Retained

Level 2

Parent = $\{X_1 \le c_1\}$		Parent = $\{X_2 > c_2\}$	
Split by X_2	Split by X_3	Split by X_1	Split by X_3
$L_{12} = \{X_1 \le c_1,$ $X_2 \le c_{12}\}$ Abandoned	$L_{13} = \{X_1 \le c_1,$ $X_3 \le c_{13}\}$ Retained	$L_{21} = \{X_2 > c_2,$ $X_1 \le c_{21}\}$ Abandoned	$L_{23} = \{X_2 > c_2,$ $X_3 \le c_{23}\}$ Abandoned
$H_{12} = \{X_1 \le c_1,$ $X_2 > c_{12}\}$ Retained	$H_{13} = \{X_1 \le c_1,$ $X_3 > c_{13}\}$ Abandoned	$H_{21} = \{X_2 > c_2,$ $X_1 > c_{21}\}$ Retained	$H_{23} = \{X_2 > c_2,$ $X_3 > c_{23}\}$ Retained

FIGURE 8.1
Illustration of the SIDES procedure with two promising subgroups retained for each parent ($M = 2$) and two levels of subgroup search ($L = 2$).

The two parent groups are recursively split at Level 2. Note that the biomarkers that have already been used in a parent group's definition are excluded at this stage. For example, as shown in Figure 8.1, when S_1 is a parent group at Level 2, it is split into two child subgroups using all other biomarkers but X_1. Suppose that the biomarkers X_2 and X_3 are selected as the top two splitting covariates for the first parent group and X_1 and X_3 as the top two splitting covariates for the second parent group. The biomarker-low and biomarker-high subgroups are then defined for each parent and splitting covariate as above. Consider, for example, the process of splitting the parent group $\{X_2 > c_2\}$ by the biomarker X_1. The optimal cutoff, denoted by c_{21}, is determined by maximizing the differential treatment effect between the following two subgroups:

$$L_{21} = \{X_2 > c_2 \text{ and } X_1 \le c_{21}\}, H_{21} = \{X_2 > c_2 \text{ and } X_1 > c_{21}\}.$$

The other biomarker-low and biomarker-high subgroups are constructed in a similar fashion and promising subgroups with the larger positive treatment effect are selected from each pair. The resulting four promising subgroups are identified in Figure 8.1:

$$H_{12}, L_{13}, H_{21}, H_{23}.$$

The subgroup search algorithm stops at this point because it has reached the second level ($L = 2$). Suppose that all four promising subgroups at the second level met the complexity criterion. In this case, the terminal set includes the following four subgroups:

$$\{X_1 \leq c_1 \text{ and } X_2 > c_{12}\}, \quad \{X_1 \leq c_1 \text{ and } X_3 \leq c_{13}\},$$
$$\{X_2 > c_2 \text{ and } X_1 > c_{21}\}, \quad \{X_2 > c_2 \text{ and } X_3 > c_{23}\}.$$

As seen from this example, an important property of the SIDES procedure is that it identifies multiple plausible subgroups that are typically ordered in terms of their relevance, for example, by the magnitude of the treatment effect.

8.3.3 Multiplicity Control

Once the final set of subgroups has been determined, a multiplicity adjustment is applied to evaluate the significance of the treatment effect within each subgroup. It is well known that naive subgroup search methods tend to be highly unreliable. These methods typically focus on subgroups with a significant treatment effect without any adjustment for the total number of subgroups studied (search space), which leads to spurious results. As mentioned at the beginning of this section, a distinguishing feature of SIDES is that this procedure provides explicit control of the overall probability of incorrectly discovering a subgroup. This error rate control is defined in the weak sense (Dmitrienko et al., 2009), that is, the probability of a false discovery is computed under the assumption that the treatment provides no benefit compared to the control across all possible subgroups.

The error rate is controlled by using a multiplicity adjustment based on a permutation procedure (Westfall and Young, 1993; Wang and Lagakos, 2009). Specifically, the SIDES procedure is run to define a set of final subgroups and unadjusted p-values are computed to assess the significance of the treatment effect within each subgroup. The unadjusted treatment effect p-values tend to be highly significant. However, this simply reflects the fact that most significant results were selected from a large pool of subgroups examined by the subgroup search algorithm.

To perform a multiplicity adjustment and obtain more reliable measures of treatment benefit, null data sets are constructed by permuting the treatment labels in the original data set. A set of subgroups is identified for each null data set based on the SIDES procedure and, for each given null data set, the most significant treatment effect p-value is found across the identified promising subgroups. A multiplicity-adjusted p-value is computed for each final subgroup in the original data set as the proportion of null data sets where the most significant treatment effect p-value is less than or equal to the unadjusted p-value for the selected final subgroup. The resulting multiplicity-adjusted p-values are typically much larger than the unadjusted treatment effect p-values and provide the basis for reliable inferences within each final subgroup.

8.3.4 Algorithm Parameters

To summarize, the following parameters need to be specified to run the SIDES subgroup search algorithm:

- D, splitting criterion. The criterion based on the differential effect p-value is commonly used.
- M, maximum number of child subgroups retained for each parent group. This parameter is commonly set to 5.
- L, maximum number of covariates to define a subgroup. This parameter is commonly set to 3.
- γ, complexity parameter, which defines the relative improvement in the one-sided treatment effect p-value in a child subgroup compared to the parent group. This parameter typically ranges between 0.1 and 1, and its values can be determined by cross-validation; see Lipkovich et al. (2011) for more information.
- n_{min}, minimal number of subjects within a child subgroup. This parameter is typically driven by the clinical objectives.
- p_{max}, upper bound on the one-sided treatment effect p-value in a final subgroup. The upper bound is typically specified only if the complexity criterion is disabled. In this case, the upper bound is typically much lower than 0.025 to help select subgroups with a highly beneficial treatment effect.

8.4 Case Study

A case study based on a Phase III clinical trial with an oncology indication will be used to illustrate the SIDES subgroup search procedure introduced in Section 8.3. This case study will also be used in Section 8.5 to motivate extensions of the regular SIDES procedure.

8.4.1 Phase III Clinical Trial

A Phase III trial was conducted to investigate the effect of an experimental therapy for the treatment of colorectal cancer. The subjects in the treatment arm received the best supportive care (BSC) in addition to experimental therapy, whereas the subjects in the control arm received BSC only. Unequal randomization was employed in the trial with 353 subjects allocated to the treatment arm and 177 subjects allocated to the control arm.

The setting considered in this case study serves as an example of a retrospective approach to biomarker discovery and subgroup identification. The overall outcome of the trial was negative. The experimental therapy did not demonstrate a meaningful improvement in progression-free survival (PFS) over the control. The median survival times in the treatment and control arms were 50 and 48 weeks, respectively. The associated treatment effect *p*-value computed from a Cox proportional hazards model was 0.3240 (one sided).

The trial's sponsor was interested in performing a comprehensive review of the clinical trial database to investigate the impact of relevant phenotypical, clinical, and other markers on the treatment response. This included important clinical variables, such as tumor grade and diagnostic site, and genetic markers, for example, KRAS gene mutation. In addition, several protein expression markers with a known prognostic value were included in the candidate set. For example, data from other trials suggested that higher values of X_8 and X_9 are generally correlated with tumor growth.

The final set of candidate biomarkers available at baseline is defined in Table 8.2. Most biomarkers in the candidate set were continuous. One biomarker was ordinal (X_1) and two biomarkers were measured on a nominal scale (X_2 and X_5).

A series of ad hoc subgroup analyses revealed that selected biomarkers, for example, X_4, X_6, and X_8, had significant discriminatory power and helped predict treatment-related PFS improvement. These analyses served

TABLE 8.2

Candidate Biomarkers in the Case Study (Phase III Clinical Trial in Subjects with Colorectal Cancer)

Biomarker	Description	List of Values or Range
X_1	Tumor grade	1, 2, 3, and 4
X_2	Primary diagnostic site	Colon and rectum
X_3	Time from the initial diagnosis to the metastatic disease (months)	0–126
X_4	Time from the initial diagnosis to the start of treatment (months)	12–189
X_5	KRAS mutation status	Wild type, mutated
X_6	Protein expression marker	1–32
X_7	Protein expression marker	40–236
X_8	Protein expression marker	1–38
X_9	Protein expression marker	0.6–7.4

as a starting point, and a more rigorous assessment of the predictive ability of individual biomarkers and biomarker signatures was performed using the SIDES procedure.

8.4.2 Subgroup Identification Based on SIDES Procedure

The SIDES procedure provides a systematic approach to evaluating promising biomarkers (as well as biomarker signatures) in the case study. The procedure was applied to the clinical trial database with $k = 9$ biomarkers. The following parameters were used in the subgroup search algorithm:

- The differential splitting criterion defined in Appendix A was utilized to find optimal cutoffs during the subgroup search ($D = D_1$).
- The maximum number of promising subgroups for each parent was set to 5 ($M = 5$).
- The maximum number of biomarkers in the definition of a subgroup was set to 3 ($L = 3$).
- The complexity parameter (γ) was set to 0.1 (restrictive search) and 0.5 (liberal search) was used to explore the effect of the complexity criterion on the final set of subgroups.
- The minimal number of subjects within a child subgroup was set to 50 ($n_{min} = 50$).
- The restriction based on nominal significance was not used in the subgroup selection (one-sided $p_{max} = 1$).

To speed up subgroup search, each continuous biomarker was discretized by converting it into a categorical covariate with 15 levels based on the 15 percentile groups. A grid search was utilized to find optimal cutoffs for the resulting discretized biomarkers as well as the only ordinal biomarker in the database. Exhaustive search through all possible splits was used for the two nominal covariates.

To illustrate the subgroup search algorithm, consider the decision rules used at the first level. The overall population served as the parent group. As indicated in Section 8.4, this group included 530 subjects and the treatment difference was nonsignificant (one-sided $p = 0.3240$). Using the differential splitting criterion, the optimal cutoff was determined for each biomarker in the candidate set and the child subgroups, denoted by L_j and H_j, $j = 1, \ldots, 9$, were found. The optimal values of the splitting criterion, that is, d_j, $j = 1, \ldots, 9$, were computed.

It was pointed out in Section 8.3 that any splitting rule tends to "reward" biomarkers with a larger number of possible splits. As the number of possible splits of the parent group into child subgroups increases, there are more opportunities to find a more extreme value of the splitting criterion, and thus, the unadjusted values $d_1, \ldots, d_9$ tend to be unreliable.

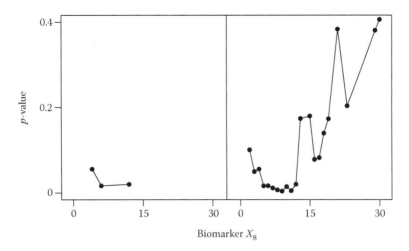

FIGURE 8.2
Value of the differential splitting criterion D_1 for two categorical covariates derived from the biomarker X_8 (categorical covariate with four levels, left panel; categorical covariate with 22 levels, right panel).

To examine the effect of the number of splits on the optimal value of a splitting criterion, Figure 8.2 shows the values of the differential splitting criterion D_1 for two categorical covariates derived from the biomarker X_8. For the sake of illustration, this continuous biomarker was converted into a categorical covariate with four levels (based on the quartiles of its distribution) and 22 levels (based on all observed values of X_8). It is clear that, with more potential splits in the right panel of the figure, the differential effect p-value used in the splitting criterion D_1 becomes more significant. Specifically, the optimal value of the criterion in the left panel is 0.0165 with the optimal cutoff at $X_8 = 6$. In the right panel, the criterion achieves the optimal value of 0.0038 at $X_8 = 9$. The optimal value in the latter case suggests a stronger differential effect, but this might be simply due to the fact that the search was performed over a finer grid.

To mitigate this problem, the optimal values of the differential splitting criterion were adjusted for the total number of possible splits of the parent group. This adjustment can be thought of as a "local" multiplicity adjustment that complements the "global" multiplicity adjustment described in Section 8.3. The local adjustment helps eliminate bias in the selection procedure, and the global adjustment helps preserve the overall probability of incorrectly discovering a subgroup. Using the general method defined in Appendix B, a multiplicity-adjusted splitting criterion was computed for the two categorical covariates defined above. The adjusted splitting criterion was 0.0362 for the categorical covariate with four levels and 0.0328 in the case of 22 levels. The two values are very close to each other and help illustrate the fact that a properly adjusted criterion is virtually independent of the number of potential splits.

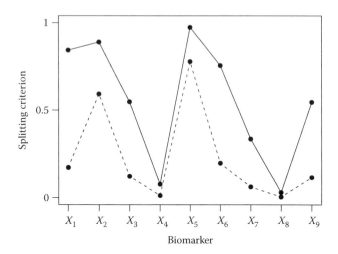

FIGURE 8.3
Original values of the splitting criterion (dashed curve) and adjusted values of the splitting criterion (solid curve) for the nine candidate biomarkers at the first level in the subgroup search algorithm.

Figure 8.3 displays the unadjusted values $(d_1, \ldots, d_9)$ as well as adjusted values $(\tilde{d}_1, \ldots, \tilde{d}_9)$ of the splitting criterion for all nine candidate biomarkers in the case study. As expected, the adjusted splitting criterion was less significant than the original splitting criterion. The lowest values of the adjusted criterion, which suggests the most pronounced differential treatment effect, were achieved for the biomarkers X_4 and X_8. The least significant value was observed for the biomarker X_5.

The candidate biomarkers were arranged according to the adjusted splitting criterion. With $M = 5$, less relevant subgroups were discarded and five best pairs of child subgroups were retained by the algorithm. The biomarker-low and biomarker-high subgroups within each pair are given below:

$$L_3 = \{X_3 \leq 33\}, \ H_3 = \{X_3 > 33\},$$
$$L_4 = \{X_4 \leq 66\}, \ H_4 = \{X_4 > 66\},$$
$$L_7 = \{X_7 \leq 127\}, \ H_7 = \{X_7 > 127\},$$
$$L_8 = \{X_8 \leq 11\}, \ H_8 = \{X_8 > 11\},$$
$$L_9 = \{X_9 \leq 1.27\}, \ H_9 = \{X_9 > 1.27\}.$$

Figure 8.4 displays the one-sided treatment effect p-value and size of each retained child subgroup. A child subgroup with the larger positive PFS effect, that is, smaller treatment effect p-value, was selected from each pair and the restriction on the size of each subgroup was checked. No subgroup was removed since the total sample size was greater than $n_{min} = 50$ in each promising subgroup. The resulting five promising subgroups were given by

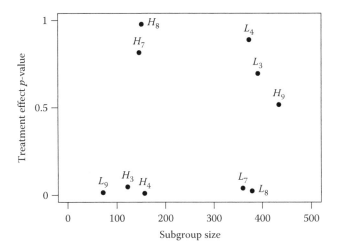

FIGURE 8.4
Treatment effect p-values and sizes of the 10 child subgroups retained at the first level in the subgroup search algorithm.

$$S_3 = H_3 = \{X_3 > 33\},$$
$$S_4 = H_4 = \{X_4 > 66\},$$
$$S_7 = L_7 = \{X_7 \leq 127\},$$
$$S_8 = L_8 = \{X_8 \leq 11\},$$
$$S_9 = L_9 = \{X_9 \leq 1.27\}.$$

Further, the complexity criterion was applied to select the subgroups with a prespecified degree of improvement in the PFS effect compared to the parent group. The assessment was performed on a p-value scale using the complexity parameters $\gamma = 0.1$ and 0.5. The higher value of γ is more liberal and results in a broader subgroup search. On the other hand, selecting a lower value of the complexity parameter γ leads to a more selective approach with a reduced search space. To illustrate the process of applying the complexity criterion, Figure 8.5 displays the five promising subgroups, that is, S_3, S_4, S_7, S_8, and S_9.

The complexity criterion imposes an upper bound on the treatment effect p-value in each promising subgroup. Since the treatment effect p-value in the parent group (overall population) was $p_0 = 0.3240$, the upper bound associated with the more liberal approach was given by

$$0.5 \cdot 0.3240 = 0.1620.$$

This upper bound is shown in Figure 8.5, and it follows from the figure that all promising subgroups satisfy the complexity criterion since the

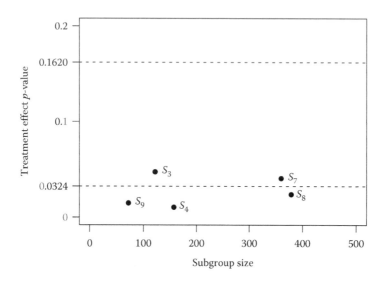

FIGURE 8.5
Application of the complexity criterion with a liberal complexity parameter ($\gamma = 0.5$) and restrictive complexity parameter ($\gamma = 0.1$) at the first level in the subgroup search algorithm.

treatment effect p-values are well below this threshold. This implies that the treatment-related improvement in the PFS rate is high enough relative to the overall population, and the five subgroups should be added to the list of parent groups. These groups will be studied and recursively split into smaller subgroups at the second level within the SIDES algorithm. These subgroups correspond to biomarker signatures with two biomarkers.

When the more restrictive approach with $\gamma = 0.1$ was considered, the upper bound on the treatment effect p-value in a subgroup was set

$$0.1 \cdot 0.3240 = 0.0324.$$

Clearly, this upper bound results in stricter complexity control, and it can be seen from Figure 8.5 that only three promising subgroups met the complexity criterion in this case, namely, S_4, S_8, and S_9. The PFS improvement was not substantially higher in S_3 and S_7 relative to the overall population and these subgroups were discarded. Consequently, fewer subgroups will be further split at the next level compared to the more liberal case with $\gamma = 0.5$. This example shows that a smaller value of γ helps control complexity and reduce the size of the search space.

Table 8.3 lists the final sets of subgroups selected by the SIDES procedure after the subgroup search algorithm reached the third level ($L = 3$) and explored biomarker signatures with up to three component biomarkers. The table includes the final sets in the settings with the more liberal and more restrictive complexity criteria ($\gamma = 0.1$ and 0.5).

TABLE 8.3

Final Subgroups Selected by the SIDES Procedure with Liberal and Restrictive Complexity Criteria

Subgroup	Size	Observed p-Value	Adjusted p-Value
Liberal Complexity Criterion ($\gamma = 0.5$)			
$\{X_6 > 3 \text{ and } X_4 > 66\}$	132	0.0022	0.66
$\{X_7 \leq 127 \text{ and } X_8 \leq 8\}$	237	0.0101	0.85
$\{X_9 \leq 1.27\}$	72	0.0147	0.87
$\{X_7 \leq 127 \text{ and } X_3 > 33\}$	95	0.0163	0.87
$\{X_7 \leq 127 \text{ and } X_4 > 57\}$	138	0.0165	0.87
$\{X_8 \leq 11\}$	379	0.0239	0.89
Restrictive Complexity Criterion ($\gamma = 0.1$)			
$\{X_4 > 66\}$	157	0.0104	0.28
$\{X_8 \leq 11\}$	379	0.0239	0.35

Table 8.3 displays the observed and multiplicity-adjusted one-sided treatment effect p-values in the selected subgroups. As was pointed out in Section 8.3, the observed p-values substantially overstate the significance of the treatment effect. On the basis of observed p-values, the treatment appears to be highly effective in all the subgroups. However, after a resampling-based multiplicity adjustment is applied, the p-values are no longer significant. Consider, for example, the first subgroup selected by the procedure based on the liberal complexity criterion, that is,

$$\{X_6 > 3 \text{ and } X_4 > 66\}.$$

The one-sided treatment effect p-value in this subgroup was 0.0022. As a quick check, 1000 null sets were generated from the Phase III trial database and the SIDES procedure was applied to each null set to determine how frequently the same or a more significant result would be observed in the best subgroup. The treatment effect achieved the same level of significance in the best subgroup in 66% of the null sets and, as a result, the multiplicity-adjusted one-sided p-value in the subgroup was set to 0.66. This highly nonsignificant p-value clearly indicates that, in truth, the treatment does not provide a meaningful PFS benefit in the selected subgroup.

It is also instructive to consider the effect of the complexity criterion on the number of subgroups in the final set. When a larger value of γ is used, the subgroup search algorithm examines more intermediate subgroups, which translate into a larger final set. Table 8.3 shows that, with $\gamma = 0.5$, the SIDES procedure selected six subgroups and, with $\gamma = 0.1$, only two subgroups were included in the final set.

To provide additional insight into the role of complexity control in subgroup search problems, Figure 8.6 plots the observed hazard ratios and sizes of the

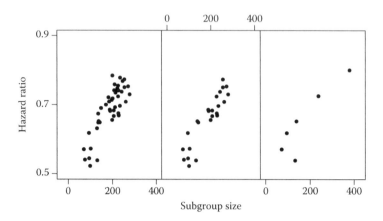

FIGURE 8.6
Hazard ratios and sizes of the final subgroups selected by the SIDES procedure with different complexity criteria ($\gamma = \infty$, left panel; $\gamma = 1$, central panel; and $\gamma = 0.5$, right panel).

final sets of subgroups identified by the SIDES procedure in three different cases (a hazard ratio <1 indicates a positive treatment effect). This includes the case where complexity is not controlled ($\gamma = \infty$) and cases where stricter complexity criteria are applied ($\gamma = 1$ and $\gamma = 0.5$). The figure demonstrates that the complexity criterion serves as a sieve that reduces the number of subgroups in the final set without changing the relationship between the two fundamental factors, namely, the magnitude of the treatment effect within a subgroup and its size. Specifically, when complexity is not explicitly controlled, the SIDES procedure identifies 45 subgroups and, as shown in the left panel of the figure, the observed hazard ratio rapidly increases with the increasing subgroup size. With $\gamma = 1$ and $\gamma = 0.5$, the number of subgroups in the final set decreases to 25 and 6, respectively. However, the overall pattern in the central and right panels of the figure is virtually identical to that in the left panel. The subgroups retained by the stricter complexity criteria are representative of the general ensemble of subgroups in the setting without complexity control. A smaller value of the complexity parameter γ essentially helps lower the level of background noise, which ultimately improves the performance of the subgroup search algorithm.

8.5 Extended Subgroup Search Procedures (SIDEScreen Procedures)

Section 8.3 introduces the regular SIDES procedure developed in Lipkovich et al. (2011). This procedure utilizes a tree-based recursive partitioning algorithm to identify biomarker-based subgroups in which the treatment effect is highly beneficial. The SIDES procedure was designed for settings with a relatively small number of candidate biomarkers; for example, for settings with up to 15–20 covariates in the candidate set. The performance of the regular SIDES procedure tends to deteriorate in high-dimensional biomarker discovery problems when this procedure faces proverbial "needle in a haystack" problems.

This section defines an extended SIDES method that suits complex biomarker selection problems better with larger candidate sets when only a small number of biomarkers are expected to be reliable predictors of treatment response. Extended SIDES procedures, known as the SIDEScreen procedures (Lipkovich and Dmitrienko, 2014), are built using a two-stage subgroup search algorithm. The first stage serves as a screening stage that helps filter out noninformative biomarkers. This screen helps reduce the level of background noise induced by noninformative covariates. The selected biomarkers are examined in the second stage to obtain the final set of subgroups with improved treatment effect.

A biomarker screen utilized in a two-stage procedure is based on the concept of *variable importance*, which has found numerous applications in machine learning procedures, for example, in random forests (Breiman, 2001). The variable importance approach helps quantify the predictive ability of a biomarker by taking advantage of the fact that only a small number of candidate biomarkers are truly predictive of treatment benefit. The resulting variable importance index serves as a reliable tool for distinguishing informative biomarkers from noninformative biomarkers, which helps improve the performance of the SIDEScreen procedures compared to the regular SIDES procedure.

8.5.1 Variable Importance

As was explained above, the regular SIDES procedure can be extended by incorporating variable importance indices that provide a quantitative assessment of the predictive value of each biomarker in the candidate set. The variable importance index can be defined as the average "contribution" of a biomarker over the set of final subgroups.

Using the general setting considered in Section 8.3, let $X_1, \ldots, X_k$ denote the candidate biomarkers and let $S_1, \ldots, S_m$ denote the final subgroups identified by the SIDES procedure. The contribution of the biomarker X_j, $j = 1, \ldots, k$, to the subgroup S_l, $l = 1, \ldots, m$, is denoted by λ_{jl}. The contribution is defined as

$$\lambda_{jl} = \begin{cases} -\log d_{jl} & \text{if } X_j \text{ contributes to the subgroup,} \\ 0 & \text{if } X_j \text{ does not contribute to the subgroup.} \end{cases}$$

Here, d_{jl} is the optimal value of the splitting criterion associated with the biomarker X_j, provided X_j is one of the splitting covariates in the subgroup. Note that the splitting criterion is transformed to ensure that a more significant value of d_{jl} translates into a larger contribution.

The variable importance score for the biomarker X_j, denoted by $VI(X_j)$, is defined as the average contribution over all sets of final subgroups, that is,

$$VI(X_j) = \frac{1}{m} \sum_{l=1}^{m} \lambda_{jl}.$$

The variable importance indices help differentiate between "important" biomarkers included in most subgroups in the final set and "unimportant" biomarkers that are used only in a handful of subgroups. Higher variable importance scores are assigned to those biomarkers that consistently appear as predictors of treatment response across multiple subgroups. On the other hand, if a biomarker serves as the splitting covariate in a few subgroups, most of its contributions to the final subgroups will be equal to 0. As a result, its variable importance score will be close to 0, which directly reflects the fact that the predictive power of this biomarker is low.

In addition, the variable importance score for a given biomarker provides a "multivariate" rather than a "marginal" characterization of the biomarker's predictive properties. The biomarker may appear to be fairly noninformative at the first level of the algorithm, that is, when the overall population is split by this biomarker. However, it may turn out to be a strong predictor of treatment benefit in subgroups identified at the subsequent levels. In this case, the biomarker's variable importance score will be updated to reflect its contributions to these subgroups.

To compute the variable importance scores for a set of biomarkers, it is recommended that the complexity criterion in the SIDES procedure be disabled by setting $\gamma = \infty$. A broad subgroup search results in a better estimate of the score and, as will be explained in the next section, two-stage subgroup search algorithms do not need to rely heavily on the complexity criterion since complexity is controlled through biomarker screening.

8.5.2 Two-Stage Subgroup Search Algorithm

As explained above, a SIDEScreen procedure is based on a two-stage subgroup search algorithm. The variable importance scores of the candidate biomarkers are computed in the first stage using the regular SIDES procedure and a *biomarker screening rule* is applied to choose the best predictors of treatment effect for the second stage of the algorithm.

An efficient biomarker screening rule helps a SIDEScreen procedure pick a few of the most important covariates out of a large set of candidate biomarkers. Following Lipkovich and Dmitrienko (2014), we will consider two classes of SIDEScreen procedures based on two different approaches to defining a screening rule:

- Fixed SIDEScreen procedures
- Adaptive SIDEScreen procedures

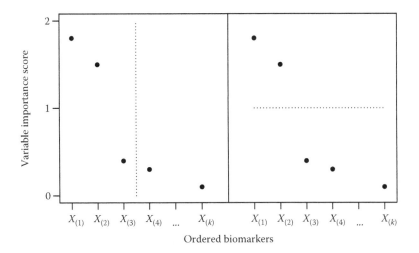

FIGURE 8.7
Examples of biomarker screens used in fixed SIDEScreen procedures (left panel) and adaptive SIDEScreen procedures (right panel).

Fixed SIDEScreen procedures utilize a simple screening rule that relies on selecting a predetermined number of biomarkers with the highest variable importance scores. The fixed biomarker screening rule is illustrated in the left panel of Figure 8.7. The regular SIDES procedure without complexity control is applied to a set of k candidate biomarkers to determine the variable importance scores. The biomarkers are then ordered from the highest variable importance score to the lowest (the ordered biomarkers are denoted by $X_{(1)}, \ldots, X_{(k)}$). A screening rule based on selecting the top three biomarkers is visualized using a vertical dotted line, that is, the ordered biomarkers $X_{(1)}$, $X_{(2)}$, and $X_{(3)}$ will be selected for the second stage of the procedure.

This and similar fixed screening rules generally look appealing. It is natural to focus on the biomarkers with the highest variable importance scores to choose the most likely predictors of treatment benefit. For this reason, a fixed SIDEScreen procedure should be expected to provide a more efficient subgroup search compared to the regular SIDES procedure. On the other hand, Figure 8.7 shows that fixed screening rules may not be reliable. First of all, in this particular case, the first two ordered biomarkers ($X_{(1)}$ and $X_{(2)}$) appear to be important, but the third one has a fairly low variable importance score. Secondly, it is unclear whether or not the variable importance scores of $X_{(1)}$ and $X_{(2)}$ suggest a strong predictive effect. In fact, all the biomarkers selected by the fixed screening rule may be noninformative. In other words, this approach may not preserve the *selection error rate*. This error rate is defined as the probability of choosing at least one biomarker for the second stage when all biomarkers are known to be noninformative. To build a sound biomarker screening rule, it will be desirable to have more control over the selection error rate.

A viable alternative to the fixed biomarker screening rule is an adaptive screening rule based on a data-dependent threshold, which helps distinguish informative biomarkers from noninformative ones. An example of a data-dependent threshold is given in the right panel of Figure 8.7. The screening rule selects a biomarker if its variable importance score exceeds the threshold represented by a horizontal dotted line, that is, the biomarkers $X_{(1)}$ and $X_{(2)}$ will be chosen in this case.

The threshold in an adaptive screening rule is chosen to guarantee that the selection error rate is protected at a specified level. The selection error rate is computed under the null case, which corresponds to the case where all k biomarkers are noninformative. As in Section 8.3, the null case is evaluated using a permutation-based approach. The maximum variable importance score, denoted by VI_{max}, is computed from each null data set and the distribution of VI_{max} is obtained from a large number of permutations. An appropriate percentile of the null distribution of VI_{max} will serve as the threshold. Since the null distribution is approximately normal, the threshold corresponding to a prespecified selection error rate is easily found from the standard normal distribution function. Specifically, let E_0 and V_0 denote the mean and variance of the null distribution of VI_{max} and let α denote the desirable selection error rate. The resulting threshold for an adaptive screening rule is given by

$$c = E_0 + Z_{1-\alpha}\sqrt{V_0},$$

where $Z_{1-\alpha}$ is the $100(1-\alpha)$th percentile of the standard normal distribution. For example, with $\alpha = 0.2$, the threshold is equal to $E_0 + 0.84\sqrt{V_0}$. With this threshold, no biomarkers will be selected for the second stage 80% of the time when all biomarkers are completely noninformative, and thus, the selection error rate is preserved at 20%.

An adaptive SIDEScreen procedure utilizes an adaptive screening rule with a specified selection error rate. The adaptive SIDEScreen procedure relies on more flexible screening rules and is generally expected to outperform fixed SIDEScreen procedures.

Multiplicity control is performed within the SIDEScreen approach by accounting for the subgroup assessment and biomarker screen in the first stage of the algorithm as well as the subgroup identification in the second stage. A permutation-based method described in Section 8.3 is applied to the entire two-stage subgroup search algorithm to compute the multiplicity-adjusted treatment effect p-values in the final set of subgroups selected after the second stage.

8.5.3 Subgroup Identification Based on SIDEScreen Procedures

The two-stage approach to subgroup search based on the concept of variable importance will be illustrated using the case study from Section 8.4.

We will begin with the computation of the variable importance scores for the nine candidate biomarkers in this case study. The SIDES subgroup search algorithm was run to estimate the predictive ability of the biomarkers based on their variable importance scores. As was recommended earlier in this section, the complexity criterion was not applied, and thus, the calculation was based on all 45 subgroups in the final set (see the left panel of Figure 8.6). The biomarkers were ordered by the variable importance scores, and the resulting sequence is displayed in Figure 8.8.

Figure 8.8 shows that the biomarker X_8 was clearly the most reliable predictor of treatment effect on PFS in the Phase III trial with a variable importance score of 1.85. The next two biomarkers (X_1 and X_7) demonstrated a comparable performance with the scores of 0.59 and 0.57, respectively. The variable importance score gradually decreased and the last biomarker in the sequence (X_5) received a variable importance score of 0. This biomarker was not used in any of the 45 final subgroups identified by the procedure.

Using the variable importance scores presented in Figure 8.8, the following fixed and adaptive SIDEScreen procedures were applied in the case study:

- Procedure 1: Fixed SIDEScreen procedure that selects the three biomarkers with the highest variable importance scores.
- Procedure 2: Adaptive SIDEScreen procedure that selects the biomarkers in the upper 20th percentile of the null distribution of the maximum variable importance score.
- Procedure 3: Adaptive SIDEScreen procedure that selects the biomarkers in the upper 10th percentile of the null distribution of the maximum variable importance score.

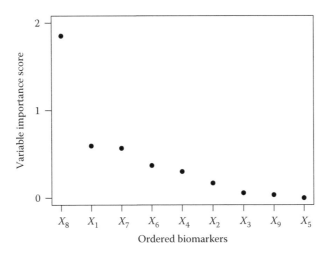

FIGURE 8.8
Ordered variable importance scores in the SIDES subgroup search algorithm.

The adaptive SIDEScreen procedures (Procedures 2 and 3) rely on the biomarker screening rules that are calibrated to guarantee the selection error rates of 20% and 10%, respectively.

The regular SIDES algorithm was employed in the second stage based on the most promising biomarkers identified by the fixed and adaptive screening rules. The fixed SIDEScreen selected the biomarkers X_1, X_7, and X_8. The adaptive SIDEScreen procedures used an adaptive rule derived from the null distribution of the maximum variable importance score. The mean and variance of the null distribution were $E_0 = 0.95$ and $V_0 = 0.57$. Thus, the thresholds used in Procedures 2 and 3 were given by

$$c_2 = E_0 + 0.84\sqrt{V_0} = 1.59,$$
$$c_3 = E_0 + 1.28\sqrt{V_0} = 1.92,$$

respectively. On the basis of these thresholds, the screening rule in Procedure 2 selected the biomarker with the highest score, that is, X_8. The screening rule in Procedure 3 turned out to be too restrictive, and therefore, no biomarker was chosen for the second stage. The final sets of subgroups identified by the fixed SIDEScreen procedure (Procedure 1) and adaptive SIDEScreen procedure (Procedure 2) are presented in Table 8.4.

Table 8.4 shows that the fixed procedure selected two subgroups defined in terms of the three biomarkers examined in the second stage. When the adaptive procedure was applied, only one biomarker was carried forward into the second stage and the procedure identified a single subgroup. It is important to note that the multiplicity-adjusted treatment effect p-values displayed in Table 8.4 are generally much lower than the adjusted p-values within the subgroups generated by the SIDES procedure (these p-values are found in Table 8.3). Most striking is the difference between the adjusted p-values associated with the subgroup $\{X_8 \leq 11\}$. On the basis of permutation-based multiplicity adjustment within the regular SIDES procedure, the treatment effect on PFS rates is highly nonsignificant ($p = 0.35$). However, with the adaptive SIDEScreen procedure, the associated treatment effect p-value

TABLE 8.4

Final Subgroups Selected by the SIDEScreen Procedures

Subgroup	Size	Observed p-Value	Adjusted p-Value
Fixed SIDEScreen Procedure (Procedure 1)			
$\{X_7 \leq 127$ and $X_8 \leq 12$ and $X_1 = 2, 3, 4\}$	227	0.0032	0.52
$\{X_7 \leq 127$ and $X_8 \leq 12\}$	239	0.0034	0.53
Adaptive SIDEScreen Procedure (Procedure 2)			
$\{X_8 \leq 11\}$	379	0.0239	0.08

becomes borderline significant ($p = 0.08$). This is a direct consequence of an efficient approach to subgroup search used in the adaptive two-stage procedure. Focusing on a small number of strong predictors in the second stage helps this SIDEScreen procedure substantially improve the signal-to-noise ratio and reduce the burden of multiplicity.

The example based on the case study demonstrates the strength of the SIDEScreen approach. In general, two-stage procedures with a biomarker screen provide a substantial improvement over the regular SIDES procedure. SIDEScreen procedures based on adaptive screening rules are particularly appealing. They offer robust tools for handling background noise and associated multiplicity issues in complex biomarker discovery problems. At the same time, as shown above, an adaptive SIDEScreen procedure with a low selection error rate may be too restrictive and no subgroups will be generated at the end of the second stage. Therefore, it is important to carefully investigate the properties of candidate subgroup search procedures to decide on the most appropriate procedure for a particular setting. The operating characteristics of the SIDES procedure and its extensions are discussed in the next section.

8.6 Operating Characteristics of SIDES and SIDEScreen Procedures

The operating characteristics of the regular and extended SIDES procedures were examined in several publications. For example, Lipkovich et al. (2011) presented the results of simulation studies that were aimed at evaluating the probabilities of false and correct subgroup discovery for the regular SIDES procedure. In addition, the reproducibility rates of the SIDES procedure were studied in a setting with training and confirmatory databases. Lipkovich and Dmitrienko (2014) performed extensive simulations to characterize the performance of the SIDEScreen procedures with biomarker screening and compare it to the performance of the regular SIDES procedure. This section provides a high-level summary of these simulation results as well as additional results that provide insights into the challenges of biomarker identification in problems with a high level of background noise.

8.6.1 Simulation Study

The simulation setting assumed in this setting is similar to the one used in Lipkovich and Dmitrienko (2014). Consider a clinical trial to evaluate the effectiveness of a single dose of an experimental treatment compared to a control based on a normally distributed primary endpoint. The total sample size is n subjects and the trial employed a balanced design with $n/2$ subjects in each treatment arm.

It is assumed that there is no beneficial treatment effect in the overall population, that is, the mean treatment difference is equal to 0. The trial's sponsor is interested in evaluating k baseline biomarkers to identify a subgroup of subjects who experience a positive effect. The biomarkers are binary and $X_j = 1$ ($X_j = 0$) indicates the presence (absence) of the biomarker X_j, $j = 1, \ldots, k$. The biomarker prevalence rates are the same across the biomarkers, that is,

$$P(X_j = 1) = \sqrt{1/2}, \quad j = 1, \ldots, k.$$

Suppose that two biomarkers in the candidate set, namely, X_1 and X_2, are true predictors of treatment benefit and the other biomarkers are completely noninformative (these biomarkers will be referred to as noise covariates). The true subgroup with a positive treatment effect is defined as follows:

$$\{X_1 = 1, X_2 = 1\}.$$

Given the assumption about the prevalence rate, the size of the true subgroup is

$$\sqrt{1/2} \cdot \sqrt{1/2} \cdot n = n/2$$

subjects.

The binary biomarkers are modeled using the same approach as in Lipkovich et al. (2011), that is, by considering a set of k continuous covariates that follow a multivariate normal distribution and defining binary covariates via dichotomization. Within this model, it is assumed that the correlation between the true predictors is 0 and the correlation between any true predictor and any noise covariate as well as between any noise covariates is ρ. Note that the assumption of a constant correlation coefficient is not very realistic and it may be more reasonable to model the correlations between the noise and predictive biomarkers as random quantities. However, this would certainly dilute the effect of collinearity, and a worst-case scenario in which all noninformative biomarkers are equicorrelated with the two predictive biomarkers was considered in this simulation study.

Let y_i denote the response for the ith subject, $i = 1, \ldots, n$. As before, $\mathbf{x}_i$ denotes the vector of biomarker values, that is, $\mathbf{x}_i = (x_{i1}, \ldots, x_{ik})$, where $x_{ij} = 1$ if X_j is present in the ith subject and 0 otherwise, $j = 1, \ldots, k$. The following treatment effect model is assumed:

$$y(\mathbf{x}_i) = \delta(\mu + \alpha_1 x_{i1} + \alpha_2 x_{i2})t_i + \varepsilon_i.$$

Here, $t_i = 1$ if the ith subject is assigned to the treatment arm and 0 otherwise. Further, δ determines the effect size in the true subgroup and is chosen to guarantee 95% power of detecting a significant treatment effect within this subgroup. The other three parameters are calibrated to ensure that the mean treatment difference is equal to 0, that is,

$$\mu = \sqrt{2}, \quad \alpha_1 = 1, \quad \alpha_2 = 1.$$

Lastly, ε_i is an error term that follows a standard normal distribution. Thus, the mean treatment effect for the ith subject is

$$t(\mathbf{x}_i) = \delta(\sqrt{2} + x_{i1} + x_{i2})t_i.$$

Three procedures were applied to search for the true subgroup in this problem:

- Regular SIDES procedure with a strict complexity parameter ($\gamma = 0.1$).
- Fixed SIDEScreen procedure with a biomarker screen that selects three biomarkers with the highest variable importance scores.
- Adaptive SIDEScreen procedure with a biomarker screen that guarantees a 16% selection error rate (the screen chooses the biomarkers in the upper 16th percentile of the null distribution of the maximum variable importance score).

The operating characteristics of these procedures were evaluated for the following values of the trial parameters:

- Total sample size, $n = 300$.
- Total number of candidate biomarkers, $k = 20, 60,$ and 100.
- Correlation between a true predictor and a noise covariate, $\rho = 0, 0.1,$ $0.2,$ and 0.3.

The simulation-based evaluation was performed using 10,000 runs.

The settings with a large number of candidate biomarkers ($k = 60$ or 100) and positively correlated covariates ($\rho = 0.2$ or 0.3) are the most challenging cases in this simulation study with a very high signal-to-noise ratio.

8.6.2 Correct Subgroup Identification

The first objective of the simulation study was to estimate the probability of correctly identifying the true subgroup. This probability was defined as the percent of all simulation runs in which $\{X_1 = 1, X_2 = 1\}$ was the top subgroup in the final set identified by each procedure. Figure 8.9 examines the effect of the common correlation between the predictive biomarkers and noise biomarkers (ρ) and total number of biomarkers in the candidate set (k) on the probability of correct subgroup identification for the three procedures. To streamline the comparison of the procedures, this figure focuses on the scenarios where the correlation coefficient is either 0 or 0.2.

The results presented in Figure 8.9 provide important insight into the performance of the regular SIDES procedure compared to the two-stage SIDEScreen procedures that employ biomarker screens to select the best

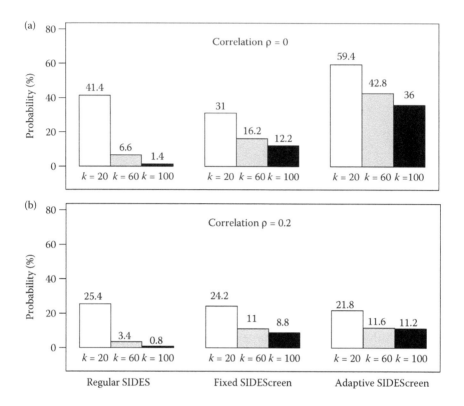

FIGURE 8.9
Probability of correctly identifying the true subgroup for the regular SIDES and SIDEScreen procedures as a function of the correlation between the predictive and noise biomarkers (ρ) and total number of biomarkers (k).

predictors of treatment response. In the case of the SIDES procedure, the probability of correct subgroup identification decreased very rapidly with the increasing number of noise biomarkers (k). As the signal-to-noise ratio decreased, the probability of identifying the true subgroup dropped from 41% with $k = 20$ to 1.4% with $k = 100$ in the more favorable case of independent covariates ($\rho = 0$). When the noise covariates were assumed to be positively correlated with the true predictors ($\rho = 0.2$), the regular SIDES procedure performed fairly poorly with $k = 20$ and the probability of selecting the true subgroup approached 1% with $k = 100$.

The two SIDEScreen procedures performed much better in the case of independent covariates. With the adaptive SIDEScreen procedure, the probability of correct subgroup identification was 59% in the scenario with 20 biomarkers and 36% with 100 biomarkers. This implies that, with $k = 100$, the adaptive SIDEScreen performed almost as reliably as the regular SIDES with $k = 20$. The fixed SIDEScreen procedure also demonstrated an improvement over the regular SIDES procedure but was clearly much more sensitive to the number of noise biomarkers than the adaptive procedure. For example, the fixed procedure correctly selected the true subgroup only 12% of the time when the candidate set included 100 biomarkers.

The case of correlated covariates was fairly challenging for both SIDEScreen procedures. The true subgroup was identified less frequently than in the independent case. However, the drop in the probability of correct subgroup identification was smaller compared to the regular SIDES. In the setting with the highest level of background noise ($k = 100$), the success rate for the fixed and adaptive SIDEScreen procedures was 9% and 12%, respectively.

To understand the performance of the fixed and adaptive SIDEScreen procedures better in this simulation study, Figure 8.10 summarizes the key characteristics of the biomarker screens, namely, the probabilities of selecting the predictive biomarkers after the first stage of each procedure. Specifically, the probabilities of the following two outcomes are displayed in the figure:

- Outcome 1: Select the true predictors (X_1 and X_2) and potentially other biomarkers.

- Outcome 2: Select only the true predictors (X_1 and X_2).

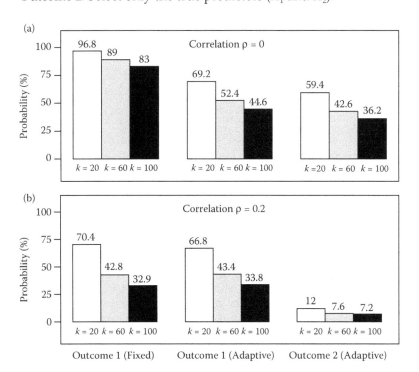

FIGURE 8.10
Probability of Outcomes 1 and 2 for the fixed and adaptive SIDEScreen procedures as a function of the correlation between the predictive and noise biomarkers (ρ) and total number of biomarkers (k).

Recall that the fixed SIDEScreen procedure always carried forward three biomarkers into the second stage, and thus, the probability of Outcome 2 was computed only for the adaptive SIDEScreen procedure.

Figure 8.10 shows that it was relatively easy for the fixed SIDEScreen procedure to select the two true predictors (along with other covariates) in the case of independent biomarkers ($\rho = 0$). The selection probability was above 80% even in the scenario with 100 biomarkers. With a more selective screen used in the adaptive procedure, the probability of Outcome 1 was lower and quickly decreased with the total number of biomarkers. Note that the probability of an exact biomarker selection (Outcome 2) was lower by <10 percentage points. This means that the adaptive screen worked quite well, that is, whenever X_1 and X_2 were included in the set of biomarkers examined in the second stage, most of the time, only the two true predictors were selected.

As expected, the probability of Outcome 1 decreased for both procedures when the case of positive correlation was studied ($\rho = 0.2$). A more dramatic change was observed for the probability of an exact selection. With the higher level of background noise, it was increasingly difficult for the adaptive procedure to filter out the noise biomarkers and correctly identify the true predictors.

8.6.3 Effect of Collinearity on Variable Importance

Figure 8.9 demonstrates that the performance of all subgroup search procedures, even the adaptive SIDEScreen procedure, deteriorated in the settings where the predictive and noise biomarkers were positively correlated. Challenges of variable selection in the presence of correlated predictors, which is fairly common in clinical trial applications, have been recognized and investigated in the machine learning literature (Fan and Lv, 2008, 2010). As stated in Fan and Lv (2010, p. 102),

> A notorious difficulty of high dimensional model selection comes from the collinearity among the predictors. The collinearity can easily be spurious in high dimensional geometry which can make us select a wrong model … As a result, any variable can be well approximated even by a couple of spurious variables, and can even be replaced by them when the dimensionality is much higher than the sample size. If that variable is a signature predictor and is replaced by spurious variables, we choose wrong variables to associate the covariates with the response and, even worse, the spurious variables can be independent of the response at population level, leading to completely wrong scientific conclusions.

An additional simulation was performed to understand the effect of collinearity better among candidate biomarkers on the variable importance indices, which ultimately affects the performance of the SIDEScreen procedures. Figure 8.11 displays several measures of variable importance computed at the end of the first stage in the two-stage procedures:

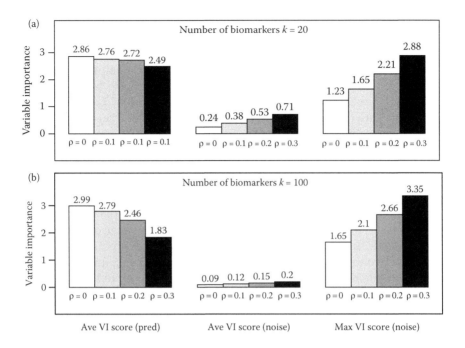

FIGURE 8.11
Measures of variable importance as a function of the correlation between the predictive and noise biomarkers (ρ) and total number of biomarkers (*k*).

- Ave VI score (pred): Average of the VI scores of the predictive bio-markers (X_1 and X_2).
- Ave VI score (noise): Average of the VI scores of the noise biomarkers ($X_3, \ldots, X_k$).
- Max VI score (noise): Maximum over the VI scores of all noise bio-markers ($X_3, \ldots, X_k$).

Note that the evaluation was performed before biomarker screening, and thus, the conclusions apply to the fixed and adaptive procedures.

The average VI score for the noise biomarkers helps quantify the predictive strength of the noninformative biomarkers induced by a positive correlation with the true predictors. In other words, a positive correlation with strong predictive biomarkers leads to an appearance of a predictive effect. When the noise biomarkers are considered one at a time, this effect is rather weak. Figure 8.11 shows that the average VI score for the noise biomarkers was much lower compared to the average VI score for the two predictive biomarkers X_1 and X_2. Further, a quick comparison of the top and bottom panels shows that the contribution of the noise biomarkers, measured by their variable importance, decreased as the number of candidate biomarkers increased. The average VI score for the noise biomarkers was clearly lower with 100 biomarkers.

The maximal VI score summarizes the synergistic effect of a large number of noninformative biomarkers. This measure provides helpful insight into the joint effect of two key factors that greatly complicate biomarker identification in problems with collinear covariates. The first factor is positive correlation with the predictive biomarkers and the second factor is multiplicity inherent in biomarker selection. Even though the VI score was low for each noise biomarker, the true predictors had to compete with the strongest covariate chosen from a large set of noise biomarkers. In other words, for a subgroup search procedure to successfully distinguish true predictors from "phantom" predictors, the VI score for a predictive biomarker needed to be greater than the maximal VI score computed over multiple noise biomarkers. It is shown in Figure 8.11 that, as the correlation and size of the candidate set increased, the maximal VI score grew rapidly and the strongest noise biomarker eventually overcame the true predictors. For example, in the case of 20 candidate biomarkers, the average VI score for the predictive biomarkers was slightly greater than the maximal VI score when the correlation was 0.2 (2.72 vs. 2.21). With $k = 100$, the maximal VI score exceeded the average VI score for the predictive biomarkers when $\rho = 0.2$ (2.66 vs. 2.46). In this setting, it would be quite challenging even for the most powerful biomarker identification procedure to pick the true predictors out of a large set of covariates and identify the true subgroup.

8.6.4 Treatment Effect Fraction

The performance of the SIDES and SIDEScreen procedures was evaluated in Figure 8.9 using the probability of identifying the true subgroup. This approach relies on a simple dichotomous decision rule and no credit is given for selecting a subgroup that is close to the true one and includes subjects who experience treatment benefit. It is also helpful to consider other approaches that account for the treatment response in the subgroups identified by the individual procedures. It was pointed out in Lipkovich et al. (2011, p. 2614) that this approach is relevant in the context of personalized medicine:

> Assessing the performance using the fraction of the treatment effect retained is highly relevant in the context of clinical tailored therapeutics. The purer scientific objective of exactly identifying the covariates is important and closely related, but in terms of clinical practice, the more empirical objective of identifying the right patients is the key. From a practical standpoint, given that in real data sets many important covariates are highly intercorrelated, and therefore virtually identical subgroups may be defined by alternative descriptors, so, identifying the right patients may be more relevant than identifying "the right covariates."

Two continuous metrics to estimate the average treatment response in a subgroup were proposed in Lipkovich et al. (2011) and Lipkovich and Dmitrienko (2014). Both metrics are based on the ratio of the treatment effect per subject in the correct subgroup to that in the most promising subgroup selected by a procedure. Here, we will focus on the metric, termed the *treatment effect fraction* introduced in Lipkovich and Dmitrienko (2014).

The treatment effect fraction is defined as

$$R = 100 \frac{\sum_{i=1}^{n} I_i^* t(\mathbf{x}_i)}{\sum_{i=1}^{n} I_i t(\mathbf{x}_i)},$$

where $I_i^* = 1$ or 0 if the ith subject is included or not included in the true subgroup and $I_i = 1$ or 0 if the ith subject is included or not included in the top subgroup identified by a procedure, $i = 1, \ldots, n$. Further, $t(\mathbf{x}_i)$ is the mean treatment effect defined earlier in this section.

This metric quantifies the "distance" between the two subgroups. The treatment effect fraction is equal to 100% if and only if the procedure selects the true subgroup and introduces penalties for identifying subsets or supersets of the true subgroup. For example, if a procedure selects either $\{X_1 = 1, X_2 = 1, X_3 = 1\}$ (subset) or $\{X_1 = 1\}$ (superset) in the simulation study, it is easy to verify that the treatment effect fraction is reduced to $100/\sqrt{2}\% = 70.7\%$. In general, if a subgroup search procedure achieves the treatment effect fraction of 90%, this means that the best subgroup on average retains 90% of the treatment benefit in the true subgroup.

The treatment effect fractions were computed for the three subgroup search procedures under the scenarios used in Figure 8.9, that is, the correlation between the predictive and noise biomarkers was set to $\rho = 0$ and 0.2, and the candidate set included $k = 20$, 60, and 100 biomarkers. The results are presented in Figure 8.12. The adaptive SIDEScreen procedure maintained a uniformly higher treatment effect fraction compared to the other two procedures in the case of independent biomarkers ($\rho = 0$). In addition, the performance of the two SIDEScreen procedures was not considerably affected by the number of biomarkers. The treatment effect fraction decreased by only 5 and 4 percentage points for the fixed and adaptive procedures, respectively, when the number of covariates increased from $k = 20$ to $k = 100$. In contrast, the treatment effect fraction for the regular SIDES procedure dropped by almost 20%, which is mostly due to the procedure's inability to efficiently deal with the decreasing signal-to-noise ratio. Further, the advantage of the SIDEScreen procedures over the regular SIDES diminished in the case of positively correlated biomarkers ($\rho = 0.2$). However, in the more challenging scenarios with 60 and 100 biomarkers, the fixed and adaptive SIDEScreen procedure still achieved a higher treatment effect fraction than the regular SIDES procedure.

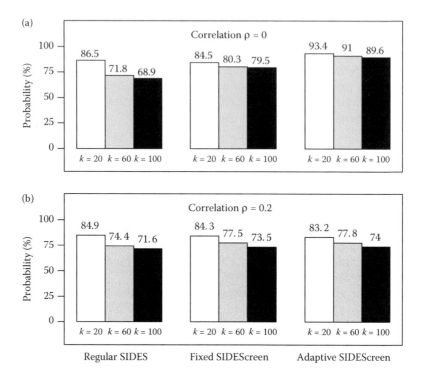

FIGURE 8.12

Treatment effect fraction for the regular SIDES and SIDEScreen procedures as a function of the correlation between the predictive and noise biomarkers (ρ) and total number of biomarkers (k).

Appendix A: Splitting Criteria

In this section, we introduce popular splitting criteria used in the SIDES subgroup search algorithm. To simplify notation, we will focus on a single biomarker, say, X_j, and drop the biomarker index j from the formulas. Let $Z_L(c)$ and $Z_H(c)$ denote the test statistics for testing the one-sided null hypothesis of no treatment effect based on the primary efficacy variable in the biomarker-low and biomarker-high subgroups, that is, $L(c)$ and $H(c)$. A one-sided test is carried out since the sponsor is interested in identifying subgroups of subjects with a positive treatment effect. A larger value of the test statistic indicates clinical improvement within a subgroup.

The test statistics are based on the treatment contrast for the experimental therapy ($T = 1$) versus control ($T = 0$). For example, if the outcome variable Y is continuous and larger values of Y indicate a beneficial effect, the treatment contrast in the overall sample is an estimate of the true mean difference

$$E(Y|T = 1) - E(Y|T = 0).$$

The statistical significance of this treatment effect is evaluated using the standard approach, that is, the test statistic is computed from the sample treatment difference normalized by the common standard error. Similarly, for a binary outcome, the treatment contrast is typically the difference in the probability of a desirable outcome ($Y = 1$) between the treatment arms, that is,

$$P(Y = 1|T = 1) - P(Y = 1|T = 0)$$

and

$$E(Y|T = 1, \mathbf{x} \in S) - E(Y|T = 0, \mathbf{x} \in S),$$

when evaluated in the subgroup S.

The corresponding test statistic is based on the difference in proportions normalized by the common standard error. For a survival outcome variable, the treatment contrast reflects the difference in underlying hazards between the two treatment arms. The log-rank statistic can be used for testing the null hypothesis of no treatment effect in this case.

The most commonly used splitting criterion is the *differential* splitting criterion. This criterion is given by

$$D_1(c) = 2\left[1 - \Phi\left(\frac{|Z_H(c) - Z_L(c)|}{\sqrt{2}}\right)\right],$$

where $\Phi(x)$ is the cumulative distribution function of the standard normal distribution. This splitting criterion is measured on a "*p-value*" scale, and a smaller value of D_1 indicates a stronger differential effect between the two child subgroups.

It is important to note that the *p*-value used in the differential splitting criterion is different from the *p*-value obtained from a standard interaction test statistic. To illustrate the difference, let d_H and d_L denote the appropriate estimates of the treatment effect in the biomarker-low and biomarker-high subgroups, for example, the sample mean treatment differences. Further, let s_H and s_L denote the sample standard errors of d_H and d_L, respectively. The standard interaction effect statistic is given by

$$D = \frac{|d_H - d_L|}{\sqrt{(s_H)^2 + (s_L)^2}}.$$

It is easy to see that the relative sizes of the two child groups are only taken into account for the computation of the pooled variance in the denominator of this formula but do not affect the between-subgroup contrast in the numerator. In contrast, the weights assigned to the treatment effect estimates within the two child groups in the differential splitting criterion are proportional to their relative variance, which depends on the subgroup size and inherent sampling variability in each subgroup. To see this, note that D_1 is a function of a "weighted interaction" test statistic, which is given by

$$\left| \frac{d_H}{s_H} - \frac{d_L}{s_L} \right|.$$

The difference between the two approaches becomes important when evaluating child subgroups based on cutoffs that are close to the extreme values of the biomarker. The interaction test statistic may behave erratically on the boundaries, as it may be driven by outliers in the smaller group. However, the differential splitting criterion will appropriately downweight or suppress a (possibly spurious) treatment effect in the smaller subgroup and focus on the treatment effect in the larger subgroup, which may indeed be the key subgroup. The volatility of the interaction test statistic may also contribute to its low power for detecting subgroups, especially when the true split is not close to the median of the biomarker distribution.

One limitation of the differential splitting criterion is that it focuses on the absolute treatment difference between the two child subgroups. As a result, it will fail to discriminate between the splits associated with a large positive treatment effect in one of the subgroups and those associated with a large negative effect. For instance, in an active-controlled trial, a biomarker may be classified as promising if it helps select subjects who benefit from the control rather than the experimental therapy. To help address this potential problem, a sponsor may consider a criterion that combines the differential splitting criterion with the smallest of the treatment effect p-values in the two child groups. This criterion was termed the *hybrid* splitting criterion in Lipkovich et al. (2011), and it was defined as

$$D_3 = \max(D_1, D_2)$$

where

$$D_2(c) = 2\min\left[1 - \Phi(Z_H(c)), 1 - \Phi(Z_L(c))\right].$$

Note that unlike D_1, D_2 explicitly favors subgroups with a positive treatment effect. However, it is not clear whether the two criteria are comparable and the hybrid splitting criterion may be difficult to interpret.

Another, and perhaps a more natural, extension of the differential splitting criterion D_1 is based on reducing the contribution of the child subgroup with a large negative treatment effect. Let $Z_{\min}(c)$ and $Z_{\max}(c)$ denote the ordered test statistics in the two child subgroups, that is,

$$Z_{\min}(c) = \min[Z_L(c), Z_H(c)], \quad Z_{\max}(c_j) = \max[Z_L(c), Z_H(c)].$$

The *directional* splitting criterion is defined as follows:

$$D_4(c) = 2\left[1 - \Phi\left(\frac{Z_{max}(c) + \min[-Z_{min}(c), \delta]}{s}\right)\right] \quad \text{if } Z_{max}(c) \geq 0$$

and

$$D_4(c) = 1 \quad \text{if } Z_{max}(c) < 0.$$

Here, s is the standard deviation of $Z_{max}(c) + \min[-Z_{min}(c), \delta]$ under the null distribution. Further, δ is a prespecified non-negative constant that helps control the contribution of a subgroup with a large negative effect. First, if $\delta = 0$ and $Z_{min}(c)$ is negative, D_4 simplifies to the greedy criterion D_2, which ignores the subgroup with the smaller treatment effect. However, if $Z_{min}(c)$ is positive, it will be subtracted from $Z_{max}(c)$. This will reduce the value of the criterion and diminish the attractiveness of the split, which leads to selection of the subgroup with a larger treatment effect. Lastly, D_4 addresses the limitation of the differential splitting criterion described above; namely, D_4 is directional and discards splits where a negative treatment effect is observed in the better child group, which is consistent with the ultimate goal of subgroup search.

Appendix B: Adjusted Splitting Criteria

This section defines a "local" multiplicity adjustment for the splitting criterion in the SIDES subgroup search algorithm. When considering the commonly used splitting criteria defined in Appendix A, it is important to realize that the optimal value of a criterion for a given biomarker is driven not only by a relevant measure of the differential treatment effect but also by the total number of possible splits.

As explained in Section 8.3, for every candidate biomarker, each possible split is evaluated using an appropriate splitting criterion D and the optimal split is identified. The candidate biomarkers are then ordered by the criterion value associated with the best split and a prespecified number of top biomarkers is retained. All other things being equal, the optimal value of D will be lower for a biomarker with a larger number of possible splits. This leads to selection bias favoring biomarkers with more potential splits. For example, if m denotes the number of distinct values of a biomarker, there are $G = 2^{m-1} - 1$ possible nontrivial splits if the biomarker is nominal. Further, if the biomarker is measured on an ordinal scale, there are $G = m - 1$ possible splits.

This problem can be addressed by considering a splitting criterion adjusted for the total number of possible splits. Recall that the splitting criteria are defined on a p-value scale; thus, an adjusted criterion can be constructed by applying a standard multiplicity adjustment. In this section, we define a multiplicity adjustment based on a Šidák-type test (Dmitrienko et al., 2009), which accounts for the correlation among the p-values associated with all possible splits for a given biomarker.

Using the same setting as in Appendix A, consider a biomarker X and let $Z_L(c_i)$ and $Z_H(c_i)$ denote the test statistics for testing the hypothesis of no treatment effect in the biomarker-low and biomarker-high subgroups associated with the cutoff c_i, $i = 1, \ldots, G$. Select an appropriate splitting criterion and let p_i denote the value of this criterion for the ith split. This value represents a differential treatment effect p-value and the adjusted criterion for the ith split can be defined as the multiplicity-adjusted p-value based on the regular Šidák test, that is,

$$q_i = 1 - (1 - p_i)^G, \quad i = 1, \ldots, G,$$

where G is the total number of possible splits.

The Šidák test is known to become conservative when the p-values are positively correlated and positive correlation is naturally induced in the selection of optimal splits for an ordinal covariate. To account for the positive correlation and improve the performance of the Šidák test, the modified multiplicity-adjusted p-value is defined as

$$q_i = 1 - (1 - p_i)^{G^*}, \quad i = 1, \ldots, G,$$

where G^* is the "effective" number of possible splits, which accounts for the correlation among the p-values. The effective number of splits is given by

$$G^* = G^{1 - \bar{\rho}},$$

where $\bar{\rho}$ is the average correlation across the $G(G - 1)/2$ test statistics resulting from the evaluation of the splitting criterion on the G splits. This form of adjustment was first proposed as an "ad hoc" approximation method in Dubey (1985). Note that the average correlation depends on the splitting criterion and covariate type (ordinal or nominal) and can be evaluated directly under the assumption of multivariate normality. However, instead of evaluating multivariate integrals, it is sufficient, for our purposes, to approximate the average correlation.

As an example, consider the differential splitting criterion D_1 defined in Appendix A. This criterion is equal to the two-tailed p-value for the differential test statistic, that is, the normalized difference between the test statistics in the biomarker-low and biomarker-high subgroups, that is,

$$Z_i = \frac{Z_H(c_i) - Z_L(c_i)}{\sqrt{2}}, \quad i = 1, \ldots, G.$$

Under the null hypothesis of no difference between the treatment effects in the two subgroups, Z_i follows a standard normal distribution. We are interested in evaluating the correlation between the absolute values of Z_i and Z_j, $i \neq j$. It can be shown that this correlation is given by

$$h(r) = \frac{2(\sqrt{1 - r^2} + \arcsin(r)r - 1)}{\pi - 2},$$

where r is the correlation between the differential test statistics Z_i and Z_j. Therefore, we need to obtain a reasonable approximation for r.

We will need the following notation. Without loss of generality, suppose that $i = 1$ and $j = 2$. Each split of the biomarker X is indexed by an m-dimensional indicator vector

$$\mathbf{J} = (J_1, \ldots, J_m).$$

The ith element of this vector, that is, J_i, is set to 1 or 0 depending on whether the observations in the ith category are allocated to the biomarker-low or biomarker-high subgroup, respectively. Further, $\tilde{\mathbf{J}}$ denotes the complementary vector with the biomarker-low and biomarker-high subgroups switched. For example, if X is an ordinal biomarker with seven distinct values, the split that defines the following pair of subgroups

$$\{X \leq 2 \ X > 2\}$$

corresponds to the vectors

$$\mathbf{J} = (1,1,0,0,0,0,0), \quad \tilde{\mathbf{J}} = (0,0,1,1,1,1,1).$$

The correlation between the differential test statistics Z_1 and Z_2 depends on the allocation of observations into the two child subgroups and associated variances of the outcome variable. However, under the simplifying assumption that the variance of the outcome variable is equal to σ^2 across the subgroups formed by the m levels of the biomarker and the sample sizes in the treatment and control groups within each level are equal to n_1 and n_0, respectively; this correlation depends only on $\mathbf{J}_i$ and $\mathbf{J}_j$ and their intersection $\mathbf{J}_1^T \mathbf{J}_2$, where $\mathbf{J}^T$ is the transpose of $\mathbf{J}$.

Let $m(\mathbf{J})$ and $m(\mathbf{J}_1, \mathbf{J}_2)$ denote the sums of the elements in $\mathbf{J}$ and $\mathbf{J}_1^T \mathbf{J}_2$, respectively. Note that in the case of a continuous outcome variable, the differential test statistic can be expressed as

$$Z(\mathbf{J}) = \frac{1}{\sigma\sqrt{2}} \left(\frac{s_1(\mathbf{J})/f - s_0(\mathbf{J})}{\sqrt{n_0 m(\mathbf{J})(f + 1)/f}} - \frac{s_1(\tilde{\mathbf{J}})/f - s_0(\tilde{\mathbf{J}})}{\sqrt{n_0(m - m(\mathbf{J}))(f + 1)/f}} \right),$$

where

$$s_1(J) = \sum_{i=1}^{m} s_{i1}J_i$$

and s_{i1} is the sum of the outcome values for subjects in the treatment group within the ith level of the biomarker. Similarly,

$$s_0(J) = \sum_{i=1}^{m} s_{i0}J_i,$$

where s_{i0} is the sum of the outcome values for subjects in the control group within the ith level of the biomarker. Finally, f denotes the ratio of subjects in the treatment group versus control, that is, $f = n_1/n_0$.

It is now easy to see that the correlation between $Z_1 = Z(J_1)$ and $Z_2 = Z(J_2)$ is given by

$$r_{12} = \frac{1}{2}\left(\frac{m(J_1, J_2)}{\sqrt{m(J_1)m(J_2)}} + \frac{m(\tilde{J}_1, \tilde{J}_2)}{\sqrt{m(\tilde{J}_1)m(\tilde{J}_2)}} - \frac{m(J_1, \tilde{J}_2)}{\sqrt{m(J_1)m(\tilde{J}_2)}} - \frac{m(\tilde{J}_1, J_2)}{\sqrt{m(\tilde{J}_1)m(J_2)}} \right).$$

Note that

$$m(\tilde{J}) = m - m(J),$$
$$m(J_1, \tilde{J}_2) = m(J_1) - m(J_1, J_2),$$
$$m(\tilde{J}_1, J_2) = m(J_2) - m(J_1, J_2),$$
$$m(\tilde{J}_1, \tilde{J}_2) = m - m(J_1) - m(J_2) + m(J_1, J_2).$$

Given the correlation between the differential test statistics Z_1 and Z_2, denoted by r, the correlation between $|Z_1|$ and $|Z_2|$ is equal to $h(r)$. The average correlation $\bar{\rho}$ is computed as the weighted average of the correlations of the absolute test statistics over all $G(G-1)/2$ pairs of partitions with distinct values of the triple

$$m(J_i), m(J_j), m(J_i, J_j), \quad i \neq j.$$

The weight is defined as the number of occurrences for each distinct triple among these pairs.

Let $r_m(x, y, z)$ denote the correlation between $|Z_1|$ and $|Z_2|$ as a function of

$$x = m(J_1), \quad y = m(J_2), \quad z = m(J_1, J_2).$$

Using combinatorics, it can be shown that, if the biomarker X is nominal, the average correlation is given by

$$\bar{r} = \frac{2}{G(G-1)} \sum_{l=1}^{m-1} \left\{ \frac{1}{2} \sum_{h=\max(2l-m+1,0)}^{l-1} r_m(l,l,h)C(m-1,l)C(l,h)C(m-l-1,l-h) \right.$$

$$\left. + \sum_{i=l+1}^{m-1} \sum_{h=\max(i+l-m+1,0)}^{l} r_m(l,i,h)C(m-1,l)C(l,h)C(m-l-1,l-h) \right\}.$$

Here, $C(n, k)$ is the binomial coefficient, that is,

$$C(n,k) = \frac{n!}{k!(n-k)!}$$

If X is ordinal and assumes m distinct levels denoted by $x_{(i)} < x_{(j)}$, $i \neq j$, i, $j = 1, \ldots, m$, the correlation between the test statistics $|Z_i|$ and $|Z_j|$ based on the following pairs of child subgroups:

$$\{X \leq x_{(i)}, X > x_{(i)}\}, \quad \{X \leq x_{(j)}, X > x_{(j)}\}, \quad i < j$$

is given by

$$r_m(i,j,i) = h\left(\frac{1}{2} \left[\frac{i}{\sqrt{ij}} + \frac{m-j}{\sqrt{(m-i)(m-j)}} - \frac{j-i}{\sqrt{(m-i)j}} \right] \right).$$

Therefore, the average correlation is equal to

$$\bar{r} = \frac{2}{(m-1)(m-2)} \sum_{i=1}^{m-2} \sum_{j=i+1}^{m-1} r_m(i,j,i).$$

Note that the average correlation can be computed for each $2 < m \leq m_{max}$, where m_{max} is the maximum number of levels across all k candidate covariates in the clinical trial database, in advance and stored in the computer memory before executing the SIDES subgroup search algorithm. This is highly desirable, given that the recursive partitioning algorithm uses the average correlations whenever it needs to compute the adjusted value of the criterion associated with every split.

Table 8.5 lists the effective number of splits for ordinal and nominal covariates based on the differential splitting criterion D_1 in the balanced case (equal number of subjects within each of the m levels). It is easy to see that the effective number of splits is substantially smaller than the total number

TABLE 8.5

Effective Number of Splits Used in the Multiplicity-Adjusted Differential Splitting Criterion D_1

Number of Levels (m)	Nominal Biomarker		Ordinal Biomarker	
	Number of Splits (G)	Effective Number of Splits (G^*)	Number of Splits (G)	Effective Number of Splits (G^*)
3	3	2.4	2	1.67
4	7	5.0	3	2.22
5	15	9.7	4	2.71
6	31	18.9	5	3.16
7	63	37.0	6	3.58
8	127	72.6	7	3.98
9	255	143.6	8	4.36
10	511	285.0	9	4.73
11	1023	567.0	10	5.08
12	2047	1130.4	11	5.42
13	4095	2256.1	12	5.76
14	8191	4505.8	13	6.08
15	16,383	9002.6	14	6.40

of possible splits, especially in the case of ordinal covariates. As a result, the modified multiplicity adjustment is less conservative than the standard Šidák-based multiplicity adjustment, which leads to a less conservative adjustment of the splitting criterion.

References

Berger, J., Wang, X., Shen, L. 2014. A Bayesian approach to subgroup identification. *Journal of Biopharmaceutical Statistics*. To appear.

Breiman, L. 2001. Random forests. *Machine Learning*. 45, 5–32.

Breiman, L., Friedman, J.H., Olshen, R.A., Stone, C.J. 1984. *Classification and Regression Trees*. Wadsworth, Belmont, CA.

Brookes, S.T., Whitley, E., Peters, T.J., Mulheran, P.A., Egger, M., Davey Smith, G. 2001. Subgroup analyses in randomised controlled trials: Quantifying the risks of false-positives and false-negatives. *Health Technology Assessment*. 5, 1–56.

Cai, T., Tian, L., Wong, P., Wei, L.J. 2011. Analysis of randomized comparative clinical trial data for personalized treatment selections. *Biostatistics*. 12, 270–282.

Dixon, D.O., Simon, R. 1991. Bayesian subset analysis. *Biometrics*. 47, 871–882.

Dmitrienko, A., Bretz, F., Westfall, P.H., Troendle, J., Wiens, B.L., Tamhane, A.C., Hsu, J.C. 2009. Multiple testing methodology. *Multiple Testing Problems in Pharmaceutical Statistics*. Dmitrienko, A., Tamhane, A.C., Bretz, F. (eds). Chapman & Hall/CRC Press, New York.

Dubey, S.D. 1985. Adjustments of *p*-values for multiplicities of intercorrelating symptoms. *The Sixth International Society for Clinical Biostatisticians*. Dusseldorf, Germany.

Fan, J., Lv, J. 2008. Sure independence screening for ultrahigh dimensional feature space (with discussion). *Journal of the Royal Statistical Society. Series B*. 70, 849–911.

Fan, J., Lv, J. 2010. A selective overview of variable selection in high dimensional feature space. *Statistica Sinica*. 20, 101–148.

Food and Drug Administration. 2012. Guidance for industry: Enrichment strategies for clinical trials to support approval of human drugs and biological products. http://www.fda.gov/downloads/Drugs/GuidanceComplianceRegulatory Information/Guidances/UCM332181.pdf

Foster, J.C., Taylor, J.M.C., Ruberg, S.J. 2011. Subgroup identification from randomized clinical trial data. *Statistics in Medicine*. 30, 2867–2880.

Friedman, J.H., Fisher, N.I. 1999. Bump hunting in high-dimensional data. *Statistics and Computing*. 9, 123–143.

Gunter, L., Zhu, J., Murphy, S. 2011. Variable selection for qualitative interactions in personalized medicine while controlling the familywise error rate. *Journal of Biopharmaceutical Statistics*. 21, 1063–1078.

Hardin, D.S., Rohwer, R.D., Curtis, B.H., Zagar, A., Chen, L., Boye, K.S., Jiang, H.H., Lipkovich, I.A. 2013. Understanding heterogeneity in response to antidiabetes treatment: A post hoc analysis using SIDES, a subgroup identification algorithm. *Journal of Diabetes Science and Technology*. 7, 420–429.

Hodges, J.S., Cui, Y., Sargent, D.J., Carlin, B.P. 2007. Smoothing balanced single-error-term analysis of variance. *Technometrics*. 49, 12–25.

Imai, K., Ratcovic, M. 2013. Estimating treatment effect heterogeneity in randomized program evaluation. *The Annals of Applied Statistics*. 7, 443–470.

Jones, H.E., Ohlssen, D.I., Neuenschwander, B., Racine, A., Branson, M. 2011. Bayesian models for subgroup analysis in clinical trials. *Clinical Trials*. 8, 129–143.

Kehl, V., Ulm, K. 2006. Responder identification in clinical trials with censored data. *Computational Statistics and Data Analysis*. 50, 1338–1355.

Lipkovich, I., Dmitrienko, A. 2014. Strategies for identifying predictive biomarkers and subgroups with enhanced treatment effect in clinical trials using SIDES. *Journal of Biopharmaceutical Statistics*. To appear.

Lipkovich, I., Dmitrienko, A., Denne, J., Enas, G. 2011. Subgroup identification based on differential effect search (SIDES)—A recursive partitioning method for establishing response to treatment in subject subpopulations. *Statistics in Medicine*. 30, 2601–2621.

Loh, W.-Y., Shih, Y.-S. 1997. Split selection methods for classification trees. *Statistica Sinica*. 7, 815–840.

Negassa, A., Ciampi, A., Abrahamowicz, M., Shapiro, S., Boivin, J.-F. 2005. Tree-structured subgroup analysis for censored survival data: Validation of computationally inexpensive model selection criteria. *Statistics and Computing*. 15, 231–239.

Rothwell, P.M. 2005. Subgroup analysis in randomized controlled trials: Importance, indications, and interpretation. *Lancet*. 365, 176–186.

Schulte, P.J., Tsiatis, A.A, Laber, E.B., Davidian, M. 2013. Q- and A-learning methods for estimating optimal dynamic treatment regimes. http://arxiv.org/pdf/1202.4177v2.pdf.

Sivaganesan, S., Laud, P.W., Mueller, P. 2011. A Bayesian subgroup analysis with a zero-enriched Polya Urn scheme. *Statistics in Medicine*. 30, 312–323.

Su, X., Tsai, C.L., Wang, H., Nickerson, D.M., Li, B. 2009. Subgroup analysis via recursive partitioning. *Journal of Machine Learning Research*. 10, 141–158.

Sun, X., Briel, M., Walter, S.D., Guyatt, G.H. 2010. Is a subgroup effect believable? Updating criteria to evaluate the credibility of subgroup analyses. *British Medical Journal*. 340, 850–854.

Tian, L., Alizaden, A.A., Gentles, A.J., Tibshirani, R. 2012. A simple method for detecting interactions between a treatment and a large number of covariates. Available at http://arxiv.org/abs/1212.2995.

Tibshirani, R. 1996. Regression shrinkage and selection via the lasso. *Journal of the Royal Statistical Society. Series B*. 58, 267–288.

Vapnik, V.N. 1995. *The Nature of Statistical Learning Theory*. Springer, New York.

Wang, R., Lagakos, S.W. 2009. Inference after variable selection using restricted permutation methods. *Canadian Journal of Statistics*. 37, 625–644.

Westfall, P.H., Young, S.S. 1993. *Resampling-Based Multiple Testing: Examples and Methods for p-Value Adjustment*. John Wiley, New York.

Zhang, B., Tsiatis, A.A., Davidian, M., Zhang, M., Laber, E. 2012a. Estimating optimal treatment regimes from a classification perspective. *Statistics*. 1, 103–114.

Zhang, B., Tsiatis, A.A., Laber, E.B., Davidian, M. 2012b. A robust method for estimating optimal treatment regimes. *Biometrics*. 68, 1010–1018.

Zhao, Y., Kosorok, M.R., Zeng, D. 2009. Reinforcement learning design for cancer clinical trials. *Statistics in Medicine*. 28, 3294–3315.

Zhao, Y., Zheng, D., Rush, A.J., Kosorok, M.R. 2012. Estimating individualized treatment rules using outcome weighted learning. *Journal of the American Statistical Association*. 107, 1106–1118.

9

Multiplicity in Pharmacogenomics

Lingyun Liu, Fredrick Immermann, and Sandeep Menon

CONTENTS

9.1 Introduction

9.1.1 Pharmacogenomics and Drug Development

The main objective in pharmacogenomics is to study variation in genetic characteristics or gene expression and determine whether the variation is related to drug response. Genetic variations can influence all aspects of disease and the potential treatment of the disease. Genomic differences that are of most relevance to drug development fall into the following four categories: (1) pharmacokinetic (PK) markers: genes relevant to drug PK characteristics such as absorption, distribution, metabolism and formation of active metabolites, and excretion, (2) pharmacodynamic (PD) markers: genes that affect intended and unintended responses to a drug, (3) prognostic markers: genes that predict the course of disease development (e.g., genes that predict the likelihood of tumor development or metastasis), either without treatment or with standard-of-care treatment, and (4) predictive markers: genes that predict the course of disease development when the patient is treated with a particular drug.

FDA's draft guidance for industry on clinical pharmacogenomics (2011) recognizes that information on variations in genes in early pharmacogenomic studies can be used to guide late-phase drug development from the following aspects:

1. Identify populations to receive higher or lower doses of a drug because of excretory or metabolic differences. The metabolic differences are generally identified by genetic abnormalities defining metabolic status for enzymes with genetic polymorphisms.

2. Identify populations at higher risk of developing serious adverse effects and consequently improve the benefit–risk relationship. For example, such information could be used to identify poor metabolizers or ultrarapid metabolizers (e.g., CYP2D6) whose blood levels of parent or relevant metabolites could be dramatically affected so that such patients could be excluded from the trials or doses could be modified to account for genetic variations.

3. Identify populations with better response to the study drug therapy based on phenotypic, receptor, and/or genetic characteristics. Such strategies have been commonly used in oncology. Such predictive biomarkers can be used to enrich a study population and enhance the benefit–risk profile of the drug therapy.

One good example of the use of information on genetic differences to enhance the benefit–risk relationship is abacavir (Ziagen), which is an antiretroviral drug to treat HIV-1 infection. About 5–8% of trial patients experienced a hypersensitivity reaction (HSR), which is a well-recognized safety issue. HSR includes fever, rash, gastrointestinal and respiratory symptoms, and can be life threatening. Such adverse events were an important limitation to the use of abacavir. New pharmacogenomics research done after marketing approval of abacavir found that an allele (HLA-B*5701) was associated with HSR. A 6-week, randomized-controlled trial called PREDICT-1 (Mallal et al. 2008) was conducted to assess the clinical utility of HLA-B*5701. In this trial, 1956 abacavir-naive patients were equally randomized to the control arm or the experimental arm. Patients allocated to the control arm were treated by an abacavir-containing regimen and were monitored according to the standard of care. Patients allocated to the experimental arm were screened for the HLA-B*5701 allele prior to treatment. Patients with a positive test for HLA-B*5701 were excluded and only HLA-B*5701-negative patients were enrolled. The results of this trial were significant with respect to two coprimary endpoints: the rate of clinically suspected HSR and the rate of immunologically confirmed HSR. Consequently, the label of abacavir in the United States was updated in July 2008 to include a strong recommendation for HLA-B*5701 screening in clinical practice.

Pharmacogenomics has been widely used in cancer clinical research to aid the development of targeted therapy, which is the use of a medication designed to target aberrant molecular pathways present in a subset of patients with a given cancer type. For example, trastuzumab (marketed as Herceptin) is used in the treatment of women with breast cancer. Critical to the success of Herceptin was the discovery that the patients who positively respond to the treatment are those who overexpress a protein called HER2. The FDA label for trastuzumab specifies that patients with overexpression of HER2 are appropriate for drug therapy. To determine which patients will benefit from Herceptin, diagnostic tests that measure either HER2 protein levels or gene copy numbers have been developed and are used by physicians to guide treatment decisions.

9.1.2 Multiplicity Issues in Pharmacogenomics Research

In cases such as those cited above, the end result of a pharmacogenomics research effort is a diagnostic test that yields a single, well-defined result for each sample. Multiplicity may or may not be an issue in analyses involving data from such tests. However, other pharmacogenomic efforts, especially those in early or exploratory phases, yield data on many endpoints for each sample. Dealing with multiplicity is a crucial issue when analyzing these types of data.

In recent decades, many novel biotechnologies have been developed that enable identification of genetic variants (e.g., single-nucleotide polymorphisms [SNPs], insertions, deletions, and copy number variations) or differentially expressed genes, (i.e., genes for which RNA is either overexpressed or underexpressed in one group of samples relative to another group of samples). One of the most important technologies used in pharmacogenomics is based on the microarray assay platform. A microarray is an orderly arrangement of thousands of identified sequenced genes printed on an impermeable solid support, usually glass, silicon chips, or nylon membrane. Microarray technology provides scientific researchers the opportunity to quickly and accurately perform simultaneous analysis of literally thousands of genes in a massively parallel (multiplexed) manner in a single experiment, hence providing extensive and valuable information on gene interaction and function. As a typical microarray experiment analyzes and reports expression levels for thousands of genes at a time, large multiplicity problems are generated. Other types of technology, such as multiplexed quantitative polymerase chain reaction (PCR) arrays and bead-based flow cytometry methods, are also used in pharmacogenomic applications and generate data for many genes for each sample. For example, Lu et al. (2005) measured expression levels for 217 known human microRNAs (miRNAs), by a bead-based flow cytometric profiling method, in cells from 46 cancerous and 140 noncancerous tissues (n = 186 target samples in total). Dudoit and van der Lan (2008) reanalyzed the data set for 155 miRNAs using logistic regression modeling. To identify miRNAs differentially expressed between cancerous and noncancerous tissues, let Y_i be the binary outcome of cancerous status with 1 for cancer and 0 for noncancer. Let X_{ij} be the expression measures for the ith sample and jth miRNA ($i = 1,\dots,186; j = 1,\dots,155$). The following logistic regression model relating cancer status Y to expression measure X can be fitted

$$\log\left(\frac{E(Y)}{1 - E(Y)}\right) = \alpha_j + \beta_j X_j (j = 1,\dots,155)$$

where α_j is a baseline effect parameter and β_j is the main effect parameter for the expression measure X_j of the jth miRNA. The parameter of interest for the purpose of identifying differentially expressed miRNAs is $\beta_j (j = 1,\dots,155)$. To identify both over- and underexpressed miRNAs in cancerous tissues, let $H_j:\beta_j = 0$ be the null hypothesis that the jth miRNA is not related to cancer status against the two-sided alternative hypothesis $\bar{H}_j:\beta_j \neq 0$. Let $\hat{\beta}_j$ be the estimator for β_j and $\hat{\sigma}_j$ be the estimated standard error. Then the jth null hypothesis H_j can be tested using the following t statistics: $T_j = \hat{\beta}_j / \hat{\sigma}_j (j = 1,\dots,155)$.

In this example, there are 155 null hypotheses to be tested simultaneously. Without proper adjustments for multiplicity, type I error will be inflated.

9.2 Overview of Multiple Testing Procedures

9.2.1 Definitions of Type I and II Errors

If there is only one hypothesis to be evaluated, then the definition of the type I error rate is straightforward—it is the probability of rejecting the null hypothesis when it is actually true (i.e., a false-positive error). In pharmacogenomics, there are typically many null hypotheses that are tested simultaneously as the example in Section 9.1.2 shows. Generally, a multiple testing procedure should be used to control the appropriate type I error in this situation. Several possible criteria can be used to define the type I error rate. To define the type I error rate, this section introduces a few criteria that are commonly used in a multiple testing setting. To this end, the following notations are used. Let M denote the total number of null hypotheses, R be the total number of rejected hypotheses, and V be the number of rejected hypotheses that are true null (Table 9.1).

9.2.1.1 Type I Error Rates Based on the Distribution of the Number of Type I Errors

9.2.1.1.1 Familywise Error Rate

The familywise error rate (FWER) is the probability of making at least one type I error or the probability of rejecting at least one true null hypothesis in a set, or family, of hypothesis tests. Using the above notations, FWER is defined as

$$FWER = P(V > 0)$$

9.2.1.1.2 Generalized Familywise Error Rate

For some integer $k(1 \leq k \leq M)$, the generalized familywise error rate (gFWER) is defined as the probability of making at least k type I errors, that is,

$$gFWER = P(V \geq k)$$

It is easy to see that when $k = 1$, gFWER is reduced to FWER. For the example in Section 9.1.2, suppose that out of 155 genes in the study, 100 have expression levels that are truly correlated with cancer status and expression levels for the remaining 55 genes are not related to cancer status. FWER is the probability of falsely rejecting the null hypothesis for any of the 55 genes not related to cancer status. For $k = 20$, the gFWER is the probability of falsely rejecting the null hypothesis for at least 20 out of 55 genes that are not related to cancer status.

TABLE 9.1

Null Hypotheses and Decisions

	Rejected	Accepted	
True Null	V	W	N_0
False Null	U	S	N_1
	R	A	M

9.2.1.2 Type I Error Rates Based on the Distribution of the Proportion of Type I Errors among the Rejected Hypotheses

9.2.1.2.1 False Discovery Rate

The false discovery rate (FDR) is defined as the expected value of the proportion of type I errors among the rejected hypotheses, that is,

$$FDR = E\left(\frac{V}{R}\right)$$

where we define $V/R = 0$ if $R = 0$.

9.2.1.2.2 False Discovery Proportion

For a user-specified constant $\gamma \in (0,1)$, the false discovery proportion (FDP) is the criterion to control the tail probability for the proportion of type I errors among the rejected hypotheses, that is,

$$FDP = P(V/R > \gamma)$$

Note that FDR can be expressed as $FDR = E(V/R)P(V > 0)$. Under the global null hypothesis (i.e., all hypotheses are true null hypotheses), all rejected hypotheses are type I errors, which imply $V/R = 1$ and $FDR = FWER = P(V > 0)$. In general, $FDR \leq FWER$ for any given multiple testing procedure since $V/R \leq 1$.

9.2.1.2.3 Weak Control versus Strong Control of Type I Error Rate

Hochberg and Tamhane (1987) and Westfall and Young (1993) introduced two concepts regarding the type I error control in multiple testing: weak and strong control of the type I error rate. Weak control of the type I error rate refers to control under the global null hypothesis. For the example in Section 9.1.2, this means control of type I error under the scenario where none of the 155 genes are differentially expressed between the cancer and noncancer samples. On the other hand, strong control of the type I error rate refers to control under all configurations of the true null and false null hypotheses. For example, in Section 9.1.2, there are in total 2^{155} possible configurations. Strong control of type I error implies that the type I error rate is controlled under any of the 2^{155} scenarios. It is easy to see that any multiple testing procedure that strongly controls the type I error rate also provides weak control of the type I error rate. The reverse is not true.

9.2.1.2.4 Power

For a single-hypothesis test, a type II error is the probability of accepting the null hypothesis when it is actually false (i.e., a false-negative error), and power is defined as 1-type II error. In the multiple-test setting, as in the case of the type I error rate, there is no unique definition of power. In other words, the criteria used to define the probability of correctly rejecting the null hypotheses are not unique. A widely used approach is the probability of rejecting at least one false null hypothesis, which is often referred to as disjunctive power.

Multiplicity adjustment may reduce study power dramatically. This is the so-called multiplicity penalty. The general approach is to control the type I error rate at some small level and optimize power. The appropriate power definition needs to be considered on a case-by-case basis depending on the study objectives. Please refer to Hommel and Bretz (2008) for general considerations of trade-offs between power and other aspects in a multiple testing setting, and Dudoit et al. (2003) for a discussion of power considerations in microarray applications. Software to compute power is generally not available. In most cases, extensive simulations need to be performed to assess power. See Section C in the Appendix for a description of software that computes power estimates for different multiplicity adjustment procedures.

9.2.2 Multiple Testing Procedures for Controlling FWER

Hochberg and Tamhane (1987), and Dmitrienko et al. (2010) review many of the FWER-controlling procedures based on marginal p-values. Such procedures make no or very mild assumptions on the joint distribution of the test statistics, and hence are widely used in practice. On the basis of whether the decision of one particular hypothesis depends on the decisions of other hypotheses, these procedures are classified into single-step or stepwise multiple testing procedures. In single-step multiple testing procedures, the decision on any hypothesis can be made independent of the decisions on other hypotheses. In contrast, in stepwise multiple testing procedures, the acceptance of any hypothesis is dependent on the test results for other hypotheses. This section will review some of the commonly used single-step and stepwise multiple testing procedures based on marginal unadjusted p-values. Single-step multiple testing procedures include the Bonferroni and Šidák procedures. Stepwise multiple testing procedures include the Holm, stepdown Šidák, and Hochberg tests. There are many other tests proposed in the literature to address more complex multiplicity issues with strong control of FWER (see Maurer et al. 1995, Westfall and Krishen 2001, Wiens and Dmitrienko 2005, Hommel and Bretz 2008, Bretz et al. 2009, Dmitrienko and Tamhane 2007). The following notations are introduced to discuss these tests. Let $H_1, H_2, \ldots, H_M$ be the null hypotheses of interest, which could represent no difference in the expression measures for the M genes. Let $p_1, p_2, \ldots, p_M$ be the marginal unadjusted p-values of the test statistics for testing these hypotheses. Let $p_{(1)} \leq p_{(2)} \cdots \leq p_{(M)}$ be the ordered p-values and $H_{(1)}, H_{(2)}, \ldots, H_{(M)}$ be the associated hypotheses.

9.2.2.1 Single-Step Multiple Testing Procedures for Controlling FWER

9.2.2.1.1 Bonferroni Procedure

The Bonferroni procedure (1936) for FWER control is a well-known multiple testing procedure. It provides strong control of FWER for arbitrary joint null distribution of the test statistics. The Bonferroni procedure rejects any hypothesis $H_i (i = 1,...,M)$ if and only if $p_i \leq \alpha/M$. The adjusted p-values for the Bonferroni procedure are given by $\tilde{p}_i = \min\{Mp_i, 1\}$.

9.2.2.1.2 Šidák Procedure

The single-step Šidák procedure (1967) rejects any hypothesis $H_i (i = 1,...,M)$ if and only if $p_i \leq 1 - (1-\alpha)^{\frac{1}{M}}$. The corresponding adjusted p-value is given by $\tilde{p}_i = 1 - (1-p_i)^M$. The Šidák procedure does not control FWER for the arbitrary joint null distribution of test statistics. In particular, it provides exact control of FWER under the global null hypothesis and for independent test statistics. It provides strong control of FWER for multivariate normal distribution with arbitrary covariance matrices. It also strongly controls FWER for some multivariate t- and F-distributions (Jogdeo 1977).

9.2.2.1.3 Stepwise Procedures for Controlling FWER

The single-step multiple testing procedures such as the Bonferroni and Šidák tests are simple to implement since each elementary hypothesis is tested using the same adjusted significance level. However, they tend to be conservative. The stepwise procedures improve the power by sequentially testing each elementary hypothesis. The step-down procedures start with the most significant hypothesis with the smallest p-value and work downward to the least significant hypothesis with the largest p-value. The testing procedure stops when one fails to reject a null hypothesis and all the remaining hypotheses are retained without being tested. Holm's procedure is a step-down multiple testing procedure. Step-up multiple testing procedures start with the least significant hypothesis with the largest p-value and work upward to the most significant hypothesis with the smallest p-value. The test procedure stops when one rejects a null hypothesis and all the remaining hypotheses are rejected without being tested explicitly.

9.2.2.1.4 Holm Step-Down Procedure

The Holm (1979) step-down procedure is carried out as follows:

- Step 1: If $p_{(1)} \leq \dfrac{\alpha}{M}$, reject $H_{(1)}$ and go to the next step. Otherwise, retain all hypotheses and stop.

- Step $i = 2,...,M-1$: If $p_{(i)} \leq \dfrac{\alpha}{M-i+1}$, reject $H_{(i)}$ and go to the next step. Otherwise, retain $H_{(i)},...,H_{(M)}$ and stop.

- Step M: If $p_{(M)} \leq \alpha$, reject $H_{(M)}$ and stop. Otherwise, retain $H_{(M)}$ and stop.

The adjusted *p*-value for the individual hypothesis $H_{(i)}(i = 1,2,\ldots,M)$ is given by

$$\tilde{p}_{(i)} = \begin{cases} \min(1, Mp_{(i)}) & \text{if } i = 1 \\ \max(\tilde{p}_{(i-1)}, \min\{(M - i + 1)p_{(i)}, 1\}) & \text{if } i = 2,\ldots, M \end{cases}$$

The Holm step-down procedure also controls FWER for arbitrary joint null distributions of the test statistics as the Bonferroni procedure does. Note that the critical values for the Holm procedure (except for the first step) are all greater than those for the Bonferroni procedure, which implies that the Holm procedure is uniformly more powerful than the single-step Bonferroni procedure. That is, the Holm procedure tends to reject more hypotheses than the Bonferroni procedure.

9.2.2.1.5 *Šidák Step-Down Procedure*

The Šidák step-down (Šidák-SD) procedure improves the power of the single-step Šidák test in a similar way as the Holm test does with the Bonferroni test. The step-down Šidák test is carried out as follows:

- Step 1: If $p_{(1)} \leq 1 - (1 - \alpha)^{\frac{1}{M}}$, reject $H_{(1)}$ and go to the next step. Otherwise, retain all hypotheses and stop.

- Step $i = 2,\ldots,M - 1$: If $p_{(i)} \leq 1 - (1 - \alpha)^{\frac{1}{M-i+1}}$, reject $H_{(i)}$ and go to the next step. Otherwise, retain $H_{(i)},\ldots,H_{(M)}$ and stop.
- Step M: If $p_{(M)} \leq \alpha$, reject $H_{(M)}$ and stop. Otherwise, retain $H_{(M)}$ and stop.

The adjusted *p*-value for $H_{(i)}$ ($i = 1,2,\ldots,M$) is given by

$$\tilde{p}_{(i)} = \begin{cases} 1 - (1 - p_{(i)})^M & \text{if } i = 1 \\ \max\left(\tilde{p}_{(i-1)}, 1 - (1 - p_{(i)})^{M-i+1}\right) & \text{if } i = 2,\ldots, M \end{cases}$$

The step-down Šidák procedure does not provide strong control of FWER for an arbitrary joint distribution of test statistics. It strongly controls FWER under the same assumptions as those for the single-step Šidák procedure. For example, it provides exact control of FWER under the global null hypothesis and for independent test statistics. It also provides strong control of FWER for multivariate normal distribution with arbitrary covariance matrices.

9.2.2.1.6 *Hochberg Step-Up Procedure*

The Hochberg (1988) step-up procedure is carried out as follows:

- Step 1: If $p_{(M)} > \alpha$, retain $H_{(M)}$ and go to the next step. Otherwise, reject all hypotheses and stop.

- Step $i = 2, \ldots, M - 1$: If $p_{(M-i+1)} > \dfrac{\alpha}{i}$, retain H_{M-i+1} and go to the next step. Otherwise, reject all remaining hypotheses and stop.

- Step M: If $p_{(1)} > \dfrac{\alpha}{M}$, retain $H_{(1)}$ and stop. Otherwise, reject $H_{(1)}$ and stop.

The adjusted p-value for $H_{(i)}$ ($i = 1, 2, \ldots, M$) is given by

$$\tilde{p}_{(i)} = \begin{cases} p_{(i)} & \text{if } i = M \\ \min(\tilde{p}_{(i+1)}, (M - i + 1)p_{(i)}) & \text{if } i = M - 1, M - 2, \ldots, 1 \end{cases}$$

Note that the step-up Hochberg procedure uses the same critical values as those for the Holm step-down procedure. Since it starts with the least significant hypothesis and rejects all remaining hypotheses as soon as one rejects a null hypothesis, it is uniformly more powerful than the Holm step-down procedure. However, the Hochberg procedure does not guarantee strong control of FWER for an arbitrary joint distribution of the test statistics. It only provides control of FWER under assumptions that are needed for the Simes (1986) inequality to hold. Simes (1986) proved that the equality holds for independent test statistics. Sarkar and Chang (1997) show that the Simes inequality holds for test statistics with exchangeable, positively dependent multivariate distributions such as equally correlated multivariate normal distributions. Sarkar (1998) further shows that the Simes inequality holds if the joint distribution is multivariate totally positive of order two such as central multivariate t-distributions with a common non-negative correlation coefficient.

9.2.2.1.7 Comparison of Critical Values for FWER-Controlling Procedures

Consider a simple example with 10 hypotheses of interest. Let $p_{(1)} \le p_{(2)} \le \cdots \le p_{(10)}$ be the ordered p-values. The following table displays the critical values for the Bonferroni, Šidák single-step (Šidák-SS), Holm, Sidak-SD, and Hochberg procedures at significance level 0.05.

	C_1	C_2	C_3	C_4	C_5	C_6	C_7	C_8	C_9	C_{10}
Bonferroni	0.005	0.005	0.005	0.005	0.005	0.005	0.005	0.005	0.005	0.005
Šidák-SS	0.0051	0.0051	0.0051	0.0051	0.0051	0.0051	0.0051	0.0051	0.0051	0.0051
Holm	0.005	0.0056	0.0062	0.0071	0.0083	0.0100	0.0125	0.0167	0.0250	0.0500
Šidák-SD	0.0051	0.0057	0.0064	0.0073	0.0085	0.0102	0.0127	0.017	0.0253	0.0500
Hochberg	0.005	0.0056	0.0062	0.0071	0.0083	0.0100	0.0125	0.0167	0.0250	0.0500

where $C_1, \ldots, C_{10}$ are the critical values for $p_{(1)}, p_{(2)}, \ldots, p_{(10)}$.

9.2.3 Multiple Testing Procedures for Controlling gFWER

In this section, two gFWER-controlling procedures are presented, namely, a single-step Bonferroni-like procedure and a step-down Holm-like procedure introduced by Lehmann and Romano (LR) (2005).

For controlling the gFWER making at least k type I errors, the single-step Bonferroni-like procedure rejects any null hypothesis $H_i (i = 1,2,...,M)$ if $p_i \leq k/M\alpha$. The corresponding adjusted p-values are given by $\tilde{p}_i = \min\{M/k\, p_i, 1\}$. Note that for the special case when $k = 1$, this procedure is reduced to the regular single-step Bonferroni procedure for controlling FWER with a cutoff α/M.

The step-down Holm-like procedure for controlling gFWER with parameter k is carried out as follows:

- Step 1: If $p_{(1)} \leq \dfrac{k}{M}\alpha$, reject $H_{(1)}$ and go to the next step. Otherwise, retain all hypotheses and stop.

- Step 2: If $p_{(2)} \leq \dfrac{k}{M}\alpha$, reject $H_{(2)}$ and go to the next step. Otherwise, retain all remaining hypotheses $H_{(2)}, H_{(3)},...,H_{(M)}$ and stop.

- Step k: If $p_{(k)} \leq \dfrac{k}{M}\alpha$, reject $H_{(k)}$ and go to the next step. Otherwise, retain all remaining hypotheses $H_{(k)}, H_{(k+1)},...,H_{(M)}$ and stop.

- Step $i = k, k+1,...,M$: If $p_{(i)} \leq \dfrac{k}{M+k-i}\alpha$, reject $H_{(i)}$ and go to the next step. Otherwise, retain $H_{(i)},...,H_{(M)}$ and stop.

The adjusted p-value for the individual hypothesis $H_{(i)}(i = 1,2,...,M)$ is given by

$$
\tilde{p}_{(i)} = \begin{cases} \min\left(1, \dfrac{M}{k}p_{(i)}\right) & \text{if } i \leq k \\[3mm] \max\left(\tilde{p}_{(i-1)}, \min\left\{\dfrac{M-i+1}{k}p_{(i)}, 1\right\}\right) & \text{if } i > k \end{cases}
$$

To compare the Holm-like procedure for controlling gFWER and the Holm procedure for controlling FWER, let $\alpha_{(1)}, \alpha_{(2)},...,\alpha_{(M)}$ be the critical values for the Holm procedure for controlling gFWER and let $\alpha^*_{(1)}, \alpha^*_{(2)},...,\alpha^*_{(M)}$ be the critical values for the Holm procedure for controlling FWER. Then we have

$$
\alpha_{(i)} = \begin{cases} \dfrac{k}{M}\alpha & \text{if } i \leq k \\[3mm] \dfrac{k}{M+k-i}\alpha & \text{if } i > k \end{cases}
$$

and

$$\alpha^*_{(i)} = \frac{\alpha}{M + 1 - i} (i = 1, 2, \ldots, M)$$

It is easy to see that when $k = 1$, the critical values of the Holm-like procedure for controlling gFWER reduce to the Holm procedure for controlling FWER. The Holm-like procedure for controlling gFWER is uniformly more powerful than the single-step Bonferroni-like procedure for controlling gFWER since the critical values for the Holm-like procedure are greater than or equal to those for the single-step Bonferroni-like procedure.

The following table displays the critical values for testing 10 hypotheses for the Bonferroni and Holm-like procedures at significance level 0.05 for $k = 1,2,3$.

	k	C_1	C_2	C_3	C_4	C_5	C_6	C_7	C_8	C_9	C_{10}
Bonferroni	1	0.005	0.005	0.005	0.005	0.005	0.005	0.005	0.005	0.005	0.005
	2	0.01	0.01	0.01	0.01	0.01	0.01	0.01	0.01	0.01	0.01
	3	0.015	0.015	0.015	0.015	0.015	0.015	0.015	0.015	0.015	0.015
Holm	1	0.005	0.0056	0.0062	0.0071	0.0083	0.0100	0.0125	0.0167	0.0250	0.0500
	2	0.01	0.01	0.011	0.012	0.014	0.017	0.02	0.025	0.0333	0.05
	3	0.015	0.015	0.015	0.0167	0.0188	0.0214	0.025	0.03	0.0375	0.05

9.2.4 Multiple Testing Procedures for Controlling FDR

The multiple testing procedures to control FWER or gFWER are generally conservative, especially for massive multiple testing problems such as gene expression analysis in microarray experiments. To see this, consider testing M elementary hypotheses with independent p-values. Assume that each elementary hypothesis is tested at the marginal type I error level α. Under the global null hypothesis where all M hypotheses are true null, FWER is given by

$$P(V_n \geq 1) = 1 - P(V_n = 0)$$

$$= 1 - P(p_i > \alpha) \quad \text{for all } i = 1, 2, \ldots, M$$

$$= 1 - \Pi_{i=1}^{M} P(p_i > \alpha)$$

$$= 1 - \Pi_{i=1}^{M} \{1 - P(p_i \leq \alpha)\}$$

$$= 1 - (1 - \alpha)^M$$

Hence, even if the marginal significance level is kept fixed, the overall FWER increases dramatically with the number of hypotheses. To strongly control FWER at a desirable level for a large number of hypotheses, each elementary hypothesis needs to be tested at a very low adjusted level, which leads to conservative testing procedures. FDR methods are generally less conservative than FWER methods and are now widely adopted in pharmacogenomic work.

To control FDR at level α, the step-up Benjamini and Hochberg (BH) procedure (1995) is carried out as follows:

- Step 1: If $p_{(M)} > \alpha$, retain $H_{(M)}$ and go to the next step. Otherwise, reject all hypotheses and stop.

- Step $i = 2, \ldots, M - 1$: If $p_{(M-i+1)} > \dfrac{M - i + 1}{M} \alpha$, retain $H_{(M-i+1)}$ and go to the next step. Otherwise, reject all remaining hypotheses and stop.

- Step M: If $p_{(1)} > \dfrac{\alpha}{M}$, retain $H_{(1)}$ and stop. Otherwise, reject $H_{(1)}$ and stop.

The adjusted p-values for individual hypothesis are given by

$$
\tilde{p}_{(i)} =
\begin{cases}
p_{(i)} & \text{if } i = M \\
\min\left(\tilde{p}_{(i+1)}, \dfrac{M}{M - i + 1} p_{(i)} \right) & \text{if } i = M - 1, M - 2, \ldots, 1
\end{cases}
$$

Note that the above step-up procedure for controlling FDR has some similarity to the step-up Hochberg procedure (1988) for controlling FWER. Both procedures start with the least significant hypothesis. Once the first null hypothesis is rejected, all the remaining hypotheses are automatically rejected without further being tested explicitly. However, except for the first step and the last step, BH (1995) use larger critical values than Hochberg (1988) since $M - i + 1/M\alpha \geq 1/i\alpha$. Therefore, this step-up procedure for controlling FDR is uniformly more powerful than Hochberg (1988) for controlling FWER. BH (1995) prove that the above procedure controls FDR for independent test statistics. Benjamini and Yekutieli (BY) (2001) prove that this procedure also controls FDR when the test statistics have positive regression dependency on each of the test statistics corresponding to the true null hypotheses. Many practical problems satisfy this positive dependency condition, including comparisons of many treatments with a single control, multivariate normal test statistics with positive correlation, and multivariate t-test statistics. For arbitrary joint distribution of test statistics, BY (2001) propose a conservative modification of the procedure to control FDR, which is given below.

To control FDR at level α, denote $C = \sum_{j=1}^{M} \frac{1}{j}$. Then the step-up BY procedure (2001) is carried out as follows:

- Step 1: If $p_{(M)} > \dfrac{\alpha}{C}$, retain $H_{(M)}$ and go to the next step. Otherwise, reject all hypotheses and stop.

- Step $i = 2,\ldots,M-1$: If $p_{(M-i+1)} > \dfrac{M-i+1}{M*C}\alpha$, retain H_{M-i+1} and go to the next step. Otherwise, reject all remaining hypotheses and stop.

- Step M: If $p_{(1)} > \dfrac{\alpha}{M*C}$, retain $H_{(1)}$ and stop. Otherwise, reject $H_{(1)}$ and stop.

The adjusted p-values for the individual hypothesis are given by

$$\tilde{p}_{(i)} = \begin{cases} Cp_{(i)} & \text{if } i = M \\ \min\left(\tilde{p}_{(i+1)}, \dfrac{M*C}{M-i+1}p_{(i)}\right) & \text{if } i = M-1, M-2,\ldots,1 \end{cases}$$

The following table displays the critical values for testing 10 hypotheses for the BH and BY procedures at significance level 0.05.

	C_1	C_2	C_3	C_4	C_5	C_6	C_7	C_8	C_9	C_{10}
BH	0.005	0.01	0.015	0.02	0.025	0.03	0.035	0.04	0.045	0.05
BY	0.0017	0.0034	0.0051	0.0068	0.0085	0.0102	0.0119	0.0137	0.0154	0.0171

9.2.5 Multiple Testing Procedures for Controlling FDP

Although the FDR-controlling procedures try to control the expected proportion of false positives among the rejected hypotheses, it does not prohibit the proportion of false positives from varying. This means that it is still possible to end up with a large proportion of false positives in a particular study. LR (2005) propose procedures controlling the probability that the proportion of false positives is bounded below a certain threshold γ.

For a given $\gamma \in (0,1)$, the step-down LR (2005) procedure is carried out as follows:

- Step 1: If $p_{(1)} \leq \dfrac{(\lfloor \gamma \rfloor + 1)\alpha}{M + \lfloor \gamma \rfloor}$, reject $H_{(1)}$ and go to the next step. Otherwise, retain all hypotheses and stop.

- Step $i = 2,\ldots,M-1$: If $p_{(i)} \leq \dfrac{(\lfloor \gamma i \rfloor + 1)\alpha}{M + \lfloor \gamma i \rfloor + 1 - i}$, reject $H_{(i)}$ and go to the next step. Otherwise, retain $H_{(i)},\ldots,H_{(M)}$ and stop.

- Step M: If $p_{(M)} \leq \alpha$, reject $H_{(M)}$ and stop. Otherwise, retain $H_{(M)}$ and stop.

Where $\lfloor x \rfloor$ denotes the largest integer less than or equal to x.

The adjusted p-value for the individual hypothesis $H_{(i)}(i = 1,2,\ldots,M)$ is given by

$$\tilde{p}_{(i)} = \begin{cases} \min\left(1, \dfrac{M + \lfloor \gamma \rfloor}{\lfloor \gamma \rfloor + 1} p_{(i)}\right) & \text{if } i = 1 \\[2em] \max\left(\tilde{p}_{(i-1)}, \min\left\{\dfrac{M + \lfloor \gamma i \rfloor + 1 - i}{\lfloor \gamma i \rfloor + 1} p_{(i)}, 1\right\}\right) & \text{if } i = 2,\ldots,M \end{cases}$$

LR (2005) prove that the above procedure controls FDP under either one of the following two assumptions on the joint distribution of the marginal unadjusted p-values.

Assumption 1: Let H denote the set of true null hypotheses and H^c denote the set of false null hypotheses. For any true null hypothesis $H_i \in$ H, the conditional distribution of the marginal unadjusted p-value p_i, given the marginal unadjusted p-values for all the false null hypotheses, dominates the uniform distribution, that is,

$$P(p_i \leq u \mid \text{all } p_j \in \text{H}^c) \leq u \quad \text{for any } u \in [0,1]$$

Assumption 2: The joint distribution of the marginal unadjusted p-values for the true null hypotheses in H satisfies the Simes inequality (1986).

The above procedure controls FDP under any of the two assumptions. LR (2005) also propose another modified procedure that is more conservative but controls FDP for the arbitrary joint null distribution of the marginal p-values.

For a given γ, the alternative step-down LR (2005) procedure is carried out as follows:

- Step 1: If $p_{(1)} \leq \dfrac{(\lfloor \gamma \rfloor + 1)\alpha}{(M + \lfloor \gamma \rfloor)C_{(\lfloor \gamma M \rfloor + 1)}}$, reject $H_{(1)}$ and go to the next step. Otherwise, retain all hypotheses and stop.

- Step $i = 2,\ldots,M-1$: If $p_{(i)} \leq \dfrac{(\lfloor \gamma i \rfloor + 1)\alpha}{(M + \lfloor \gamma i \rfloor + 1 - i)C_{(\lfloor \gamma M \rfloor + 1)}}$, reject $H_{(i)}$ and go to the next step. Otherwise, retain $H_{(i)},\ldots,H_{(M)}$ and stop.

- Step M: If $p_{(M)} \leq \dfrac{\alpha}{C_{(\lfloor \gamma M \rfloor + 1)}}$, reject $H_{(M)}$ and stop. Otherwise, retain $H_{(M)}$ and stop.

Where $C_{(\lfloor \gamma M \rfloor + 1)} = \sum_{j=1}^{\lfloor \gamma M \rfloor + 1} \frac{1}{j}$.

The adjusted p-value for the individual hypothesis $H_{(i)} (i = 1,2,...,M)$ is given by

$$
\tilde{p}_{(i)} = \begin{cases} \min\left(1, \dfrac{(M + \lfloor \gamma \rfloor) C_{(\lfloor \gamma M \rfloor + 1)}}{\lfloor \gamma \rfloor + 1} p_{(i)}\right) & \text{if } i = 1 \\[2em] \max\left(\tilde{p}_{(i-1)}, \min\left\{\dfrac{(M + \lfloor \gamma i \rfloor + 1 - i) C_{(\lfloor \gamma M \rfloor + 1)}}{\lfloor \gamma i \rfloor + 1} p_{(i)}, 1\right\}\right) & \text{if } i = 2,...,M \end{cases}
$$

Note that if $\gamma = 0$, the above two procedures for controlling FDP reduce to the step-down Holm procedure for controlling FWER.

The following table displays the critical values for testing 10 hypotheses for the step-down LR and the modified step-down Lehmann and Romano (MLR) procedures for $\gamma = 0, 0.05, 0.1, 0.2$ at significance level 0.05.

	γ	C_1	C_2	C_3	C_4	C_5	C_6	C_7	C_8	C_9	C_{10}
LR	0	0.005	0.0056	0.0062	0.0071	0.0083	0.0100	0.0125	0.0167	0.0250	0.0500
	0.05	0.0050	0.0056	0.0062	0.0071	0.0083	0.0100	0.0125	0.0167	0.0250	0.0500
	0.1	0.0050	0.0056	0.0062	0.0071	0.0083	0.0100	0.0125	0.0167	0.0250	0.0500
	0.2	0.0050	0.0056	0.0062	0.0071	0.0143	0.0167	0.0200	0.0250	0.0333	0.0500
MLR	0	0.0050	0.0056	0.0062	0.0071	0.0083	0.0100	0.0125	0.0167	0.0250	0.0500
	0.05	0.0050	0.0056	0.0062	0.0071	0.0083	0.0100	0.0125	0.0167	0.0250	0.0500
	0.1	0.0033	0.0037	0.0042	0.0048	0.0056	0.0067	0.0083	0.0111	0.0167	0.0333
	0.2	0.0027	0.0030	0.0034	0.0039	0.0078	0.0091	0.0109	0.0136	0.0182	0.0273

9.3 Addressing the Impact of Multiplicity in Pharmacogenomics

High-dimensional pharmacogenomic data analysis is often used more for screening and hypothesis generation than for hypothesis confirmation purposes. In an exploratory setting, some numbers of false positives are tolerable, and further work in subsequent experiments will sort out which rejected null hypotheses holdup. There is also concern in an exploratory setting with low statistical power and the dismissal of false negatives from further investigation. This has led to the relatively widespread use of FDR-controlling methods due to their increased power relative to FWER-controlling methods in these high-dimensional data sets.

In an exploratory setting, the significance levels may be varied to address different analytical or decision-making needs. A more conservative significance level (e.g., 0.05) might be used to identify genes worthy of follow-up in a subsequent study, while a more relaxed level (e.g., 0.20) might be used to develop a list of genes to submit for pathway analysis to identify biological pathways of importance. Significance test results may be combined with minimum thresholds for effect size to further reduce the number of genes passed along for follow-up.

Several approaches have been used to reduce the level of multiplicity in microarray and other high-dimensional data-analysis applications prior to hypothesis testing. One approach uses some type of nonstatistical filtering defined prior to data analysis to eliminate genes with very low or no detectable expression, or genes assayed but not of interest (e.g., genes on a commercially available microarray but of no interest for the particular study). Another approach uses some multivariate dimension reduction technique such as principal components to limit the number of hypothesis tests. Such an approach may be very effective at reducing dimensionality, but makes interpretation of results more challenging.

In a pharmacogenomics setting, many of the genes tested will be coregulated and so, will have correlated expression patterns and nonindependent test statistics. Therefore, multiplicity adjustments that accommodate nonindependent test statistics should be preferred for use in pharmacogenomics applications.

In some pharmacogenomic experiments, there may be multiple hypothesis tests for each gene (e.g., multiple treatments compared to control and comparisons to baseline at multiple time points). This leads to a need to specify what defines the set of hypotheses that will be regarded as the "family" for multiplicity purposes. One approach, perhaps, the most appropriate in the high-dimensional exploratory setting, is to regard the multiple hypotheses tested for a gene as each generating different families and, within each family, to adjust only for multiplicity across genes. Alternatively, in a more confirmatory setting, the multiple hypotheses within a gene as well as across genes could be considered as one whole family for type I error control. They might form different subfamilies depending on the study objective. For example, a hypothetical situation could be to compare three doses (high, medium, and low) of a new treatment to control with respect to many genes. A lower dose will be assessed only if a higher dose shows a significant effect over control with respect to at least one gene. In such a situation, more complex multiple testing procedures, for example, gatekeeping procedures (Dmitrienko and Tamhane 2007), can be used where tests of all genes with respect to specific doses form subfamilies. However, when one talks about the overall type I error control, all the tests should be treated as one family.

9.4 Discussion and Recommendations

This chapter reviews multiple testing procedures for controlling the number of type I errors and the proportion of type I errors in the context of pharmacogenomics. Procedures to control the FWER and the gFWER are designed to control the number of type I errors. On the other hand, procedures to control the FDR and the FDP are designed to control the proportion of type I errors among the rejected hypotheses. The procedures to control FWER are generally more conservative than other procedures and more applicable to situations with a small number of hypotheses. When the number of hypotheses is intermediate or large, the FWER-controlling procedures are too conservative and lack the power to detect significant differences. The procedures for gFWER are more tolerant of a small number of type I errors and hence, less conservative than those for FWER, which might be more suitable to an intermediate number of hypotheses. For situations in which a very large number of hypotheses are tested, more liberal procedures such as FDR and FDP are more suitable. The Appendix also provides examples on how to perform multiplicity adjustment in R and SAS and how to do power analysis using East® with some of the multiple comparison procedures.

Acknowledgments

The authors would like to thank Professor Ajit C. Tamhane and Dr. David Li for providing technical review and insightful comments. We would also like to thank Siyan Xu and Dong Xi for assisting us with the SAS and R codes, as well as Dr. Yannis Jemiai and Dr. Pralay Senchaudhuri for their comments about East® for the software implementation section.

Appendix Software Implementation

A. R Implementation

There are several packages in R that implement the multiple testing procedures introduced in Sections 2.2 through 2.5. The Bioconductor R package *multtest* provides single-step and stepwise multiple testing procedures for controlling FWER and gFWER: Bonferroni, Šidák (1967), Holm (1979), and Hochberg (1988). It also contains procedures that control FDR: Benjamini and Hochberg (1995) and Benjamini and Yekutieli (2001) step-up procedures. Adjusted p-values are used to summarize the results of these procedures.

The gene with a smaller adjusted p-value than the overall significance level is declared differentially expressed.

This section provides a tutorial for relevant functions in the *multtest* package. For complete references, see Pollard et al. (2013).

Installing *multtest*
Start R and enter:

> *source ("http ://bioconductor. org/biocLite.R")*
> *biocLite ("multtest")*

Loading *multtest*
> *library (multtest)*

Help files
Detailed information on functions in *multtest* can be obtained from *help* files.

For instance, to view the help file for the function *mt.rawp2adjp* in a browser, use *help.start* followed by *?mt.rawp2adjp*.

Case Study

We will illustrate some of the multtest functions via the microarray experiments on Colon tissue samples of Alon et al. (1999). The gene expression data set Colon in the package *plsgenomics* consists of expression levels of 2000 genes from 62 samples of which there are 42 tumor tissues and 20 normal tissues. The goal is to identify genes that are differentially expressed in patients with tumor tissues (class 2) and normal tissues (class 1). The data can be freely downloaded from

<http://microarray.princeton.edu/oncology/affydata/index.html >
Load data set Colon
> *library (plsgenomics)*
> *data (Colon)*
Colon$X : a 2000*62 matrix of gene expression levels
> *dim (Colon$X)*
[1] 62 2000
A snapshot of Colon$X
> Colon$X [1:5,1:5]

	1	2	3	4	5
1	8589.416	5468.241	4263.408	4064.936	1997.893
2	9164.254	6719.529	4883.449	3718.159	2015.221
3	3825.705	6970.361	5369.969	4705.650	1166.554
4	6246.449	7823.534	5955.835	3975.564	2002.613
5	3230.329	3694.450	3400.740	3463.586	2181.420

```
# Colon$Y : a vector of tissue labels (2 for tumor tissues and 1 for nor-
mal tissues)
> Colon$Y
[1] 2 1 2 1 2 1 2 1 2 1 2 1 2 1 2 1 2 1 2 1 2 1 2 2 2 2 2 2 2 2 2 2 2 2
[39] 1 2 2 1 1 2 2 2 2 1 2 1 1 2 2 1 1 2 2 2 2 1 2 1
```

```
# To apply multtest functions, manipulate the data set
# Transform Colon$X
> gene <- t(Colon$X)
# gene.cl: a vector of tissue labels (1 for tumor tissues and 0 for normal
tissues)
> gene.cl <- Colon$Y -1
```

---

mt.teststat

The multtest function mt.teststat produces test statistics for each column (gene) of the data frame including two-sample Welch t-statistics, Wilcoxon statistics, F-statistics, paired t-statistics, and block F-statistics. For each gene, to compute two-sample t-statistics comparing normal tissues to tumor tissues

```
> stat <- mt. teststat (gene, gene. cl)
# stat: a vector of 2000 test statistics for 2000 genes
> length (stat)
[1] 2000
```

mt.rawp2adjp

The *multtest* function *mt.rawp2adjp* computes adjusted p-values of single-step and stepwise multiple testing procedures, given a vector of raw p-values. Available procedures include the Bonferroni, Šidák (1967), Holm (1979), and Hochberg (1988) procedures for strong control of the FWER, Benjamini and Hochberg (1995), and Benjamini and Yekutieli (2001) step-up procedures for control of FDR.

To compute the raw 2-sided p-values with 2000 test statistics using the standard normal distribution.

```
> rawp <- 2*(1 - pnorm(abs (stat)))
```

To compare the Bonferroni, Šidák, Holm, Šidák step-down, Hochberg, Benjamini and Hochberg, and the Benjamini and Yekutieli procedures

```
> procedure <- c (" Bonferroni ", " Šidák SS ", "Holm", " Šidák SD", + "Hochberg ", "BH", "BY")
```

To compute the adjusted p-values and store in the original gene order *order (results$index)}*. The default order is the increasing order in the raw p-values

```
> result <- mt.rawp2adjp(rawp,procedure)
> adjpvalue <- result$adjp[order(result$index),]
```

To see the adjusted *p*-values of the first 10 genes
> *round(adjpvalue[1:10,], 2)*

	rawp	Bonferroni	Šidák SS	Holm	Šidák SD	Hochberg	BH	BY
[1,]	0.09	1	1	1	1	1	0.30	1
[2,]	0.15	1	1	1	1	1	0.39	1
[3,]	0.03	1	1	1	1	1	0.16	1
[4,]	0.34	1	1	1	1	1	0.64	1
[5,]	0.07	1	1	1	1	1	0.26	1
[6,]	0.16	1	1	1	1	1	0.40	1
[7,]	0.05	1	1	1	1	1	0.20	1
[8,]	0.12	1	1	1	1	1	0.35	1
[9,]	0.04	1	1	1	1	1	0.17	1
[10,]	0.15	1	1	1	1	1	0.39	1

For the first 10 genes, the adjusted *p*-values of the Benjamini and Hochberg procedure are less than those of all the other procedures. Thus, controlling FWER is more conservative than controlling FDR.

mt.reject
The *multtest* function *mt.reject* returns the number and identities of the rejected hypotheses for multiple testing procedures at some overall significance level. For example, the number of rejected hypotheses at level 0.05 is given by.

> *mt.reject(adjpvalue,0.05)$r*

	rawp	Bonferroni	Šidák SS	Holm	Šidák SD	Hochberg	BH	BY
0.05	502	36	37	36	38	36	215	75

Out of 2000 genes, there are 502 raw *p*-values less than 0.05 without multiplicity adjustment. For the FWER controlling procedures (Bonferroni, Šidák, Holm, Šidák step-down, and Hochberg), only about 37 genes are differentially expressed. The Benjamini and Hochberg procedure is most liberal with 215 adjusted *p*-values less than 0.05. The Benjamini and Yekutieli procedure is a more conservative procedure controlling FDR with 75 rejected hypotheses. But it is less conservative than all the FWER-controlling procedures.

The order of differentially expressed genes can be obtained as follows.
Decision on hypotheses using the Bonferroni procedure (1 for rejected and 0 for unrejected)
> *decision.Bonferroni <- mt. reject (adjpvalue, 0.05) $which [, "Bonferroni"]*
Original gene order of rejected hypotheses
> *which (decision. Bonferroni)*

[1] 26 43 47 62 66 72 75 127 138 245 249 267 365 377 399
[16] 467 493 513 515 625 652 765 780 964 1002 1042 1060 1067 1153 1293
[31] 1325 1346 1423 1582 1771 1772

mt.plot

The multtest function mt.plot provides graphical illustrations of multiple testing procedures introduced above (Bonferroni, Šidák, Holm, Šidák step-down, Hochberg, Benjamini and Yekutieli, Benjamini and Benjamini, and Hochberg procedures). Adjusted *p*-values calculated from *mt.rawp2adjp* are used to produce a number of plots.

```
# Define line types
> ltype <- c(1:7)
# Define line color
> color <-c(1:7)
# Remove raw p-values from adjpvalue
> adjpvalue <- adjpvalue[,-1]
# Legend location
> legend <- c(0.05,2000)
# Number of rejected hypotheses versus the overall significance level
    (plottype = "rvsa")
> mt.plot(adjpvalue, stat, plottype = "rvsa", proc = procedure, leg = legend,
    lty = ltype, col = color, lwd = 2)
```

The resulting plot is given in Figure 9.1 and it is clear that for any significance level, the FWER-controlling procedures (Bonferroni, Šidák, Holm, Šidák step-down, and Hochberg procedures) are more conservative than the Benjamini and Yekutieli procedure, which is more conservative than the Benjamini and Hochberg procedure.

Other types of plots can be produced by specifying the plot type. For plottype = "pvsr", "pvst", "pvsi", plots of the ordered adjusted p-values, adjusted *p*-values against test statistics, and adjusted *p*-values in the original data order are produced, respectively.

B. SAS Implementation

The *multtest* procedure in SAS can perform a number of multiple testing procedures. It works with raw data for ANOVA models, and can also accept a list of *p*-values. This section will use the same data set for the microarray experiments of the Colon tissue samples of Alon et al. (1999) to illustrate how to take a list of raw *p*-values and adjust for multiplicity using different multiple procedures. Suppose the file with the raw *p*-values is stored in

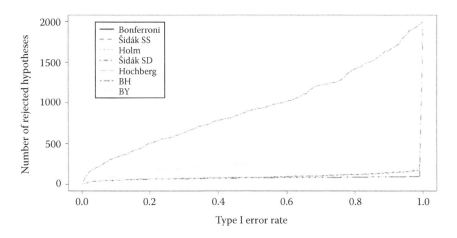

FIGURE 9.1
Number of rejected hypotheses against significance levels using the Colon data set for multiple testing procedures.

the following directory: 'D:\raw pvalues.txt'. To import the file and create a temporary SAS data set named WORK.RAWR, use PROC IMPORT as follows:

```
proc import datafile = datain out = rawp
  dbms = dlm replace;
  delimiter = '09'x;
  getnames = YES ;
run;
```

To check the data set and make sure it is correct, use PROC PRINT. For example, the raw p-values for the first 10 genes can be printed out.

```
proc print data = rawp (obs = 10)
run;
```

```
  The SAS System
Obs    Raw_p
1      0.094354853
2      0.1521451967
3      0.0332323798
4      0.3443736779
5      0.0742242309
6      0.1551772754
7      0.0512963493
8      0.1231212741
9      0.0362760023
10     0.153819513
```

To obtain the adjusted p-values for selected multiple comparison procedures such as Bonferroni, Šidák, Holm, Step-down Šidák, Hochberg, FDR (Benjamini and Hochberg 1995), and FDR (Benjamini and Yekateuli 2001), use PROC MULTTEST as follows,

```
proc multtest inpvalues = rawp bonferroni sidak holm stepsid
hochberg fdr dependentfdr out = adjp;
run;
```

Part of the SAS output is as follows. It first displays the p-value adjustment methods followed by the raw p-values and corresponding adjusted p-values based on each method.

```
        The SAS System
     The Multtest Procedure

P-Value Adjustment   Information
P-Value Adjustment   Bonferroni
P-Value Adjustment   Step-down Bonferroni
P-Value Adjustment   Sidak
P-Value Adjustment   Step-down Sidak
P-Value Adjustment   Hochberg
P-Value Adjustment   False Discovery Rate
P-Value Adjustment   Dependent FDR
```

p-Values

Test	Raw	Bonfer-roni	Step-down Bonfer-roni	Sidak	Step-down Sidak	Hoch-berg	False Discovery Rate
1	0.0944	1.0000	1.0000	1.0000	1.0000	0.9993	0.3005
2	0.1521	1.0000	1.0000	1.0000	1.0000	0.9993	0.3926
3	0.0332	1.0000	1.0000	1.0000	1.0000	0.9993	0.1577
4	0.3444	1.0000	1.0000	1.0000	1.0000	0.9993	0.6378
5	0.0742	1.0000	1.0000	1.0000	1.0000	0.9993	0.2591
6	0.1552	1.0000	1.0000	1.0000	1.0000	0.9993	0.3964
7	0.0513	1.0000	1.0000	1.0000	1.0000	0.9993	0.2020
8	0.1231	1.0000	1.0000	1.0000	1.0000	0.9993	0.3454
9	0.0363	1.0000	1.0000	1.0000	1.0000	0.9993	0.1672
10	0.1538	1.0000	1.0000	1.0000	1.0000	0.9993	0.3940
11	0.0072	1.0000	1.0000	1.0000	1.0000	0.9993	0.0595
12	0.0945	1.0000	1.0000	1.0000	1.0000	0.9993	0.3005
13	0.2238	1.0000	1.0000	1.0000	1.0000	0.9993	0.4932

```
  p-Values

 Dependent
Test      FDR

 1      1.0000
 2      1.0000
 3      1.0000
 4      1.0000
 5      1.0000
 6      1.0000
 7      1.0000
 8      1.0000
 9      1.0000
10      1.0000
11      0.4870
12      1.0000
13      1.0000
```

The adjusted *p*-values are stored in the file named WORK. ADJP. To check the output, print the adjusted *p*-values for the first 10 genes as follows,

```
proc print data = adjp (obs = 10)
run;
```

Obs	Raw_p	dfdr _p	bon _p	stpbon _p	sid _p	stpsid _p	hoc_p	fdr_p
1	0.094354853	1	1	1	1	1	0.99929	0.30049
2	0.1521451967	1	1	1	1	1	0.99929	0.39263
3	0.0332323798	1	1	1	1	1	0.99929	0.15765
4	0.3443736779	1	1	1	1	1	0.99929	0.63785
5	0.0742242309	1	1	1	1	1	0.99929	0.25907
6	0.1551772754	1	1	1	1	1	0.99929	0.39637
7	0.0512963493	1	1	1	1	1	0.99929	0.20204
8	0.1231212741	1	1	1	1	1	0.99929	0.34536
9	0.0362760023	1	1	1	1	1	0.99929	0.16719
10	0.153819513	1	1	1	1	1	0.99929	0.39400

To reorder and make appropriate labels for columns,

```
data adjp;
  retain raw_p bon_p sid_p stpbon_p stpsid_p hoc_p fdr_p dfdr_p;
  set adjp;
  label bon_p = 'Bonferroni' sid_p = 'SidakSS' stpbon_p =
  'Holm' stpsid_p = 'SidakSD' hoc_p = 'Hochberg' fdr_p = 'BH'
  dfdr_p = 'BY';
run;
```

To see the adjusted *p*-values for the first 10 genes,

```
proc print data = adjp (obs = 10) label;
format raw_p bon_p sid_p stpbon_p stpsid_p hoc_p fdr_p dfdr_p
6.2;
run;
```

The SAS System

Obs	Raw _p	Dependency False Discovery Rate p-value	Bonfer- roni p-value	Step-down Bonfer- roni p-value	Sidak p-value	Step- down Sidak p-value	Hochberg p-value	False Discovery Rate p-value
1	0.09	1.00	1.00	1.00	1.00	1.00	1.00	0.30
2	0.15	1.00	1.00	1.00	1.00	1.00	1.00	0.39
3	0.03	1.00	1.00	1.00	1.00	1.00	1.00	0.16
4	0.34	1.00	1.00	1.00	1.00	1.00	1.00	0.64
5	0.07	1.00	1.00	1.00	1.00	1.00	1.00	0.26
6	0.16	1.00	1.00	1.00	1.00	1.00	1.00	0.40
7	0.05	1.00	1.00	1.00	1.00	1.00	1.00	0.20
8	0.12	1.00	1.00	1.00	1.00	1.00	1.00	0.35
9	0.04	1.00	1.00	1.00	1.00	1.00	1.00	0.17
10	0.15	1.00	1.00	1.00	1.00	1.00	1.00	0.39

The following macro can be used to calculate the number of rejected hypotheses at any nominal level alpha.

```
%macro test(alpha =);
data adjp;
  set adjp;
  if raw_p<=&alpha then rawprej = 1;else rawprej = 0;
  if bon_p<=&alpha then bonprej = 1;else bonprej = 0;
  if sid_p<=&alpha then sidssprej = 1;else sidssprej = 0;
  if stpbon_p<=&alpha then holmprej = 1;else holmprej = 0;
  if stpsid_p<=&alpha then sidsdprej = 1;else sidsdprej = 0;
  if hoc_p<=&alpha then hocprej = 1;else hocprej = 0;
  if fdr_p<=&alpha then bhprej = 1;else bhprej = 0;
  if dfdr_p<=&alpha then byprej = 1;else byprej = 0;
run;

proc means data = adjp sum maxdec = 0;
 var rawprej bonprej sidssprej holmprej sidsdprej hocprej
  bhprej byprej;
 output out = nj sum(rawprej bonprej sidssprej holmprej
  sidsdprej hocprej bhprej byprej) = ;
run;
```

```
data nj (drop = _TYPE_ _FREQ_ );
  set nj;
  alpha = α
  label alpha = 'Alpha' rawprej = 'rawp' bonprej = 'Bonferroni'
sidssprej = 'SidakSS' holmprej = 'Holm' sidsdprej = 'SidakSD'
hocprej = 'Hochberg' bhprej = 'BH' byprej = 'BY';
run;
%mend
```

For example, the number of rejected hypotheses at level 0.05 can be computed by calling the above macro as follows:

```
%test(alpha = 0.05);
```

```
                 The MEANS Procedure
            Variable                      Sum

            rawprej                       502
            bonprej                        36
            sidssprej                      37
            holmprej                       36
            sidsdprej                      38
            hocprej                        36
            bhprej                        215
            byprej                         75
```

Out of 2000 genes, there are 502 genes with significantly different expression at marginal significance level 0.05 without multiplicity adjustment. For the FWER controlling procedures (Bonferroni, Šidák, Holm, Šidák step-down, and Hochberg), only about 36 genes are differentially expressed. The Benjamini and Hochberg procedure is the most liberal procedure which detected 215 differentially expressed genes while controlling FDR at level 0.05. The Benjamini and Yekutieli procedure is a more conservative procedure controlling FDR with 75 genes detected. But it is less conservative than all the FWER-controlling procedures.

To see which genes are detected by a particular multiplicity adjustment method, one could print the flags of rejection or acceptance. For example, the genes which have significantly different expressions after the Bonferroni procedure are as follows:

```
proc print data = adjp;
  var bonprej;
  where bonprej eq 1;
run;
```

C. Power Analysis Using Multiple Comparison Procedures in East®

East® is a trial design software package that offers an intuitive graphical user-interface to perform power analysis using multiple comparison procedures discussed in this chapter. Multiple comparison procedures for controlling

FWER, such as Bonferroni, Holm, Sidak, and Hochberg, can be evaluated and compared through simulation.

For a specific design, the software first generates the response data and then analyzes the data using a specified multiple comparison procedure. This is repeated over thousands of simulation runs, then summarized in a power analysis across all the replicated simulations.

For example, suppose that a study is designed to compare a new treatment to an existing treatment with respect to four continuous outcomes. Furthermore, assume that the means for the new treatment and for the existing treatment with respect to the four endpoints are as follows.

Endpoint ID	Mean for Existing Treatment	Mean for New Treatment
Endpoint 1	0.1	0.3
Endpoint 2	0.2	0.4
Endpoint 3	0.3	0.5
Endpoint 4	0.4	0.6

However, there are uncertainties about the correlations among these endpoints. The objectives are to evaluate the performance of different multiple comparison procedures such as the Bonferroni, Holm, Hochberg, and Hommel tests and to also investigate the impact of the magnitude of the correlation on power. To this end, one first needs to ensure that the software is installed. To open East, click the East 6 icon on the desktop. The open window will look as follows:

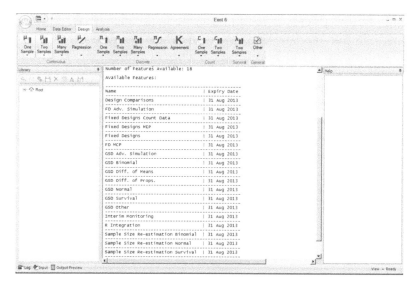

Next, click the menu for continuous endpoint > two samples as in the following screen and select multiple comparisons in the drop-down list:

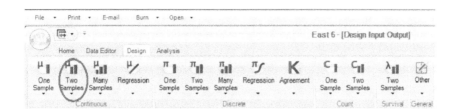

Now, the input window will appear with options for simulating the power using different multiple comparison procedures. On this window, specify the nominal FWER, the total sample size, and finally select the multiple comparison procedures to be used in the analysis.

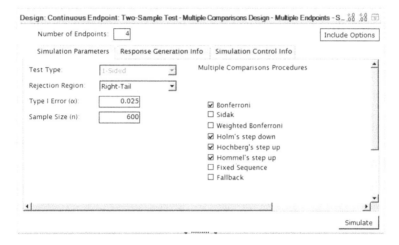

The underlying means and covariance matrix for each group must also be specified, as seen in the following window, which represents the scenario where all endpoints are independent:

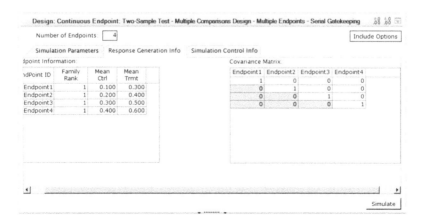

Finally, click the simulate button at the bottom right of the window to start the simulations. When all the simulations are completed, the following output summary will appear:

ID	Multiple Comparisons Procedure	Test Type	Design Type	Specified α	Overall FWER	No. of Endpoints	No. of Families	Sample Size	Rejection Region	Conjunctive Power	Disjunctive Power
Sim1	Bonferroni	1-Sided	Serial	0.025	0	4	1	600	Right-Tail	0.057	0.925
Sim2	Holm's step down	1-Sided	Serial	0.025	0	4	1	600	Right-Tail	0.202	0.925
Sim3	Hochberg's step up	1-Sided	Serial	0.025	0	4	1	600	Right-Tail	0.227	0.931
Sim4	Hommel's step up	1-Sided	Serial	0.025	0	4	1	600	Right-Tail	0.224	0.94

The output summary shows the actual FWER and different types of power including conjunctive power (probability of rejecting all false null hypotheses) and disjunctive power (probability of rejecting at least one false null hypothesis). As one can see, the four tests provide comparable disjunctive power all above 90%. However, the stepwise procedures including the Holm, Hochberg, and Hommel tests provide better conjunctive power (~20%) than the single-step Bonferroni procedure (<6%).

To see how the power is affected by the correlations among the endpoints, specify the covariance matrix as follows, which represents medium correlation among the endpoints.

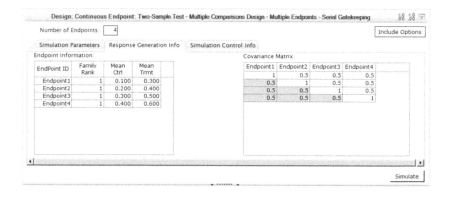

Now click the simulate button to preview the output. As one can see, the disjunctive power with medium correlation dropped by more than 10% for each specific test when compared to the situation where all the endpoints are independent. However, the conjunctive power increased by about 18%.

In conclusion, the stepwise procedures perform better than the single-step test in terms of conjunctive power. The stepwise procedures are comparable to single-step tests in terms of disjunctive power. Conjunctive power increases with an increase in correlation. In contrast, disjunctive power decreases with an increase in correlation.

ID	Multiple Comparisons Procedure	Test Type	Design Type	Specified α	Overall FWER	No. of Endpoints	No. of Families	Sample Size	Rejection Region	Conjunctive Power	Disjunctive Power
Sim1	Bonferroni	1-Sided	Serial	0.025	0	4	1	600	Right-Tail	0.18	0.784
Sim2	Holm's step down	1-Sided	Serial	0.025	0	4	1	600	Right-Tail	0.362	0.781
Sim3	Hochberg's step up	1-Sided	Serial	0.025	0	4	1	600	Right-Tail	0.392	0.787
Sim4	Hommel's step up	1-Sided	Serial	0.025	0	4	1	600	Right-Tail	0.384	0.806

For details on this multiple comparison module, please refer to the East Version 6.2 manual.

References

Benjamini, Y. and Y. Hochberg. Controlling the false discovery rate: A practical and powerful approach to multiple testing. *Journal of the Royal Statistical Society, Series B*, 57:289–300, 1995.

Benjamini, Y. and D. Yekutieli. The control of the false discovery rate in multiple testing under dependency. *Annals of Statistics*, 29(4):1165–1188, 2001.

Bretz, F., W. Maurer, W. Brannath, and M. Posch. A graphical approach to sequentially rejective multiple test procedures. *Statistics in Medicine*, 28:586–604, 2009.

Cytel Inc. East Version 6.2 User Manual. Cambridge, MA.

Dmitrienko, A. and A.C. Tamhane. Gatekeeping procedures with clinical trial applications. *Pharmaceutical Statistics*, 5:19–28, 2007.

Dmitrienko, A., A.C. Tamhane, and F. Bretz. *Multiple Testing Problems in Pharmaceutical Statistics*, Chapman and Hall/CRC Press, New York, 2010.

Dudoit, S., J.P. Shaffer, and J.C. Boldrick. Multiple hypothesis testing in microarray experiments. *Statistical Science*, 18(1):71–103, 2003.

Dudoit, S. and M.J. van der Laan. *Multiple Testing Procedures with Applications to Genomics*, Springer, New York, 2008.

FDA (Food and Drug Administration). Clinical pharmacogenomics: Premarketing evaluation in early phase clinical studies. Center for Drug Evaluation and Research, Center for Biologics Evaluation and Research, Center for Devices and Radiological Health, 2011.

Hochberg, Y. A sharper Bonferroni procedure for multiple tests of significance. *Biometrica*, 75:800–802, 1988.

Hochberg, Y. and A.C. Tamhane. *Multiple Comparison Procedures*, Wiley, New York, 1987.

Holm, S. A simple sequentially rejective multiple test procedure. *Scandinavian Journal of Statistics*, 6:65–70,1979.

Hommel, G. and F. Bretz. Aesthetics and power considerations in multiple testing-A contradiction? Biometrical Journal, 43:581–589, 2008.

Jogdeo, K. Association and probability inequalities. *Annals of Statistics*, 5:495–504,1977.

Lehmann, E.L. and J.P. Romano. Generalizations of the familywise error rate. *Annals of Statistics*, 33(3):1138–1154, 2005.

Lu, J., G. Getz, E.A. Miska, E. Alvarez-Saavedra, J. Lamb, D. Peck, A. Sweet-Cordero et al. MicroRNA expression profiles classify human cancers. *Nature*, 435(9):834–838, 2005. Available at www.broad.mit.edu/cancer/pub/miGCM.

Mallal, S. et al. _HLA-B*5701 screening for hypersensitivity to abacavir. _New England Journal of Medicine, 358(6):568–579, 2008.

Maurer, W., L.A. Hothorn, and W. Lehmacher. Multiple comparisons in drug clinical trials and preclinical assays: A priori ordered hypotheses. *Biometrie in der Chemisch-in-Pharmazeutischen Industrie. 6.* Vollman J. (editor). Fischer-Verlag, Stuttgart, 1995, 3-18.

Pollard, K. S., H. N. Gilbert, Y. Ge, S. Taylor, and S. Dudoit. multtest: Resamplingbased multiple hypothesis testing. R package version 2.16.0, 2013.

Sarkar, S.K. Probability inequalities for ordered MTP2 random variables: A proof of the Simes conjecture. *Annals of Statistics*, 26(2):494–504, 1998.

Sarkar, S.K. and C.-K. Chang. The Simes method for multiple hypothesis testing with positively dependent test statistics. *Journal of the American Statistical Association*, 92:1601–1608, 1997.

Šidák, Z. Rectangular con_dence regions for the means of multivariate normal distributions. *Journal of the American Statistical Association*, 62:626–633, 1967.

Simes, R.J. An improved Bonferroni procedure for multiple tests of significance. *Biometrika*, 73:751–754, 1986.

Westfall, P.H. and A. Krishen. Optimally weighted, fixed sequence, and gatekeeping multiple testing procedures. *Journal of Statistical Planning and Inference*, 99:25–40, 2001.

Westfall, P.H. and S.S. Young. *Resampling-Based Multiple Testing: Examples and Methods for p-value Adjustment.* Wiley, New York, 1993.

Wiens, B. and A. Dmitrienko. The fallback procedure for evaluating a single family of hypotheses. *Journal of Biopharmaceutical Statistics*, 15: 929–942, 2005.

10

Patient-Reported Outcomes in Personalized Medicine

Demissie Alemayehu and Joseph C. Cappelleri

CONTENTS

10.1 Introduction

In this chapter, we discuss the role of outcomes research in customizing health care while incorporating genomic information. An abbreviated version on some of the material discussed in this chapter may also be found in Alemayehu and Cappelleri (2012). Central to the discussion is the argument that information solicited directly from the patients about their health-related quality of life (QOL), disease burden, or other aspects of the treatment they receive is an essential component of any treatment paradigm that relies on genetic information to ensure optimal healthcare delivery. Indeed, there is growing evidence for the impact of genetics on QOL, whether the individual is a patient or not (Sprangers et al. 2010). For example, Shi et al. (2010) considered the genetic modulation of pain perception and response to analgesics, and underscored the challenges of personalized analgesic treatments. In the context of oncology, Barsevick et al. (2010) discussed cancer-associated fatigue in relation to potential biological and genetic causal mechanisms. Sprangers et al. (2010) performed a survey of the literature relating to the genetic susceptibility of negative and positive emotions. Raat et al. (2010) describe the value of a population-based prospective cohort study, from fetal life onward in Rotterdam, as a template that enables a candidate gene study and a genome-wide association study to inform about health-related QOL of mothers and their young children.

Despite the growing importance of patient-reported outcomes (PROs) in medical research, their role in customizing health care is not widely recognized. Information solicited directly from patients about their patient-reported health status or health-related QOL, disease burden, or other aspects of their disease or treatment should be an essential component of any treatment paradigm that relies on genetic and other patient-specific information to ensure optimal care delivery for the individual patient. Broadly defined, a PRO is any report on the status of a patient's clinical condition that comes directly from the patient, without interpretation of the patient's response by a clinician or by anyone else. "PROs" is an umbrella term that includes a variety of subjective outcomes, such as pain, fatigue, depression, aspects of well-being (e.g., physical, functional, psychological), treatment satisfaction, health-related QOL, and physical symptoms, such as nausea and vomiting. PROs are often relevant for studying different conditions—such as pain, erectile dysfunction, fatigue, migraine, anxiety, and depression—that cannot be assessed adequately without input from patients on the impact of the disease or the treatment.

Effective use of PROs data in the context of personalized medicine entails a careful evaluation of both conceptual and methodological issues associated with both PROs and personalized medicine. There are guidelines and best practices that have been developed to strengthen the value of the data from those two fields. The issues surrounding PRO data, including but not restricted to patient-reported health-related QoL, have in particular been a focus of extensive research (Sloan et al. 2007). Regulatory guidelines and other guidance documents have been developed to address some of the issues (see Bottomley et al. 2009, Acquadro et al. 2003). Incidentally, genetic research shares some of the commonly encountered issues that arise in QOL studies, including multiplicity of endpoints, handling of missing data, reliability, and validity (see Hüebner et al. 2007). For genetic research, similar documents are available as resources for researchers (Bogardus et al. 1999, Pelias 2001).

In recent years, the role of QOL in personalized medicine has continued to gain increasing attention, owing in part to the activities of such organizations as the GeneQol Consortium (http://www.geneqol.org), which aims to promote research on biological mechanisms, potential genes, and genetic variants involved in QOL (Sprangers et al. 2009). Advances in the area include summaries on the genetic background of common symptoms and overall well-being (see Sprangers et al. 2009).

With the growing interest in comparative effectiveness research (CER), the role of PROs in personalized medicine is expected to get correspondingly increased attention. The field of CER involves a comprehensive and patient-centered assessment of alternative treatment options using all available methods and sources of information. In a recent evaluation, Alemayehu et al. (2011) provided a detailed discussion of the challenges and opportunities of PROs in the context of CER. Similarly, there are compelling arguments for the need to align CER and personalized medicine to properly account for the effects of individual patient differences in the study of alternative treatment options. In addition to the commonly studied attributes (e.g., severity of disease, comorbidities, and risk factors), these include genetic characteristics. A valid study of heterogeneity of treatment effects in the context of CER, therefore, should incorporate both elements of personalized medicine and PROs. An exposition of personalized medication in relation to CER can be found elsewhere (http://www.lewin.com/~/media/lewin/cer/site_shell/images/lewin_cer-pm.pdf).

The rest of the chapter is organized as follows. In Section 10.2, the role of PRO data in personalized medicine is addressed. In Section 10.3, analytical issues with PRO data are highlighted, with particular reference to multiplicity problems, handling of missing values, and commonly used statistical models, including factor analytic, mediation, longitudinal, and item response theory (IRT) models.

10.2 PROs in Personalized Medicine

PRO instruments are designed to quantify concepts pertaining to how a patient feels or functions and help generate evidence of a treatment benefit or harm from the patient's perspective. Accordingly, they can provide complementary information to other clinical endpoints for use in personalized medicine. Indeed, accumulating data from recent studies suggests the existence of an association between the genetic disposition of patients and their QOL. For example, in one study, Rijsdijk and colleagues (2003) noted that the overall heritability of psychosocial distress ranged from 20% to 44%. In other studies (Romeis et al. 2000, Leinonen et al. 2005), evidence of genetic influences has been reported for PROs. While much research is still needed to determine the precise proportion of variability in PRO that is explained by genetic factors, there is considerable progress in some areas such as oncology to quantify the association between polymorphisms and PROs (see Yang et al. 2009).

The role of PROs in the assessment of heterogeneity of treatment effects is well recognized (Horn and Gassaway 2010). In addition, baseline PRO values may provide useful information about subgroup differences in ways not captured by other baseline clinical variables (Cella et al. 2009). The integration of PROs in personalized medicine requires the formulation of a framework that addresses theoretical, analytical, and operational issues pertinent to both areas. Below, we discuss some of the major points that need to be considered.

10.2.1 Conceptual Framework

As fully discussed in Sprangers et al. (2010), the study of the genetic disposition of PROs requires a conceptual model to establish the relationships among QOL domains, biological mechanisms, and genetic variants. A model that appears to be appropriate in this setting is one that was introduced by Wilson and Cleary (1995), which links biological factors and patient-reported QOL. The model has further been enhanced by Spranger et al. (2010) to include the genetic underpinnings of biological variables as well as other individual characteristics. Notably, the model is general enough to allow the study of interactions among patient characteristics and environment and genetic factors.

10.2.2 Instrument Development and Validation

A major step in the incorporation of PROs in personalized medicine is the establishment and use of standardized instruments, with proven reliability and validity. Although there are numerous validated instruments that measure different domains of health from the perspective of the patient, the choice of a PRO instrument is a function of the research question, the disease, and the population under study. A partial list of common PRO instruments can be found in Fayers and Machin (2007), McDowell (2006), and Salek (2004). The commonly used and cited instruments in clinical practice include the 36-item Short-Form Health Survey (Ware et al. 1993) and the Dartmouth Primary Care Cooperative Information Project Charts (Westbury 1990), both of which are generic instruments, and the Chronic Respiratory Questionnaire (Westbury et al. 1990) and the Sexual Health Inventory for Men (Rosen et al. 1999), both of which are disease-specific instruments. Frost et al. (2007) address the systematic integration of QOL assessment into the clinical setting. Operationally, a PRO protocol must be an integral part of the overall research plan. Particular attention should also be paid to the determination of which PRO concept is important to assess in a given disease area. When possible, generally accepted measures should be used within a therapeutic area rather than individually developed PROs for a specific therapy. Standardized measures not only facilitate the interpretation of results, but also allow data synthesis from different studies.

Development of a new PRO instrument for a given disease requires the establishment of a robust and theory-based conceptual framework, linking the desired outcome to the concept of interest, and subsequently linking that concept to the specific symptoms or latent variable being measured. The use of focus groups and cognitive interviews with patients can provide the considerable input needed to establish face and content validity and to ensure that the instrument covers what patients consider important. Standard psychometric methods should be applied to test reliability, validity, and responsiveness of the PRO measure. Among them, exploratory factor analysis and confirmatory factor analysis, discussed below, should be considered to examine the factor structure of which items go with what domains.

10.3 Analytical Issues with PRO Data Analysis

Analytical approaches for genetic data are addressed in earlier chapters. Some of the issues that arise in the context of genetic data also arise in the context of PRO data analysis. These include problems of multiplicity, missing values, and dimensionality reduction. In addition, PRO data may require specialized approaches that facilitate the interpretation of results as well as the handling of nonstandard data structures. In the following, we provide a brief summary of some of the methodological approaches and the problems that are generally associated with PRO data analysis.

10.3.1 Models for Longitudinal Data

The main objective of longitudinal analysis is to describe systematic patterns of within-individual changes in the response variable, and to relate these changes to interindividual differences in selected covariates (e.g., treatment group). A single statistical model for longitudinal data, which incorporates all available data (i.e., all available observations from all available participants), can be used to capture both how individuals change over time and how to relate within-individual changes to selected covariates. Several models are used for different types of analyses, the specific type of longitudinal model depending on the objective of the study. For example, the mean of a PRO, when the measures are considered continuous, may be analyzed using linear mixed effect models when time is taken as continuous (quantitative covariate) or repeated measure models (response profiles) when time is taken as categorical (qualitative covariate).

When treatment effects are studies in the context of a parallel multiple-group design, the data may be analyzed using one of two approaches, generally referred to as random coefficients models and repeated measures models. Other approaches, which may be used for quantitative or discrete outcomes, include generalized estimating equations and generalized linear mixed-effects models are available. For more detail on longitudinal analysis, especially on the topics covered in this chapter, several books can be consulted (Singer and Willett 2003, Hedeker and Gibbons 2006, Fairclough 2010, Fitzmaurice et al. 2011).

To fix ideas, consider a two-arm study in which n_k subjects are randomized to the kth treatment group. One simple form of a repeated measures model is given by

$$Y_{ijk} = a + b_j + r_k + e_{ijk},$$

where Y_{ijk} is the PRO response for subject i at the measurement occasion j on treatment k ($i = 1, 2,..., n_k$; $j = 1, 2, 3, ..., t$; $k = 1, 2$); a is the overall mean; b_j is the fixed time effect at week j; r_k is the fixed effect of the treatment k; and e_{ijk} is the error term associated with outcome measurement Y_{ijk}. It is assumed that errors e_{ijk} are independent between subjects but are correlated within a subject. This approach has an important advantage in that it does not impose any functional relationship between outcome and time. However, the model requires specification of the correlation structure of the observations within a subject.

A more general formulation involves hierarchical linear models that provide considerable flexibility in analyzing PRO data. These linear mixed effects models can estimate individual-specific response trajectories over time. In particular, this setting permits handling of subjects with a different time assessment and a varying number of assessments (and, by implication, missing data at different time points), thereby avoiding the need to exclude such patients from analysis. It also allows estimation of changes in individual responses across time (which is taken as a continuous covariate), in addition to the usual population averages. The model may be given as

$$\mathbf{y}_i = \mathbf{X}_i \beta + \mathbf{Z}_i \upsilon_i + \varepsilon_i$$

where $\mathbf{y}_i$ ($n_i \times 1$ vector) denotes the response of the ith individual ($i = 1, ...,N$); $\mathbf{X}_i$ is an $n_i \times p$ *matrix of* covariates for individual i, β is the $p \times 1$ vector of fixed effects, $\mathbf{Z}_i(n_i \times r)$ is the design matrix corresponding to random effects; υ_i ($r \times 1$) a vector of random individual effects; and ε_i is the $n_i \times 1$ vector of error terms. For the random components, the following assumptions are typically made

$$\varepsilon_i \sim N(0, \Omega_i)$$
$$\upsilon_i \sim N(0, \Sigma_\upsilon)$$

10.3.2 Factor Analysis

A factor is a latent or unobserved variable: a hypothetical construct that affects certain observed variables (or manifest variables) that can be measured directly. Factor analysis is concerned with detecting and analyzing patterns based on the correlations among quantitative variables. In factor analysis, a set of measured variables is reduced into a smaller, more manageable set of unobservable factors that underlie the measured variables. The objective is to identify the number and the nature of the factors that are responsible for covariation in the data and to determine the domain structure of a questionnaire, which may be unidimensional or multidimensional with several subscales.

In *exploratory factor analysis*, there is initial uncertainty as to the number of factors being measured, and the results of the analysis are used to help solve for the number of factors. Exploratory factor analysis is suitable for generating hypotheses about the structure of the data. It can be used to lend structure and validity to the data (Hatcher 1994). In addition, it can further refine an instrument by revealing what items may be dropped from the questionnaire because they contribute little to the presumed underlying factors.

Figure 10.1 depicts a simplified path model where responses to questions 1 through 6 of a hypothetical PRO instrument are represented as six squares labeled V1 through V6. This path model suggests that variables V1, V2, and V3 are correlated with each other because they are influenced by the same underlying common factor (labeled anxiety). Similarly, the items V4, V5, and V6 are correlated with each other because they are influenced by the same underlying factor (labeled depression). In this setting, only one common factor is assumed to have a significant loading for a variable; for example, V1 displays a significant loading for factor 1 (through the coefficient b1) but not for factor 2.

The double-headed arrow (a bidirectional arrow) connecting the two ovals indicates that the two constructs, anxiety and depression, are correlated (and said to be oblique). Notice that the two common factors in Figure 10.1 are not the only factors that influence the observed variables. For example, two factors actually influence variable V1: the common factor, factor 1, and a second factor labeled "U1." Here U1 is a unique factor that only influences V1 (through the coefficient d1) and represents all of the independent factors

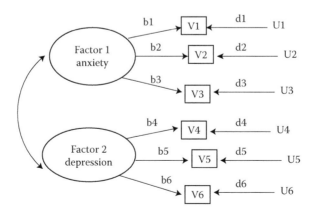

FIGURE 10.1
(See color insert.) Path model for a six-variable, two-factor model with correlated factors.

that are unique to V1 (including its error component). The unique factor U1 affects only V1, U2 affects only V2, and so on.

A rotation is a linear transformation that is performed on the factor solution for the purpose of making the solution easier to interpret. In exploratory factor analysis, an orthogonal rotation is one in which the (common) factors are taken as uncorrelated. An oblique rotation, on the other hand, is one in which the factors are taken as correlated or associated.

One recommendation on how many factors (latent variables) to retain is to use the scree test. The scree test is a rule-of-thumb criterion and involves the plot of the eigenvalue (i.e., the amount of variance that is accounted for by a given factor) associated with each factor. The objective of a scree plot is to look for a break between factors with relatively large eigenvalues and those with smaller eigenvalues; factors that appear before the break are taken to be meaningful and retained. Researchers often refer to the break as the elbow in the curve of the scree plot.

Three other criteria can be used to evaluate the number of factors and their content for suitability: (1) items that load on a given factor are assumed to have a shared conceptual meaning; (2) items that have high-standardized factor pattern loadings or standardized regression coefficients (≥ 0.40 in absolute value) on one factor and low loadings on the other factors; and (3) consistency of results across assessment time points (Hatcher 1994).

Exploratory factor analysis is often confused with principal component analysis. Both exploratory factor analysis and principal component analysis are variable reduction procedures, reducing a number of variables to a smaller number, and they have been applied to determine item reduction and factor structure in the analysis of PROs. But the two procedures are generally different and not conceptually identical. In exploratory factor analysis, the observed variables are linear combinations of the underlying factors. In principal components analysis, however, the principal components are linear combinations of the observed variables. Because principal component analysis makes no attempt to separate the common component from the unique component of each item's (variable's) variance, and exploratory factor analysis does, exploratory factor analysis is more appropriate than principal component analysis in identifying the factor structure of the data.

While exploratory factor analysis explores the patterns in the correlations of items (or variables), *confirmatory factor analysis* tests whether the correlations conform to an anticipated or expected scale structure given in particular research hypotheses (Hatcher 1994, Brown 2006). In confirmatory factor analysis, there must be not only a prespecified number of unobserved factors (latent variables) being assessed, but also a theoretical framework of which observable (manifest) variables are related and not related to which factors. A more important distinction is that confirmatory factor analysis, unlike exploratory factor analysis, tests for a specified relationship between latent factors and, in doing so, allows for testing hypotheses on which factors affect other factors. A confirmatory factor analysis, for example, may be used to evaluate in advance, *a priori* in a confirmatory fashion, that a particular set of three items related to anxiety and another particular set of three items related to depression, and that anxiety and depression are related.

In using knowledge of theory, previous empirical evidence, or both, researchers can postulate and examine an *a priori* relationship on what items belong with what factors and then test the fit of this model statistically. Model fit indices, such as Bentler's comparative fit index, are used to determine whether the sample data are consistent with the imposed constraints (e.g., that certain items belong to certain factors but not others) or, in other words, whether the data confirm the substantively generated model. It is in this sense that the model is thought of as confirmatory.

In confirmatory factor analysis, as well as in exploratory factor analysis, factor loadings are coefficients that indicate the importance of a variable to each factor. These coefficients are important because they signify the nature of the variables that most strongly relate to a factor; the nature of the variables helps to capture the nature and meaning of a factor.

10.3.3 Mediation Models

A mediation model is one that seeks to identify and explain the mechanism that underlies an observed relationship between an independent variable (e.g., treatment) and a dependent variable (e.g., sleep disturbance) via the inclusion of a third explanatory variable (e.g., pain), known as a mediator variable (MacKinnon 2008). Rather than hypothesizing a direct causal relationship between the independent variable and the dependent variable, a mediation model hypothesizes that the independent variable influences the mediator variable, which in turn influences the dependent variable. The mediator variable therefore serves to clarify the nature of the relationship between the independent and dependent variables.

Most research has focused on the relations between two variables, say, X and Y. Such research includes situations where the explanatory (predictor) variable X can be considered a possible cause of the outcome (dependent) variable Y as when, for example, subjects are randomized to interventions of the treatment group variable X. In this simple bivariate case, the coefficient (say, c) relating X to Y represents the total effect of X on Y. This total effect is the sum of the direct effect of X on Y and indirect effect of X on Y through an intervening or mediating variable.

A theoretical premise posits that an intervening (mediator) variable is an indicative measure of the process through which an independent variable is thought to affect a dependent variable. The objective is to assess the extent to which the effect of the independent variable on the dependent variable is direct or, alternatively, indirect via the mediator. Mediation, in its simplest form, represents the addition of a third variable (M, the mediator) to this X and Y relation, so that X causes or at least influences M, which in turn causes or at least influences Y ($X \rightarrow M \rightarrow Y$). In studies in which mediation is posited

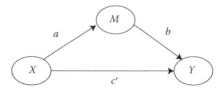

FIGURE 10.2
A simple and standard mediation model. X = independent variable, M = mediator, Y = dependent variable.

and tested, therefore, the question is to what extent the effect of X is direct ($X \rightarrow Y$) and indirect as mediated through the mediator M ($X \rightarrow M \rightarrow Y$).

In Figure 10.2, the coefficient a represents the relation of X to M, b represents the relation of M to Y adjusted for X, and c' represents the relation of X to Y adjusted for M. The path coefficient c' is called the direct effect of X on Y. Complete mediation is the case in which the variable X no longer affects Y when M has been controlled and so the path coefficient c' is zero. The cross-product of a and b (ab) refers to the indirect effect of X on Y. No mediation occurs when the total effect of X on Y exists entirely through the direct effect, so that c' is nonzero and ab is zero. Partial mediation is the case in which the direct path (c') and indirect path (ab) are both nonzero.

10.3.4 Item Response Theory

IRT is a statistical theory consisting of nonlinear logistic models to express the probability of a particular response to a scale item as a function of the quantitative attribute of interest (called a latent or "unobservable" trait or concept, like depression) (Hambleton et al. 1991, de Ayala 2005). The mathematical description for the item response is called an item characteristic curve, which gives the probability of responding to a particular category of an item for an individual with an estimated amount on the attribute. Each item typically has its own level of difficulty (items that are more difficult are harder to endorse) and can have its own level of discrimination (items with more discrimination are more likely to distinguish among persons with varying levels on the attribute).

The application and relevance of IRT for PROs has increased considerably over the last several years. For instance, IRT has been the cornerstone of the Patient-Reported Outcomes Measurement Information System (PROMIS), a large initiative of the National Institute of Health (NIH), which aims to revolutionize the way PROs are selected and employed in clinical research and practice evaluation. The broad objectives of the NIH PROMIS network are to develop and test a large bank of items measuring PROs; create a computerized adaptive testing system that allows for an efficient, psychometrically robust assessment of PROs in clinical research involving a wide range of chronic diseases; and create a publicly available system that can be added to and modified periodically and that allows clinical researchers to access a common repository of items and computerized adaptive tests (Cella et al. 2007a,b).

10.3.5 Multiplicity Issues

Multiplicity in the context of genomic and subgroup analysis is fully discussed in Chapter 5. In PRO data analysis, multiplicity problems arise in a variety of ways. First, by virtue of the design of the instruments used to generate the data, multiple endpoints are an integral component of PRO analysis. In addition, there may be a desire to evaluate treatment effects at different time points and for different subgroups. Thus, when used in the context of personalized medicine, the problem is compounded and poses further analytical challenges.

Alternative approaches to multiplicity depend on the research objectives, endpoints, decision rules, and other factors (EMA 2005, Fayers and Machin 2007, Dmitrienko et al. 2009, FDA 2009, Fairclough 2010). The approaches may include the use of familiar standard statistical techniques (e.g., step-down, step-up, and other gate-keeping procedures), as well as definitions of composite endpoints to reduce the number of potential endpoints to be evaluated. The latter, however, requires caution and subject-matter expertise to ensure that the original intent of the instrument is preserved.

10.3.6 Missing Values

In the context of PRO analysis, missing data may arise in two major ways (FDA 2009, Fairclough 2010). Data may be missing for an entire domain or for specific items within domains. While the former is generally true for other clinical endpoints, the latter is a phenomenon more commonly associated with PRO data. In all cases, the handling of the missing values is a function of the missingness mechanism.

When it can be justified that the data that are missing are random, then there are well-established approaches to handle the problem (Little and Rubin 1987). On the other hand, if the missingness is nonrandom, then analysis of the data requires caution. While there are techniques to determine if the missing data are random or nonrandom (Little and Rubin 1987), there is no definitive way of ruling out the latter. Therefore, in case of doubt, sensitivity analysis should be performed to ensure the robustness of the findings under alternative scenarios (Little and Rubin 1987).

10.3.7 Interpretation of PROs

An inherent and fundamental issue for a PRO centers on its meaning. Interpretation of PRO scores, while distinct from validity and reliability, is central for a PRO to gain currency and usefulness. Approaches to the interpretation of PRO scores are available (Lydick et al. 1993, Marquis et al. 2004, Schünemann et al. 2006, Revicki et al. 2007, McLeod et al. 2011). Methods fall under two broad strategies—anchor-based approaches and distribution-based approaches—and the variations within them aim at enhancing the understanding and meaning of PRO scores.

Regarding the anchor-based approaches, an anchor is a measure or criterion related to the targeted PRO under examination. An anchor can be a measure different from or even part of the PRO measure under consideration. The chosen anchor should be clearly understood in context and be easier to interpret than the PRO measure of interest, and the anchor should be appreciably correlated with the targeted PRO. An anchor-based approach links the targeted concept of the PRO to the meaningful concept or criterion emanating from the anchor, such as patient-assessment on the severity of the condition. Four anchor-based methodologies include (1) percentages based on thresholds, (2) criterion-group interpretation, (3) content-based interpretation, and (4) clinically important difference (Marquis et al. 2004, Schünemann et al. 2006, Fayers and Machin 2007).

Regarding distribution-based approaches, they can offer valuable insights about the magnitude of an effect. These methods also allow for a standardization of different scales with different ranges and ways of scoring. A limitation of distribution-based methods should be noted: they do not provide information about *clinical* meaningfulness. Two useful distribution-based methods include (1) effect size, and (2) responder analysis and cumulative proportions (Fayers and Machin 2007; McLeod et al. 2011).

A third strategy, which has not been typically used for interpretation of PROs, is mediation analysis. It enriches the interpretation or meaning of PRO scores by eliciting the mechanism of action of an intervention as it relates to a PRO. Mediation analysis in the context of interpretation of PRO scores is a relatively new development.

10.4 Concluding Remarks

With the growing interest in personalized medicine, there are compelling reasons to incorporate PROs as an integral part of the research endeavor in this area. However, to ensure that PROs play an effective complementary role to traditional clinical endpoints in personalized medicine, it is essential to understand the issues that are inherent in such data and to put in place processes to guide researchers and other stakeholders.

In this chapter, we highlighted the need for a conceptual frame to incorporate PRO data in the personalized medicines and discussed methodological and analytical approaches that are relevant for the analysis and interpretation of PROs. Interestingly, some of the issues that arise in genetic data analysis are also shared by PROs. This provides both challenges and opportunities from the standpoints of application as well as methodological research. With the recent developments in the areas of patient-centered outcomes research, there is considerable opportunity to bring the two areas even closer and to advance the way treatment is attuned to address individual needs.

Acknowledgment

The authors gratefully acknowledge Jose Ma. J. Alvir of Pfizer Inc. for his thoughtful and valuable review of this chapter.

References

Acquadro C, Berzon R, Dubois D, Leidy NK, Marquis P, Revicki D, Rothman M, PRO Harmonization Group. Incorporating the patient's perspective into drug development and communication: An ad hoc task force report of the Patient-Reported Outcomes (PRO) Harmonization Group meeting at the Food and Drug Administration, February 16, 2001. *Value in Health* 2003; 6:522–31.

Alemayehu D, Cappelleri, JC. Conceptual and analytical considerations toward the use of patient-reported outcomes in personalized medicine. *American Health & Drug Benefits* 2012; 5:310–6.

Alemayehu D, Sanchez R, Cappelleri JC. Considerations on the use of patient-reported outcomes in comparative effectiveness research. *Journal of Managed Care Pharmacy* 2011; 17 (9-a):S27–33.

Barsevick A, Frost M, Zwinderman A, Hall P, Halyard M, and the GENEQOL Consortium. I am so tired: Biological and genetic mechanisms of cancer-related fatigue. *Quality of Life Research* 2010; 19:1419–27.

Bogardus ST Jr, Concato J, Feinstein AR. Clinical epidemiological quality in molecular genetic research: The need for methodological standards. *Journal of the American Medical Association* 1999; 281:1919–26.

Bottomley A, Jones D, Claassens L. Patient-reported outcomes: Assessment and current perspectives of the guidelines of the Food and Drug Administration and the reflection paper of the European Medicines Agency. *European Journal of Cancer* 2009; 45:347–53.

Brown, TA. *Confirmatory Factor Analysis for Applied Research.* 2006. New York, NY: Guilford Press.

Cella D, Cappelleri JC, Bushmakin A, Charbonneau C, Li JZ, Kim ST, Chen I, Michaelson MD, Motzer RJ. Quality of life predicts progression-free survival in patients with metastatic renal cell carcinoma treated with sunitinib vs. interferon-alfa. *Journal of Oncology Practice* 2009; 5:66–70.

Cella D, Gershon RC, Lai JS, Choi SW. The future of outcomes measurement: Item banking, tailored short-forms, and computerized adaptive assessment. *Quality of Life Research* 2007a; 16:133–41.

Cella D, Yount S, Rothrock N, Gershon R, Cook K, Reeve B, Ader D, Fries JF, Bruce B, Rose M for the PROMIS Cooperative Group. The Patient-Reported Outcomes Measurement Information System (PROMIS): Progress of an NIH Roadmap cooperative group during its first two years. *Medical Care* 2007b; 45 5 (Suppl 1):S3–11.

de Ayala RJ. *The Theory and Practice of Item Response Theory*. 2005. New York, NY: Guilford Press.

Dmitrienko A, Tamhane A, Bretz F (editors). *Multiple Testing Problems in Pharmaceutical Statistics*. 2009. Boca Raton, Florida: Chapman and Hall/CRC.

European Medicine Agency, Committee for Medicinal Products for Human Use. Reflection paper on the regulatory guidance for the use of health-related quality of life (HRQL) measures in the evaluation of medicinal products. 2005. http://www.ema.europa.eu/docs/en_GB/document_library/Scientific_guideline/2009/09/WC500003637.pdf (Accessed 31 August 2013).

Fairclough DL. *Design and Analysis of Quality of Life Studies in Clinical Trials*. 2010. 2nd edn. Boca Raton, Florida: Chapman & Hall/CRC.

Fayers FM, Machin D. *Quality of Life: The Assessment, Analysis and Interpretation of Patient-Reported Outcomes*. 2007. 2nd edn. Chichester, England: John Wiley & Sons Ltd.

Fitzmaurice GM, Laird NM, Ware JH. *Applied Longitudinal Analysis*. 2011. 2nd edn. Hoboken, New Jersey: John Wiley & Sons.

Food and Drug Administration. Guidance for Industry: Patient-reported Outcome Measures: Use in Medical Product Development to Support Labeling Claims. Rockville, Maryland: U.S. Department of Health and Human Services. December 2009. http://www.fda.gov/downloads/Drugs/GuidanceCompliance RegulatoryInformation/Guidances/UCM193282.pdf (Accessed 31 August 2013).

Frost M, Bonomi AE, Cappelleri JC, Schünemann HJ, Moynihan TJ, Aaronson N and the Clinical Significance Consensus Meeting Group. Applying quality-of-life data formally and systematically into clinical practice. *Mayo Clinic Proceedings* 2007; 82:1214–28.

Hambleton RK, Swaninathan HJ, Rogers HJ. *Fundamentals of Item Response Theory*. 1991. Newbury Park, CA: Sage Publications.

Hatcher L. *A Step-By-Step Approach to Using the SAS® System for Factor Analysis and Structural Equation Modeling*. 1994. Cary, North Carolina: SAS Institute Inc.

Hedeker D, Gibbons RD. *Longitudinal Data Analysis*. 2006. Hoboken, NJ: John Wiley & Sons.

Horn SD, Gassaway J. Incorporating clinical heterogeneity and patient reported outcomes for comparative effectiveness research. *Medical Care* 2010; 48 (6) suppl; s17–22.

http://www.geneqol.org.

http://www.lewin.com/~/media/lewin/cer/site_shell/images/lewin_cer-pm.pdf.

Hüebner C, Petermann I, Browning BL et al. Triallelic single nucleotide polymorphisms and genotyping error in genetic epidemiology studies: MDR1 (ABCB1) G2677/T/A as an example. *Cancer Epidemiology, Biomarkers & Prevention* 2007; 16:1185–92.

Leinonen R, Kaprio J, Jylhä M, Tolvanen A, Koskenvuo M, Heikkinen E, Rantanen T. Genetic influences underlying self-rated health in older female twins. *Journal of the American Geriatric Society* 2005; 53:1002–7.

Little RJA, Rubin DB. *Statistical Analysis with Missing Values.* 1987. New York, NY: John Wiley Sons.

Lydick E, Epstein RS. Interpretation of quality of life changes. *Quality of Life Research* 1993; 2:221–6.

MacKinnon DP. *Introduction to Statistical Mediation Analysis.* 2008. Mahwah, NJ: Erlbaum.

Marquis P, Chassany O, Abetz L. A comprehensive strategy for the interpretation of quality-of-life data based on existing methods. *Value in Health* 2004; 7:93–104.

McDowell I. *Measuring Health: A Guide to Rating and Questionnaires.* 2006. 3rd edn. New York, NY: Oxford University Press.

McLeod, LD, Coon CD, Martin SA, Fehnel SE, Hays RD. Interpreting patient-reported outcome results: US FDA guidance and emerging methods. *Expert Reviews in Pharmacoeconomics & Outcomes Research* 2011; 11:163–169.

Pelias MZ. Federal regulations and the future of research in human and medical genetics. *Journal of Continuing Education in the Health Professions* 2001; 21:238–46.

Raat H, van Rossem L, Jaddoe VWV, Landgraf JM, Feeny D, Moll HA, Hofman A, Mackenbach JP. The Generation R study: A candidate gene study and genome-wide association study (GWAS) on health-related quality of life (HRQOL) of mothers and young children. *Quality of Life Research* 2010; 19:1439–46.

Revicki D, Erickson PA, Sloan JA, Dueck A, Guess H. Santanello NC and the Mayo/FDA Patient-Reported Outcomes Consensus Meeting Group. Interpreting and reporting results based on patient-reported outcomes. *Value in Health* 2007; 10:S116–24.

Rijsdijk FV, Snieder H, Ormel J, Sham P, Goldberg DP, Spector TD Genetic and environmental influences on psychological distress in the population: General Health Questionnaire analysis in UK twins. *Psychological Medicine* 2003; 33:793–801.

Romeis JC, Scherrer JF, Xian H, Eisen SA, Bucholz K, Heath AC, Goldberg J, Lyons MJ, Henderson WG, True WR. Heritability of self-reported health. *Health Services Research* 2000; 35:995–1010.

Rosen RC, Cappelleri JC, Smith MD, Lipsky J, Pena BM. Development and evaluation of an abridged, 5-item version of the International Index of Erectile Function (IIEF-5) as a diagnostic tool for erectile dysfunction. *International Journal of Impotence Research* 1999; 11:319–26.

Salek S. *Compendium of Quality of Life Instruments: Volume 6.* 2004. Haselmere, Euromed Communications Ltd.

Schünemann HJ, Akl EA, Guyatt GH. Interpreting the results of patient reported outcomes in clinical trials: The clinician's perspective. *Health and Quality of Life Outcomes* 2006; 4:62.

Shi Q, Cleeland CS, Klepstad P, Miaskowski C, Pedersen NL. Biological pathways and genetic variables involved in pain. *Quality of Life Research* 2010; 19:1407–17.

Singer JD, Willett JB. *Applied Longitudinal Data Analysis: Modeling Change and Event Occurrence.* 2003. New York, NY: Oxford University Press.

Sloan JA, Dueck AC, Erickson PA et al. Analysis and interpretation of results based on patient-reported outcomes. *Value in Health* 2007; 10 (suppl 2):S106–15.

Sprangers MA, Bartels M, Veenhoven R et al. Which patient will feel down, which will be happy? The need to study the genetic disposition of emotional states. *Quality of Life Research* 2010; 19:1429–37.

Sprangers MA, Sloan JA, Barsevick A et al. Scientific imperatives, clinical implications, and theoretical underpinnings for the investigation of the relationship between genetic variables and patient reported quality-of-life outcomes. *Quality of Life Research* 2010; 19:1395–403.

Sprangers MAG, Sloan JA, Veenhoven R, Cleeland CS, Halyard MY, Abertnethy AM, Frank Baas F et al. The establishment of the GENEQOL consortium to investigate the genetic disposition of patient-reported quality-of-lfe outcomes. *Twin Research and Human Genetics* 2009; 12:301–11.

Ware JE, Snow KK, Kosinki M, Gandek B. *SF-36 Health Survey: Manual and Interpretation Guide*. 1993. Lincoln, RI: Quality Metric Inc.

Westbury RC. *Use of the Dartmouth COOP Charts in a Calgary Practice*. In: Lipkin M, editor. Functional status measurement in primary care. 1990. New York (NY): Springer-Verlag, 166–80.

Wilson IB. Cleary PD Linking clinical variables with health-related quality of life. A conceptual model of patient outcomes. *Journal of the American Medical Association* 1995; 273:59–65.

Yang P, Mandrekar SJ, Hillman SH, Allen Ziegler KL, Sun Z, Wampfler JA, Cunningham JM, Sloan JA, Perez E, Jett JR. Evaluation of glutathione metabolic genes on outcomes in advanced non-small cell lung cancer patients after initial treatment with platinum-based chemotherapy: An NCCTG-97–24–51 based study. *Journal of Thoracic Oncology* 2009; 12:479–85.

11

Regulatory Issues in Use of Biomarkers in Drug Development

Aloka G. Chakravarty[*]

CONTENTS

11.1 Background and Definition

In recent years, there has been an increased awareness and interest in personalized medicine. Since the efficacy of a therapeutic product is observed only in the respondents while the toxicity is universally shared by the entire intent-to-treat population, the patient exposure to agents that are not likely to be beneficial to a select genotype should be limited. Thus, careful consideration of biomarkers (and surrogate markers) plays an important role in drug development and regulatory decisions.

---

[*] This book chapter reflects the views of the author and should not be construed to represent FDA's views or policies.

A *biomarker* is a characteristic that is objectively measured and evaluated as an indicator of normal biologic processes, pathogenic processes (abnormal biologic processes), or responses to a therapeutic intervention. It is not a clinical assessment of the patient, those evaluating or closely relating to how a patient feels or functions, or survival (Biomarker Definition Working Group, 2001).

Biomarkers are categorized by how they are used in drug development and may have utility in more than one category.

- *Prognostic biomarkers* indicate the future clinical course of the patient with respect to a specified clinical outcome in the absence of an intervention. So, there is no connection to any particular new treatment. A post-therapy marker–clinical relationship may differ among treatments.
- *Predictive biomarkers* are measured prior to an intervention and identify patients susceptible to a particular drug effect vs. patients less susceptible to a certain benefit or harm. These biomarkers are developed treatment by treatment and are not necessarily prognostic of the post-treatment clinical course.
- *Pharmaco-dynamic biomarkers* (PD) or response-indicator biomarkers reveal whether, or how large, a biological response has occurred in that particular patient and may or may not be therapy specific. Development occurs in a treatment-by-treatment manner.
- *Surrogate endpoint* or efficacy-response biomarkers are a small subset of biomarkers that predict the clinical outcome of the patient at a distal time. Usually they have some prognostic utility, or else placebo group measurements cannot be interpreted. Surrogate markers have been used extensively for accelerated approval of drugs that meet an unmet medical need (Chakravarty, 2001).

Biomarkers with a predetermined scientific basis may be classified by their ability to predict the intended therapeutic response or clinical benefit endpoints as follows (Temple, 1999):

1. Biomarkers thought to be valid surrogates for clinical benefit (e.g., blood pressure, cholesterol, viral load)
2. Biomarkers thought to reflect the pathologic process and be at least candidate surrogates (e.g., brain appearance in Alzheimer's disease, brain infarct size)
3. Biomarkers reflecting drug action but of uncertain relation to clinical outcome (e.g., inhibition of ADP-dependent platelet aggregation, ACE inhibition)
4. Biomarkers that are still more remote from the clinical benefit endpoint (e.g., degree of binding to a receptor or inhibition of an agonist)

While all surrogate endpoints are biomarkers, it is likely that only a few bio-markers will be considered for use as surrogate endpoints. The term surro-gate marker applies primarily to endpoints in therapeutic intervention trials, although it may sometimes apply in natural history or epidemiological studies (Ellenberg and Hamilton, 1989).

Historically, how have biomarkers been accepted? Most often, they have been considered case by case. They are often considered within a specific IND/NDA/BLA/labeling update and for a specific drug, driven by a specific need.

General use is accepted over an extended period as scientific experience accumulates through varied uses. One of the limitations of this approach is that usually an extended time frame is required and the evidence collection may not always be cohesively directed. A guidance document on biomarker qual-ification is available, and details from it will be discussed in a later section (at http://www.fda.gov/Drugs/GuidanceComplianceRegulatoryInformation/Guidances/default.htm). (Guidance to Industry: Qualification Process).

Co-development of a drug and diagnostic test assay in companion diag-nostics is an established path and draft guidance is available detailing this regulatory path at http://www.fda.gov/Drugs/GuidanceCompliance RegulatoryInformation/Guidances/default.htm. In addition, an International Council of Harmonization (ICH) document "E16-Biomarkers related to Drug or Biotechnology product development: context, structure and format of qualification submissions" provides a regulatory paradigm (International Council of Harmonization document).

Use of biomarkers in drug development programs can be for multiple pur-poses (Temple, 1995). They can be used as a patient selection tool for enroll-ment in enrichment study designs, as prognostic or predictive biomarkers, or as a patient stratification tool to ensure balance within strata across ran-domized groups in other characteristics (Himan et al., 2006).

11.1.1 Use of Biomarkers That Are Not Surrogates in Drug Development

In Phase I studies, biomarkers demonstrate that the drug is bioactive and may indicate actions on early cellular effects rather than clinical outcome. Then it may aid in selecting the dose/regimen for later studies and help jus-tify putting resources into further development.

In Phase II studies, PD biomarkers are used to evaluate dose–response relationships, identify patient characteristics that may be predictive markers, and help design adequate and well-controlled studies. Through aiding in the selection of doses and of the patient population, as well as in the estimation of the sample size, biomarkers can play a critical role in an efficient and suc-cessful development program.

In adequate and well-controlled studies in Phase III, biomarkers may assist the primary analysis by serving as a surrogate endpoint if there is a well-established relationship to the clinical outcome. Under accelerated approval provisions of regulations, surrogate markers "reasonably likely to predict" clinical relationships can drastically cut down the time needed for conventional marketing approval.

11.1.2 Use of Surrogate Markers in Drug Development

For the concept of a surrogate endpoint to be useful, one must clearly prespecify the clinical endpoint, the intervention class, and the intended patient population in which the substitution is considered reasonable (Chakravarty, 2005). From a regulatory perspective, a biomarker is not considered an acceptable surrogate endpoint for the determination of efficacy of a new drug unless it has been empirically shown to function as a valid indicator of clinical benefit in comparative trials where the effect of the treatment or the marker can be assessed (Prentice, 1989). Theoretical justification alone does not meet the evidentiary standards for market access (Lesko and Atkinson, 2001). Many biomarkers will never undergo the rigorous statistical evaluation that would establish their value as a surrogate endpoint to determine efficacy or safety, but they can still be of use earlier in the drug development process.

11.2 Study Design Considerations in the Evaluation of Predictive Biomarkers

Often, biomarkers have to be evaluated based on retrospective analyses of completed studies (Chakravarty et al., 2011). This may be due to emerging science or due to the fact that the biomarker relationship to the clinical outcome is not preplanned. From a regulatory perspective, if prospective analysis with predefined hypotheses is not feasible, then retrospective analysis on biomarker subgroups can be used to

- Expand or restrict the use or approval of a therapeutic agent.
- Provide treatment effects and/or claims for biomarker subgroups.

In either case, we assume that the effect of the experimental agent is greatly heterogeneous across the biomarker subgroups. Conversely, if it is believed that there is very little difference in the true effects across subgroups, the study should be designed around hypotheses for the entire population. Multiplicity can occur commonly in these settings due to genomic signatures using high-dimensional genomic data, multiple candidates, and assays. Thus, control of multiplicity and false discovery rates become very important.

There are some key design elements that should be considered in order for a retrospective evaluation to be considered adequate:

- There is a predetermined, independent scientific basis to the biomarker hypothesis.

- Studies upon which retrospective analyses are planned are adequate, well controlled, and have large enough sample sizes to ensure adequate power.
- Prognostic factors not used in stratification, but considered important, are balanced across treatment arms within the subgroups being compared.
- The collection of subjects who contribute evaluable tissue and biomarker status should be representative of the entire intent-to-treat population. When the ascertainment of tissue specimens is not random, a convenience sample arises. In practice, this lack of randomness leads to a collection of subjects who contribute tissue specimens that may be quite different from the case of subjects without tissue specimens.
- The assay used to determine biomarker status should be well characterized and have acceptable analytical performance. Ideally, the same assay has been used in all the studies contributing to the retrospective analysis and will be available post-approval.
- The analysis plan that accounts for the retrospective nature of the biomarker. The integrity of the analysis is in question when the analysis plan occurs after the efficacy data have been unblinded and the biomarker status of subjects has been determined.
- The analysis plan controls for multiplicity and the study-wise false-positive rate.

Retrospective evaluation based on biomarker status should not be used to salvage a negative study. If all pre-specified hypotheses have been tested and all Type I errors exhausted, further testing would inflate the false-positive rate. The results from further testing may be useful to guide in the design of future prospective clinical trials or in the proper adaptation of an ongoing clinical trial (Wang et al., 2007). With careful alpha allocation and hierarchical hypothesis testing, a retrospective evaluation of the results in biomarker subgroups may be acceptable provided some principles are followed. Many of these principles will be discussed further in the case example that follows.

Retrospective evaluations may misidentify biomarkers as predictive markers due to two factors—(a) multiplicity and (b) lack of comparability with a randomized control group. The biomarker-related treatment effects should be consistent across meaningful subgroups to assure that the correct breakdown of the study population is achieved through the biomarker status. A biomarker may accidentally be predictive by being correlated with a factor that is truly predictive of treatment effect. There are ramifications in misidentifying the correct predictive factor:

- An incorrectly identified patient population will lead to patients taking the experimental agent, who will not be benefit. Patients who would truly benefit, on the other hand, are not treated with the experimental agent.

- The nature of the disease population may change over time, resulting in the identified biomarker becoming either more or less predictive than before.

When the ascertainment of tissue specimens is truly at random, the estimates will be unbiased. The internal and external precision will depend on the prevalence rates and the fraction of all intent-to-treat patients whose tissue specimens were ascertained. The greater the fraction, the more consistent the results are expected to be between the biomarker evaluable population and the intent-to-treat population. Estimates of treatment effects within biomarker subgroups may need to be adjusted when the results for the biomarker evaluable population are different from the results for the intent-to-treat population, even with random ascertainment of tissue specimens (Cui et al., 2002).

In randomized clinical trials, the patient's genomic biomarker status should be determined by baseline genomic materials such as blood or tissue samples prior to initiation of a therapy. Care must be taken to obtain samples prospectively as universally as possible to avoid *convenience sampling*. In current practice, genomic testing requires an optional consent, which patients may refuse, and collection of samples may only be from certain clinical sites, groups, or treatments. Such a nonrandomized sample is statistically problematic, yielding a biased estimate with unknown characterization of the bias.

Owing to the exploratory nature of retrospective evaluations, there should be a highly statistically significant interaction between the biomarker subgroup and the treatment that is not due to sub-sampling or multiple testing. Analysis plans that assume a common treatment effect may be inappropriate when the effects are different across subgroups. If the true effects are similar across subgroups, evaluations by subgroup are probably not necessary and may lead to estimates that are less precise. The greater the heterogeneity of the effects across subgroups, the more important it is to separately evaluate and describe the subgroup effects (Fleming, 1995).

The integrity of the randomization and the intent-to-treat principle should be preserved even in the retrospective analyses. There are certain basic principles that should be considered:

- Testing within biomarker subgroups should be adequately powered, and the study-wise Type I error rate should be maintained at the required level.
- The results should be robust and not sensitive to limitations of the data, including the possibility of a legitimate amount of misclassification.

- The results should be internally consistent across primary and secondary endpoints with the robustness checked by extensive sensitivity analyses.

- The results from all studies used to ascertain the quality of the biomarker need to be provided. As with publication bias, consideration of only the results which were positive will lead to the use of biased estimates and increase the chance of a false-positive finding.

Ideally, a clinical trial is designed with *prospective* planning of evaluating a biomarker. In this situation, the role of the biomarker is well understood as prognostic or predictive, the analytic properties of the assay are well characterized, and adequate previous knowledge is available for its clinical use. This is rarely the case in reality, and often only *retrospective* information is available on the biomarkers based on limited convenience samples. A pragmatic middle ground is a *prospective–retrospective* design. A working definition is provided in Hung et al. (2007). In this design,

- The genomic hypothesis is *prospectively specified* prior to diagnostic assay testing.

- Tissue samples are collected prior to treatment initiation, and actual biomarker classification may not have occurred for reasons such as lack of a validated assay to characterize the biomarker.

- The clinical outcome data *without genomic information* may have already been (partially) collected, unblinded, and analyzed. In this case, the genomic data analysis might be arguably "prospectively" performed with a "retrospective classifier analysis."

11.2.1 Case Example: KRAS Mutation as a Predictive Marker in Colorectal Cancer

KRAS (also known as the Kirsten rat sarcoma viral oncogene homolog) is a protein that is encoded by the *KRAS* gene in humans. The protein product of the normal KRAS gene performs an essential function in normal tissue signaling, and the mutation of a KRAS gene is a step in the development of many cancers (Kalikaki et al., 2008). KRAS mutational status in third-line metastatic colorectal cancer, as a predictive and/or prognostic biomarker, was discussed at an Oncologic Drugs Advisory Committee meeting in December 2008. The sponsors proposed restricting the existing indications in two biologic products—cetuximab (commercial name: Erbitux) and panitumumab (commercial name: Vectibix)—based on the biomarker (FDA Oncologic Drug Advisory Committee, 2008).

The motivation was to limit drug exposure to those who benefit, avoid drug use in those who will be harmed, and optimize the dosing (Chakravarty et al., 2011). The sponsors were advised that a retrospective biomarker analysis could be considered under the following conditions:

- Adequate and well-conducted, well-controlled studies of appropriate size were conducted.
- The KRAS genomic status was ascertained in a large portion of randomized subjects.
- The assay had an acceptable analytical performance.
- An acceptable prespecified analysis plan was in place.

The trials had the following disposition (Table 11.1).

Some features in the trial conduct, design, and analysis of the six studies made integrating results across studies challenging.

- Not all the studies considered were positive—only two of the four cetuximab studies and one of the two panitumumab studies met their prespecified objectives. Of these three positive studies, only one met all the prespecified objectives with respect to its secondary endpoints. Hence, there was a concern for a possible inflation of the Type I error.
- The assays to determine biomarker status were not identical. Both panitumumab studies used PCR-based assays. Two of the four cetuximab studies used PCR-based assays, and the other two used a sequencing assay. Assays with different analytical performance may have differences in the identified biomarker-positive (biomarker-negative) subgroup, possibly leading to different treatment effects within the identified biomarker-positive (biomarker-negative) subgroup.
- There was a wide range in the percentage of patients assayed for KRAS status—from 23% in the EPIC (European Prospective Investigation into Cancer and Nutrition) study (collected in the US sites only) to 92% in Study 20020408. There was concern that this may lead to internally biased estimates for the KRAS subgroups.

TABLE 11.1

Trial Summary

Trials	Line	Addl Therapy	Patients Tested for KRAS			Assay	Primary Endpoint	Met Primary Objective (*p*-Value)
			n	ITT	% ITT			
Cetuximab								
Crystal	1st	FOLFIRI	540	1198	45	PCR based	PFS	Yes (0.048)
NCIC-017	3rd	BSC	394	572	69	Sequencing	OS	Yes (0.005)
EPIC	2nd	Irinotecan	300	1298	23	Sequencing	OS	No (0.71)
OPUS	1st	FOLFOX	233	337	69	PCR based	RR	No (0.06)
Panitumumab								
20020408	3rd	BSC	427	463	92	PCR based	PFS	Yes (<0.0001)
PACCE	1st	Chemo/bev	863	1053	82	PCR based	PFS	No (inferior, 0.002)

- The studies had very different patient populations than the one for which the indication was sought. Three studies were conducted in first-line patients, one in second-line patients, and two in third-line patients. There were differences in the background therapies used in the first-line studies as well.

If the treatment effect is qualitatively different in the biomarker-positive subgroup than in the biomarker-negative subgroup, we have to be cautious in interpreting the overall efficacy results. If we use an overall treatment effect to characterize efficacy, this can be misleading. Use of this average effect would understate the effect within the biomarker-positive subgroup and overstate the effect within the biomarker-negative subgroup.

The KRAS subgroup results were not consistent across studies and endpoints, thus raising doubts that they do represent a true finding with general applicability. Five studies had overall survival (OS) results available (Table 11.2). In the mutant KRAS evaluable subgroup, none had a positive observed treatment effect and one study had a negative observed treatment effect. Within the wild-type KRAS evaluable subgroup, two studies had a positive observed treatment effect with only one having a nominal p-value <0.05, one study had no observed treatment difference, and two studies had a negative observed treatment effect. Two of the five studies had larger observed treatment effects for the wild-type KRAS evaluable subgroup than for the mutant KRAS evaluable subgroup, and one study had similar treatment effects.

Progression-free survival (PFS), defined as the time from randomization to disease progression or death, had results from all six studies. Within the mutant KRAS evaluable subgroup, none of the six studies had a positive observed treatment effect; two studies had a negative observed treatment effect. Within the wild-type KRAS evaluable subgroup, five studies had a positive observed treatment effect with multiple studies having a nominal p-value <0.5 and one study had a negative observed treatment effect.

TABLE 11.2

Overall Survival and PFS Hazard Ratios by KRAS Evaluable Subgroups

Study	Background Therapy	OS HR KRAS[a] Wild Type vs. Mutant		PFS HR KRAS[a] Wild Type vs. Mutant	
Cetuximab Trials					
Crystal	FOLFIRI	0.84	1.03	0.68	1.07
OPUS	FOLFOX	—	—	0.57	1.83
EPIC	Irinotecan	1.29	2.28	0.77	1.00
CA225025	BSC	0.55	0.98	0.40	0.99
Panitumumab Trials					
PACCE	Chemo/bev	1.89	1.02	1.36	1.25
20020408	BSC	0.99	1.02	0.45	0.99

[a] Hazard ratios: cetuximab vs. no cetuximab or panitumumab vs. no panitumumab.

Five studies had larger observed treatment effects for the wild-type KRAS evaluable subgroup than for the mutant KRAS evaluable subgroup, and one study had a slightly greater detrimental effect for the WT KRAS subgroup.

While an interaction between treatment effect and the biomarker subgroup is demonstrated for the primary endpoints of studies CA225025 and 20020408, such an interaction on OS or PFS is nonexistent or in the reverse direction in many other studies of cetuximab and panitumumab in metastatic colorectal cancer. Also, the results for the WT KRAS subgroup are unimpressive or negative in the other four studies in metastatic colorectal cancer. Only study CA225025 suggested a survival advantage within the WT KRAS population. The issue thus arises as to whether the existence of an interaction is real, or whether the direction of the interaction is truly different across clinical trial settings.

There are several critical issues that arise in unplanned, post hoc, and biomarker-based subgroup analyses. To highlight these concerns, the EPIC study will be discussed further. The EPIC study was a randomized, comparative open-label study of irinotecan and cetuximab vs. irinotecan as second-line treatment in 1298 patients with metastatic, EGFR-positive colorectal cancer. The primary endpoint was OS. After 874 deaths, the cetuximab + irinotecan vs. irinotecan OS hazard ratio was 0.98 (p-value = 0.71) (Table 11.3).

Several points are to be noted:

- The results within EPIC were different for analyses based on the ITT population and the KRAS evaluable population.
- Within each biomarker subgroup within the KRAS evaluable population, the results are inconsistent across efficacy endpoints.
- For OS, the hazard ratio of 1.25 in the KRAS evaluable subgroup was quite different from that of 0.98 for the ITT population, and the results were consistent in the two biomarker subgroups.

TABLE 11.3

Results on Endpoints across Patient Groups in EPIC Study

	OS		Progression-Free Survival		Objective Response Rate
	HR[a]	95% CI	HR[1]	95% CI	C-mab/no C-mab
ITT $n = 1298$	0.98	(0.85, 1.11)	0.69	(0.62, 0.78) # events = 1208	16%/4%
KRAS evaluable $n = 300$	1.25	(0.95, 1.66) # events = 198	0.84	(0.66, 1.07) # events = 276	11%/6.5%
Wild type $n = 198$	1.29	(0.89, 1.85)	0.77	(0.57, 1.04)	10%/7%
Mutant $n = 102$	1.28	(0.81, 2.01)	1.00	(0.67, 1.49)	12%/5%

[a] HR: cetuximab + irinotecan vs. irinotecan hazard ratio.

- For PFS, the hazard ratio in the KRAS evaluable subgroup was 22% higher than in the ITT population, as well as inconsistent between the two biomarker subgroups.
- For the observed objective response (ORR) rates, the response rate in the cetuximab containing arm was 5% lower in the KRAS evaluable subgroup than in the ITT population (16% vs. 11%), but it was 2.5% higher in the mutant KRAS subgroup. A larger difference in ORR was observed in the mutant KRAS subgroup than in the WT KRAS subgroup.
- For the wild-type KRAS evaluable subgroup, there was a negative observed treatment effect on OS (29% increase in the instantaneous risk of death), a positive observed treatment effect on PFS (a 23% decrease in the instantaneous risk of an event), and a small negative treatment effect (3% increase) on response rate.
- For the mutant KRAS evaluable subgroup, there was a negative observed treatment effect on OS (28% increase in the instantaneous risk of death), no observed treatment effect on PFS (no change in the instantaneous risk of an event), and an observed treatment effect (7% increase) on response rate.
- Tumor samples were ascertained and evaluated for KRAS status from approximately 23% (300 of 1298 subjects) of the ITT population. All evaluable tumor samples came from subjects at sites within the United States only.
- For the endpoints of OS, PFS, and objective response rate, there were inconsistent results on the KRAS evaluable population and the ITT population.

As a result, the cetuximab product label was updated with the following wording—"retrospective subset analyses of metastatic or advanced colorectal cancer trials have not shown a treatment benefit for Erbitux in patients whose tumors had KRAS mutations in codon 12 or 13. Use of Erbitux is not recommended for the treatment of colorectal cancer with these mutations."

Similarly, the panitumumab label update reads—"retrospective subset analyses of metastatic colorectal cancer trials have not shown a treatment benefit for Vectibix in patients whose tumors had KRAS mutations in codon 12 or 13. Use of Vectibix is not recommended for the treatment of colorectal cancer with these mutations."

11.3 Biomarker Qualification Process

Biomarker qualification is a process undertaken to conclude that, within a carefully and specifically stated "context of use," the biomarker can reliably support a specified manner of interpretation and application in drug development. The biomarker's utility in regulatory decisions is central to the qualification process. Biomarkers are expected to have applications in multiple drug development programs. A qualified biomarker can be applied as a drug development tool (DDT) without the need for submission of extensive biomarker-supportive information in each IND or reevaluation to confirm that application is justified. Qualification may make the biomarker more attractive to use and with the potential to accelerate the drug development program (Chakravarty, 2012).

The Biomarker Qualification Process (BQP), a developing program within CDER, is an outgrowth of the Critical Path Initiative. The Center for Drug Evaluation and Research (CDER) at FDA has published draft guidance on this DDT process. This guidance discusses the qualification process for both biomarkers as well as clinical outcome assessments (PROs and other rating scales). The full guidance is available at http://www.fda.gov/downloads/Drugs/GuidanceComplianceRegulatoryInformation/Guidances/UCM230597.pdf.

What becomes "qualified"? A biomarker is a patho-physiological measurement or an analyte. Assay methods are needed to measure the biomarker, but the assay method is not the biomarker. A biomarker can have multiple assays that are capable of measuring the biomarker. Assay method performance characteristics are important, and the Center for Devices and Radiological Health (CDRH) within FDA has the regulatory authority to clear or approve commercial testing devices for clinical measurements. Note that CDRH clearance does not equal CDER qualification, as they are for two very different purposes.

How do biomarkers become developed? Disease biochemistry, pathophysiology, and natural history may serve as a guide to select assessments to develop. Collection of scientific data related to a particular context of use justifies relying on the biomarker. A substantial amount of effort may be required and a collaborative model for this work, including the pharmaceutical industry in the "pre-competitive" space, is being evaluated. This model reduces the resources per participant; however, development resources are needed well in advance of applying a biomarker in drug development.

11.3.1 Context of Use and Its Elements

Biomarkers are qualified for a specific context of use (CoU). A CoU is a regulatory statement of the manner and purpose of use, including how to apply results to decision making and the impact on drug development. The CoU identifies the boundaries of known reliability as shown by evidence, and not all boundaries of nonreliability are known. A biomarker may also have utility outside the currently qualified CoU, accepted on a case-by-case (IND specific) basis and then expanded as further data justify.

CoU depends on when and how the biomarker is sampled, how the samples are assayed, how the data are analyzed and interpreted, and what decision is made based on the data. It is also important to consider how drug development is altered by the biomarker subgroup results. Adequately specifying the CoU is often a difficult first step toward qualification since it determines what kind of data are needed. Comparative claim to another biomarker is not a CoU.

There are several elements of a CoU that play an important role in the design and analysis of the trial. Identification of an individual biomarker (or a composite of several) that fully describes the purported clinical effect is critical. If, for example, a composite imaging biomarker is considered, then the lesion length or volume, number of lesions, or change from baseline should be considered. If serum protein biomarkers are considered, then the steady-state level, peak, and area under the curve (AUC) play important roles. If thresholds are used in characterizing treatment effect, prespecification on the categorization (such as greater than a specific threshold value or a certain percent change from baseline) should be done. The species of measurement is also important—is it being measured in humans or in a specific pre-clinical species? The patient population plays an important role—is it being done in a clinical setting with healthy volunteers or in a specific disease or disease subset or is it being done in a preclinical setting being measured in healthy animals or in a disease model?

The elements of a CoU can be considered in two categories—general purpose and specific drug development decisions made based on the biomarker.

- The general purpose elements identify the intended interpretation, subject selection or categories for stratification, pharmaco-dynamic measurement for proof of concept study as well as the surrogate efficacy endpoint to demonstrate effectiveness.

- Specific drug development decisions made based on the biomarker such as eligibility criterion in a clinical trial, selection of doses to be tested in a Phase 3 study, assurance of absence of toxicity to permit dose escalation and identifying study subjects experiencing toxicity for special patient management.

11.3.2 Biomarker Qualification in Drug Development Program

Qualification is intended for biomarkers that will be used in multiple drug development programs, and public knowledge and availability are essential. Consortia or collaborative groups are the most likely entities to sponsor biomarkers for qualification. Qualification is not required in all situations; a case-by-case approach for accepting use in a single IND/NDA/BLA program remains a viable path. Qualification is a voluntary activity as the holder of biomarker data can choose to pursue or not pursue qualification.

The qualification process has three major parts:

1. Initial evaluation for agreement to collaborate
2. Interactive consultation and advice stage
3. In-depth review stage

In the first phase, with initial high-level evaluation, the submitter proposes the project to FDA with a "letter of intent." In this document, they identify the biomarker and the proposed context of use as well as information on the current state of development. The FDA decides to collaborate based on whether the potential is sufficient to justify the Agency resources. An interdisciplinary working team is then assembled to guide the submitter and ultimately review the complete evidence.

The second phase, which is the advice and consultation stage, begins when summaries of available information are reviewed, and advice on how to advance development for intended use is provided. Additional studies may need to be conducted and summary results are discussed with the submitter as they become available. Advice on next steps for development usually involves iterative cycles of briefing documents, meetings, and completing next steps until ultimately development is thought to be complete.

The third phase, which is the biomarker review stage, commences with the submission of the full data package. A full review and the CDER decision on qualification are discussed and communicated to the submitter. Formal qualification is granted if appropriate. The qualification statements are made public on the FDA website. Subsequent to the qualification, any sponsor (not just the original submitter) can use the qualified biomarker in the approved CoU for their drug development process without any further justification.

11.3.3 Biomarker Qualification: A Case Example

The tests used to determine drug safety have remained unchanged for decades. Some of the newer safety testing methods have not been generally accepted by regulators as proof of safety due to differing platforms and lack of a consistent benchmark standard. This discrepancy leaves scientists uncertain about which methods should be preferred in a regulatory context. Another key factor is that the tests are not always independently validated.

The first formal qualification of safety biomarkers for regulatory decision was in renal toxicity, undertaken by a consortium of scientists in Predictive Safety Testing Consortium (PSTC). Over 250 participating scientists from regulatory agencies, pharmaceutical companies, and academia are part of this consortium. This initiative is meant to share and validate each other's safety testing methods under the advisory role of the FDA, the EMA (European Medicines Agency), and the PMDA (Pharmaceutical and Medical Devices Agency, Japan). Details of the project can be found at http://c-path.org/pstc.cfm.

The PSTC serves as a neutral third party to assess drug safety tests; the members share their internally developed methods and test these methods developed by one another across the consortium. The testing is being done with preclinical and clinical safety biomarkers in six working groups: cardiac hypertrophy, kidney, liver, skeletal muscle, testicular toxicity, and vascular injury. All biomarker research programs have a strong translational focus to select new safety tools that are applicable across the drug development spectrum.

This sharing of data by the industry has facilitated regulatory agencies to receive, review, and approve new methods as qualified for use in drug development. The new tests can now be used in laboratory research to predict the safety of experimental drugs, leading to accelerated drug development. The project is the first in which a group of drug companies worked together to propose and qualify new safety tests and then present them jointly to the FDA and EMA for consideration. The FDA and EMA laid the groundwork for these specific joint-agency biomarker reviews in 2004 with the development of a framework called the Voluntary Exploratory Data Submission review process. The new process allowed the submission of a single biomarker data application to both regulatory agencies, followed by a joint meeting to discuss it in detail and address additional scientific questions posed by the regulators. Each regulatory agency then reviewed the application separately and made independent decisions on the use of the new biomarkers.

Biomarker qualification was used to qualify seven novel laboratory tests on urine which signal kidney injury. The FDA and EMA jointly announced qualification in May 2008. In May 2010, PMDA announced the first-ever biomarker qualification decision for use in Japan (Dieterle et al., 2010).

Figure 11.1 shows the current state of various biomarkers in the regulatory pipeline.

Traditionally, two blood tests, called blood urea nitrogen (BUN) and serum creatinine, were reviewed to evaluate renal toxicity. The two traditional tests can only detect kidney damage a week after it has begun to occur. Scientists believe that seven new tests may provide important advantages over the BUN and creatinine tests. The tests measure the levels of seven key proteins or "biomarkers" found in urine that can provide additional information about drug-induced damage to kidney cells, also known as renal toxicity. The new biomarkers are KIM-1, Albumin, Total Protein, β2-microglobulin, Cystatin C, Clusterin, and Trefoil Factor-3.

In reviewing the kidney qualification data, the regulatory agencies (FDA, EMA, and PMDA) came to the conclusion that:

- The kidney biomarkers are acceptable in the context of nonclinical drug development for the detection of acute drug-induced kidney toxicity.
- The kidney biomarkers provide additional and complementary information to the currently available standards.

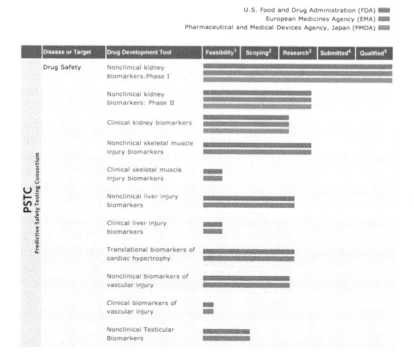

U.S. Food and Drug Administration (FDA) ▉
European Medicines Agency (EMA) ▉
Pharmaceutical and Medical Devices Agency, Japan (PMDA) ▉

FIGURE 11.1
(**See color insert.**) Drug Safety Biomarkers submitted by the Predictive Safety Testing Consortium (PSTC). (From http://www.fda.gov/NewsEvents/Newsroom/PressAnnouncements/2008/ucm116911.htm, reproduced with permission from PSTC.)

- The use of kidney biomarkers in clinical trials is to be considered on a case-by-case basis in order to gather further data to qualify their usefulness in monitoring drug-induced kidney toxicity in humans.
- Research is ongoing to further qualify biomarkers for use in clinical drug development.

In addition to the traditional tests, the regulatory agencies now consider results from the seven new tests as part of their respective drug review processes. Although a decision by the sponsor to collect information using the new tests is voluntary, if collected, it must be submitted. The new tests, however, are more sensitive and can detect cellular damage within hours. And while BUN and serum creatinine show that damage has occurred somewhere in the kidneys, the new tests can pinpoint which parts of the kidney have been affected. It is expected that the development of these and other biomarkers can result in important tools for better understanding the safety profile of new drugs, lead to human tests that detect drug-induced kidney injury in people earlier than is now possible, and help health-care professionals better manage potential kidney damage.

Biomarker qualification is an evolving science, so quick reassessments through early and frequent contacts with the regulatory agencies will be needed to ensure a successful outcome. Active collaboration in a precompetitive space cuts down on redundancies and streamlines the drug development process.

11.4 Discussion

The concept of minimizing risk and maximizing benefit by identifying the target patient population is gaining momentum in drug development (Chakravarty et al., 2008). It is seen that patients with apparently similar characteristics, such as age or gender, respond differently to the treatment with a wide range of benefit and risk from the therapy.

With increasing recognition of this heterogeneity, exploratory subgroup analyses from completed randomized clinical trials are being performed on a routine basis. However, there are several challenges, and thus it is advisable to preplan the analyses with a statistical model that includes tests of the possible subgroup by treatment interactions.

Interpretation of subgroup analyses is complex. The heterogeneity is not well understood prior to the initiation of a clinical trial, and therefore very few trials are conducted with predefined hypotheses to be tested within subgroups. The reliability and reproducibility of subgroup analyses are also difficult to assess. Confirmatory evidence is necessary for regulatory decision making and approval of a drug product. While the goal is to find tailored therapies, effects observed from small studies and/or based on convenience samples are of necessity viewed cautiously, as these may often portray false-positive or false-negative results.

Without a predefined hypothesis and allocation of the Type I error rate, it is difficult to estimate or interpret the true effect of a therapy. Prospective and retrospective observations are often not replicated. When a study results in a one-sided p-value of 0.025 from testing a predefined hypothesis, there is only a 50% probability that a second identical study will result in a one-sided p-value <0.025 when the true effect equals the observed effect in the first study. Conclusions based on convenience samples can also be problematic, as subgroups may not represent the overall population of patients with the disease under consideration. Examination of subgroups is not intended to "salvage" an otherwise failed study.

Often the diagnostic assay which is used in identifying the subgroups is not validated or FDA approved. In such a case, any approval of a drug product will depend on the reliability and performance characteristics of the assay. The process for drug-diagnostic co-development, where the safety and effectiveness of the investigational therapeutic agent and the diagnostic assay are simultaneously investigated, is often pursued.

The concept of "targeted therapy" is very appealing. It is an ideal situation if a patient can derive maximum benefit with minimum toxicity for a given therapy. With the identification of an explosion of new molecular biomarkers, there is hope that such targeted therapies are a wave of the future. As we move into this new era, we need to understand the biology of the disease and the mechanism of action of new therapy. In order to design efficient studies, we need careful planning to provide relevant, adequate, and interpretable data and information adequate for individualized informed decision making. Nevertheless, these studies are complex and the costs of such studies are likely to be substantial. As we are learning more about the differences in the biomarker as well as change of biomarker status over the course of disease, the source of tissue samples and the handling of samples and assay methodology to classify the biomarkers are becoming increasingly important. Meticulous planning and execution of well-designed studies, especially multiregional global studies, is essential.

Acknowledgments

The author would like to thank Drs. Mark Rothmann and Rajeshwari Sridhara for permission to excerpt parts of her joint work with them; to Dr. Lisa LaVange for her thoughtful comments; to the Predictive Safety Testing Consortium for use of information on their website, and to Dr. Marc Walton for his valuable discussions.

References

Biomarkers Definitions Working Group: Biomarkers and surrogate endpoints: Preferred definitions and conceptual framework. *Clin Pharmacol Ther*, 2001; 69:89–95.

Chakravarty, A.: Surrogate markers: Their role in the regulatory decision process. *Proceedings of Eighth Annual Biopharmaceutical Applied Statistics Symposium*, Savannah, Georgia, 2001.

Chakravarty, A.: Regulatory aspects in using surrogate markers in clinical trials. In: Burzykowski, Molenberghs, Buyse (Eds), *The Evaluation of Surrogate Endpoints*, Springer 2005; 13–51.

Chakravarty, A.: Biomarker qualification: FDA experience, *Proceedings of Joint Statistical Meetings*, American Statistical Association, San Diego, 2012.

Chakravarty, A., Rothmann, M., Sridhara, R.: Regulatory issues in use of biomarkers in oncology trials. *Stat Biopharm Res*, 2011; 3(4):569–576.

Chakravarty, A., Sridhara, R.: Use of progression-free survival as a surrogate marker in oncology trials: Some regulatory issues. *Stat Methods Med Res*, October 2008; 17(5):515–518.

Cui, L., Hung, H.M.J., Wang, S.J., Tsong, Y.: Issues related to subgroup analysis in clinical trials. *J Biopharm Stat*, 2002; 12:347–58.

Dieterle, F. et al.: Renal biomarker qualification submission: A dialog between the FDA-EMEA and predictive safety testing consortium. *Nat Biotechnol*, 2010; 28(5): 455–62.

Ellenberg, S.S., Hamilton, J.M.: Surrogate endpoints in clinical trials: Cancer. *Stat Med*, 1989; 8:405–13.

FDA Oncologic Drugs Advisory Committee, Dec 16, 2008; transcript and slides available at http://www.fda.gov/ohrms/dockets/ac/08/agenda/2008-4409a1-final-agenda.pdf

Fleming, T.: Interpretation of subgroup analyses in clinical trials. *Drug Inf J*, 1995; 29:1681S–7S.

Guidance for Industry: Providing Clinical Evidence of Effectiveness for Human Drugs and Biological Products: http://www.fda.gov/Drugs/GuidanceCompliance RegulatoryInformation/Guidances/ucm064981.htm.

Guidance to Industry: Qualification Process for Drug Development Tools http://www. fda.gov/downloads/Drugs/GuidanceComplianceREgulatoryInformation/ Guidances/UCM230597.pdf

Himan, L.M., Huang, S.M., Hackett, J., Koch, W.H., Love, P.Y., Pennello, G., Torres-Cabessa, A., Webster, C.: The drug diagnostic co-development concept paper. Commentary from the *3rd FDA-DIA-PWG-PhRMA-BIO Pharmacogenomics Workshop. The Pharmacogn J*, 2006; 6:375–80.

Hung, H.M., Wang, S.J., O'Neill, R.T.: Statistical considerations for testing multiple endpoints in group sequential or adaptive clinical trials. *J Biopharm Stat*, 2007; 17(6):1201–10.

International Council of Harmonization (ICH) document: E16-Biomarkers related to Drug or Biotechnology product development: Context, structure and format of qualification http://www.fda.gov/downloads/Drugs/ GuidanceComplianceRegulatoryInformation/Guidances/UCM267449.pdf.

Kalikaki, A., Koutsopoulos, A., Trypaki, M., Souglakos, J., Stathopoulos, E., Georgoulias, V., Mavroudis, D., Voutsina, A.: Comparison of EGFR and K-RAS gene status between primary tumors and corresponding metastases in NSCLC. *Br J Cancer*, 2008; 99(6):923–9.

Lesko, L.J., Atkinson, A.J.: Use of biomarkers and surrogate endpoints in drug development and regulatory decision making: Criteria, validation, strategies. *Ann Rev Pharmacol Toxicol*, 2001; 41:347–66.

Predictive Safety Testing Consortium http://c-path.org/pstc.cfm and http://c-path. org/PredictiveSafetyTestingConsortium/tabid/219/Default.aspx.

Prentice, R.L.: Surrogate endpoints in clinical trials: definitions and operational criteria. *Stat Med*, 1989; 8:431–40.

Temple, R.J.: A Regulatory authority's opinion about surrogate endpoints. In: W.S. Nimmo and G.T. Tucker (Eds), *Clinical Measurement in Drug Evaluation*, 1995; 3–22.

Temple, R.J.: Are surrogate markers adequate to assess cardiovascular disease drugs? *JAMA*, 1999; 282:790–5.

Wang, S.J., O'Neill, R.T., Hung, H.M.: Approaches to evaluation of treatment effect in randomized clinical trial with genomic subset, *Pharmaceut Stat*, 2007; 6:227–44.

Index

T - #0353 - 071024 - C16 - 234/156/17 - PB - 9780367378769 - Gloss Lamination